Illustrative Case Studies in Haematology

Red Cell Riddles

Lucio Luzzatto

David Roper

WILEY

This edition first published 2027

Registered Office(s)
John Wiley & Sons, Inc., 111 River Street, Hoboken, NJ 07030, USA
John Wiley & Sons Ltd. New Era House, 8 Oldlands Way, Bognor Regis, West Sussex, PO22 9NQ, UK

For details of our global editorial offices, customer services, and more information about Wiley products visit us at www.wiley.com.

The manufacturer's authorized representative according to the EU General Product Safety Regulation is Wiley-VCH GmbH, Boschstr. 12, 69469 Weinheim, Germany, e-mail: Product_Safety@wiley.com.

Wiley also publishes its books in a variety of electronic formats and by print-on-demand. Some content that appears in standard print versions of this book may not be available in other formats.

Library of Congress Cataloging-in-Publication Data has been applied for:

Print ISBN: 9781394354573
ePDF ISBN: 9781394354597
ePUB ISBN: 9781394354580
oBook ISBN: 9781394354603

Cover Design: Wiley
Cover Images: Courtesy of David Roper and Lucio Luzzatto, Courtesy of Professor Francesco Angelucci, Bruce Wetzel and Harry Schaefer/National Cancer Institute

Set in 11.5/14pt STIXTwoText by Lumina Datamatics

Printed in Singapore
M135699280526

Brief Table of Contents

For a few of the titles in this list (only a few) we received help from ChatGPT*, that we openly acknowledge. Initially we were surprised that AI could be witty: but of course AI has acquired "data" from e.g. Terry Pratchett and P G Wodehouse, not just from Dante Alighieri and William Shakespeare.

*This brings up a sticky issue: in the realm of science, is it advisable or even permissible to use ChatGPT at all? Our short answer is yes. A more articulate answer includes the following. (1) You can ask simple or complex questions, but you must always check ChatGPT's replies by finding and reading the original sources in the scientific literature. (2) You can broach a topic with ChatGPT just for the purpose of elaborating on your own ideas. (3) If you disagree with ChatGPT, consider it may be wrong: stick to your guns. Artificial intelligence should stimulate, not thwart natural intelligence.

Foreword

The authors Lucio Luzzatto and David Roper insist that this is not a textbook and I agree. Rather, it is a wonderful collection of real-life diagnostic puzzles arising from disorders of red blood cells. Together they solved these cases via a combination of clinical history, physical examination, and carefully targeted laboratory tests. They then managed each patient carefully considering the most appropriate treatment and applied their expert knowledge and experience to each case. The various cases were then followed often for decades usually with good outcomes and most importantly avoided action that might have *seemed* obvious to the unwary but would have been inappropriate or deleterious. These cases are not simply anecdotes but go to the very heart of the principles by which generations of trainees have been taught to practice medicine. In the words of the great physician Sir William Osler, "The good physician treats the disease; the great physician treats the patient who has the disease." The cases collected here do just that: they place the patient at the centre of diagnostic thinking, and they illustrate how clinicians through the years have been taught to use such thoughtful, stepwise approaches.

Nearly all cases presented here were first seen or referred to one of the world's leading centres of haematology located at the Royal Postgraduate Medical School (RPMS) in Hammersmith, London. This outstanding department was established by Sir John Dacie who was for decades the unchallenged leader and teacher of haematology in Britain. He was notable for his ability to extract maximum information about a patient's clinical state from the microscopic appearances of a blood film and simple laboratory tests.

Sir John Dacie was succeeded in the same vein by another internationally eminent haematologist and teacher Professor Lucio Luzzatto, the co-author of this book. Throughout his long career, Lucio Luzzatto has made unique contributions to our understanding of red cell disorders including the haemoglobinopathies, enzymopathies, and membrane disorders. David Roper, the other co-author, was a principal biomedical scientist and teacher at the RPMS with a deep expertise in analyzing red cell disorders. In a career spanning over 40 years, he reviewed cases with Sir John Dacie and worked hand in hand with Lucio Luzzatto.

The messages from these cases include those of clinical relevance; for example, illustrating the variable clinical course of patients with sickle cell disease ranging from symptomless to life-threatening, even in the same patient (Case 16). They also include the unexpected; a young *female* (Case 6) with the severe consequences of kernicterus resulting from fava beans consumed by the mother causing haemolysis before birth. Some cases illustrate how very rare cases can provide the spark for medical discovery. Case 44 had alpha thalassemia and myelodysplastic syndrome (ATMDS); a rare combination caused by mutation in a gene, called ATRX. Its mutation in other similar cases of MDS provided the first evidence that this gene underlies malignancy and it has emerged that it is one of the 20 genes most commonly mutated in cancer. Finally, I found a case of personal interest. When I was a registrar in haematology, I gave a blood sample as a control only to be told that, like Case 24, I unexpectedly had haemoglobin D Punjab. Before this report, I had not realized that this probably reflects my known Welsh ancestry.

When I was a trainee in medicine, I was always drawn to diagnostic problems presented at Grand Rounds or in the leading medical journals and I still enjoy the Monday morning European Haematology Association (EHA) challenge seeing at what stage of a haematology case presentation I can narrow down and eventually reach a diagnosis. The cases presented in this book are similarly challenging, informative, and instructive. Simple laboratory investigations are still the diagnostic mainstay in many developing countries. However, where the budget allows, the diagnostic process has changed over the past 40 years since it is now possible to take a short cut and analyze the patient's DNA on a well-designed "Red Cell Panel" to diagnose both common and rare disorders. In my view, this in no way undermines the huge value of using case reports to gain the skills to "treat the patient who has the disease." In some ways, case reports are similar to the training sets we now use for developing artificial intelligence. The larger the training set the better the performance; the more cases seen the better prepared and effective the clinician will be. From this point of view, this book will be of enormous value to haematologists throughout the world.

Douglas Higgs FRS
Emeritus Professor of Haematology
MRC Weatherall Institute of Molecular Medicine

Preface

This book is dedicated primarily to the patients, medical and laboratory staff, trainees and students – both past and present – of the Haematology department, Hammersmith Hospital, formerly the site of the Royal Postgraduate Medical School in London; but of course also to all their peers anywhere else. The book has been largely compiled by selecting a few among the hundreds of blood films, clinical and laboratory data that were reviewed in the Wednesday 3 p.m. sessions held in the diagnostic lab. Many of the cases were presented at the annual "Advances in Haematology" Course (colloquially known as the *June Course*) held at the hospital over many years; and a few have been published in regular journals.

This is not a textbook; rather, it is a collection of real-life diagnostic problems that arose from patients seen in the clinic or referred by colleagues. Red cell disorders are still numerically the majority amongst those that haematologists are called upon to diagnose and treat. Therefore, we hope the collection may be of some use to haematologists and biomedical scientists.

Historically, haematology has been at the forefront of molecular medicine: today the adjective has become almost redundant, because medicine cannot be but molecular. We have been fortunate to belong to the generation that has taken part in the transition from blood film haematology to molecular haematology: in a way, this is the common thread in our 44 cases. We have adhered for each case to a simple self-explanatory format, in which investigations take off from the blood film: we hope readers will forgive us if we have sometimes indulged on rather detailed description of red cell morphology, whereby we have introduced some neologisms.

Many cases were initially investigated when molecular methodologies were mostly Southern blotting, the polymerase chain reaction (PCR), and Sanger sequencing. Many cases could thus be solved; in some cases, these methods were subsequently supplemented or replaced by some that today are used routinely, such as NGS (next generation sequencing), MLPA (multiplex ligation-dependent probe amplification), or nanopore analysis.

In the references listed at the end of each case we have included, whenever it seemed appropriate, those reflecting recent developments; but since this is not a textbook, we have refrained from including too many. Pertinent reference books are listed on a separate page at the end of this preface.

We owe so much to so many people that this preface risks becoming too long, but we wish to thank most warmly at least some of those who have in various ways made this book possible. In looking at blood and bone marrow smears, our late dear colleague David Swirsky was a final authority; and Kay Williams retrieved many of the precious slides. In the diagnostic laboratory, under the leadership of the beloved late Eleanor Lloyd, MBE, and then of Anne Bradshaw, the contributions by Sue Saunders, Alan Clarke, and Joel Lieberman were invaluable; Richard Manning, the late Corrine Jury and Tom Vulliamy provided important laboratory records; Melanie Proven kindly offered updates on current advances. The late Mitchell Lewis made the haematology laboratory at the Hammersmith a reference centre by running for years the National External Quality Assessment Scheme (NEQAS); at the same time, Ted Gordon-Smith had unrivaled experience in the clinical management of disorders of the red cell. Barbara Bain, in charge of haematology at St. Mary's, at the time a sister institution to the Hammersmith, has been a reference figure in the teaching of haematology. We thank Mike Laffan for much highly informed advice; Marc Heller and Mark Layton for clinical data and for providing long-term follow-up in some cases. Medical Records and Library personnel were always most helpful. A special bonus at the Hammersmith was the presence of high-level experts in all specialties of medicine, who freely provided advice on many patients in the wards and, over coffee, after Staff Rounds every Wednesday; Sir Keith Peters, Professor of Medicine, was a strong supporter of Haematology. Last but not least, we pay tribute to the late Sir John Dacie, a towering figure who had founded the Haematology Department.

Since patients were referred from the UK and from other countries by many colleagues, we particularly wish to thank all of them: they are named individually at the end of each of the 44 cases. The late Bruno Rotoli and Rosario Notaro have been, for one of us, lifetime precious colleagues in haematology research.

It is not for us to say how far this book may serve its educational purpose for others: speaking for ourselves, we believe that lessons we have learned from investigating these 44 cases have helped us in subsequent problem solving.

Lucio Luzzatto and David Roper

Reference Ranges

Reference Ranges (Adults)

For haematological reference intervals in children, the reader is referred to Chapter 2 (Reference Ranges and Normal Values) in *Dacie & Lewis's Practical Haematology*, 12th Edn., 2017. Age-specific ranges for analytes have been documented in individual cases where they differ from the adult ranges below. Where possible, many of the Clinical Biochemistry Reference Intervals have since been agreed by the Pathology Harmony Group (`https://www.acb.org.uk/static/eea82309-7e93-417d-9b8991b0c65c52fb/Pathology-Harmony-biochemistry.pdf`).

Haematology

Hb:	
Male	13.0–17.0 g/dl
Female	12.0–16.0 g/dl
RBC:	
Male	4.40–5.50 $\times 10^{12}$/l
Female	3.80–4.80 $\times 10^{12}$/l
Hct:	
Male	0.400–0.510 l/l
Female	0.370–0.450 l/l

MCV	82–98 fl
MCH	27.0–32.0 pg
MCHC	31.5–35.0 g/dl
RDW_{SD}	38.8–46.0
WBC	3.7–10.0 × 10^9/l
Neuts	2.0–7.0 × 10^9/l
Lymphs	1.0–3.0 × 10^9/l
Plt	130–400 × 10^9/l
Retics	0.2–2.0% (25–85 × 10^9/l)
Autohaemolysis:	
(−) glucose	0.2–2.0% lysis
(+) glucose	0.0–0.9% lysis
Cold-agglutinin titre (4 °C)	<64
2,3 BPG	10.5–16.2 μmol/gHb
Erythropoietin	5–30 mU/ml
Folate (serum)	1.8–14 μg/l
Folate (red cell)	110–700 μg/l
Globin chain biosynthetic ratio	
Normal β: α ratio 0.96 (0.78–1.14)	
G6PD	7.0–10.4 IU/gHb
Glutathione (GSH)	61.6–87.8 mg/dl rbc
GSH -Peroxidase	8.8–21.2 IU/gHb
Hb A_2	2.2–3.0%
Hb F	<1.0%
Haptoglobins	60.0–270.0 mg/dl
Methaemoglobin	0.0–2.0%
Oxygen dissociation (P50)	24.0–30.0 mmHg (3.19–3.99 Kpa)
Pyruvate kinase	6.2–14.2 IU/gHb
Pyrimidine-5′-Nucleotidase	2.7–3.52 (ratio Abs 260/Abs 280)
Vitamin B12	200–900 ng/l

Radioisotope studies:	
Blood volume:	
Red cell volume:	
Female	20–30 ml/kg
Male	25–35 ml/kg
Plasma volume	40–50 ml/kg
Red cell survival:	
Mean cell life	90–150 days
Half-life (T50)	25–33 days
Ferrokinetics:	
Plasma iron clearance	60–140 min
Plasma iron turnover	100–150 μmol/l/day
Red cell utilization	70–80% (10–14 days)

Biochemistry

Alkaline phosphatase	39–117 IU/l
Alanine-aminotransferase (ALT)	10–40 IU/l
Amylase	3–82 IU/24hr
Aspartate-aminotransferase (AST)	5–35 IU/l
Bicarbonate	24–30 mmol/l
Bilirubin (total)	2–17 μmol/l
Bilirubin (conjugated)	<5 μmol/l
Creatinine	60–140 μmol/l
Faecal fat (3 days)	<5 g/24 hr.
Ferritin:	
Female	15–200 μg/l
Male	13–300 μg/l
Gamma-glutamyl-transferase (GGT)	7–50 IU/l
Gastrin	0–40 pmol/l
Immunoglobulin A (IgA)	0.8–2.8 g/l
Immunoglobulin G (IgG)	5–16 g/l
Immunoglobulin M (IgM)	0.5–1.8 g/l
Iron (serum)	
Female	9–30 μmol/l
Male	11–30 μmol/l

Lactate	0.6–1.8 mmol/l
Lactate dehydrogenase (LDH)	120–500 IU/l
Total iron-binding capacity	45–70 μmol/l
Transferrin	1.5–3.0 g/l
Transferrin saturation index	20–45%
Trypsin	115–350 ng/ml
Urea	
Female	2.5–6.5 mmol/l
Male	2.5–7.5 mmol/l

General Reference Books that Will Aid in Solving Red Cell Riddles

Harris, R.W. (1963). *The Red Cell*. Cambridge, MA: Harvard University Press.

Beutler, E. (1984). *Red Cell Metabolism: A Manual of Biochemical Methods*. 3 ed. New York: Grune & Stratton.

Bunn, H.F. and Forget, B.G. (1986). *Hemoglobin: Molecular, Genetic, and Clinical Aspects*. Philadelphia: Saunders.

Lee, G.R., Bithell, T.C., Foerster, J. et al. (1993). *Wintrobe's Clinical Haematology*. 10 ed. Philadelphia: Lea & Febiger.

Dacie, J.V. and Lewis, S.M. (2017). *Practical Haematology*. 12 ed. London: Churchill Livingstone.

Dacie, J.V. (1985–1999). *The Haemolytic Anaemias*. Vol. 1–5, 3 ed. London: Churchill Livingston.

Steinberg, M.H., Forget, B.G., Higgs, D.R. et al. (2001). *Disorders of Hemoglobin*. Cambridge: Cambridge University Press.

Weatherall, D.J. and Clegg, J.B. (2001). *The Thalassaemia Syndromes*. 3 ed. Oxford: Blackwell.

Serjeant, G.R. and Serjeant, B.E. (2001). *Sickle Cell Disease*. 2 ed. Oxford: Oxford Medical Publications.

Orkin, S.H, Fisher, D.E., Ginsburg, D. et al. (2015). *Nathan and Oski's Hematology and Oncology of Infancy and Childhood*. 8 ed. Philadelphia: Elsevier Saunders.

Jameson, J.L., Fauci, A.S., Kasper, D.L. et al. (2025). *Harrison's Principles of Internal Medicine*. 22 ed. New York: McGraw Hill.

Red Cell Riddles

Molecular analysis of haemoglobinopathies was carried out in the Laboratory of the Haematology Department by

Jaspal S Kaeda, PhD, FRCPath

now at the Institute for Medical Immunology
Charité-Universitätsmedizin
Campus Virchow Klinikum
Berlin, Germany

Case 1
An Active Professional Health Worker with a Serious Genetic Disorder

Patient Details

Age: 44 *Sex:* F
Ethnic background: Mauritius (Creole)
Occupation: Nursing Ward Sister

Reason for Referral

Sickle cell disease.

History and Clinical Findings in Brief

At the age of 30, the patient had a hospital admission because of bone pains. She suffered similar pains on two further occasions, when aged 36 and 39. She had never received blood transfusion. This time she was admitted to hospital with a feeling of "empty-headedness," as though she was about to faint; she also had pain in her left arm, shoulder and back. On examination, the patient looked rather pale but was not jaundiced. The throat and chest were clear. She was found to have a minimally enlarged spleen.

Laboratory Findings

The patient had a moderate microcytic anaemia (see Table 1.1). The blood film confirmed a microcytic picture; i.e. most cells were smaller than normal, and a few cells were exceedingly small (see Figure 1.1). Larger polychromatic red cells (presumably reticulocytes) seemed to stand out as against the predominant hypochromic cells and target cells. "Tear-drop" poikilocytes were also present.

Initial Assessment

This patient reported having sickle cell disease, but she had had relatively mild clinical manifestations. Her level of anaemia would be compatible with homozygous haemoglobin S disease, but her reticulocytes are

Table 1.1 Haematology Data

	Patient	Mother
Hb (g/dl)	8.3	13.4
RBC ($\times 10^{12}$/l)	3.86	7.26
MCV (fl)	66	60
MCH (pg)	21.5	18.5
MCHC (g/dl)	32.7	31.0
RDW (S.D.)	52.5	36.3
Retic (%)	3.0	–
Retic ($\times 10^9$/l)	116	–
Hb A_2 (%)	3.5	4.0
Hb F (%)	20.0	1.5
Non-α:α ratio[a]	0.75	0.54 (β:α ratio[a])
($\beta^S + \beta^A$):α ratio[a]	0.57	–

[a] Globin chain biosynthetic ratio.

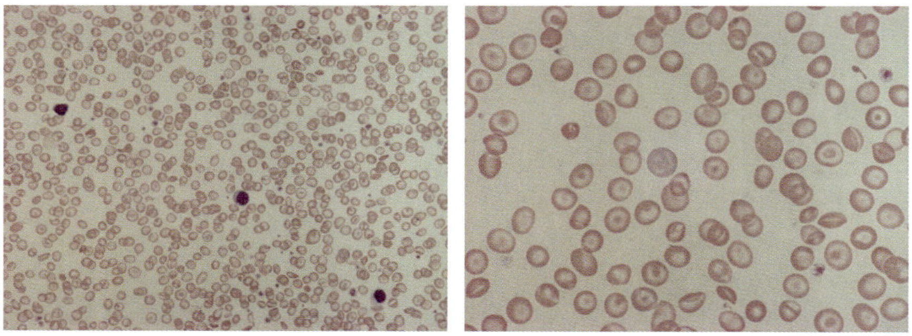

(a) (b)

Figure 1.1 Peripheral blood film: (a) medium power view; (b) high power view.

unusually low and her red cells are very microcytic. In addition, we could not find any sickle cell on the blood film. Thus, it seemed reasonable to suspect a form of sickle cell disease other than homozygosity for Hb S.

Further Investigations

Haemoglobin electrophoresis (see Figure 1.2) showed absence of Hb A with a high level of Hb F which was quantitated at 20%. The Hb A_2 was slightly increased, suggesting co-existing β-thalassaemia trait; but because it was only marginally increased, we felt we ought to confirm this suggestion by globin chain biosynthetic analysis and by testing the mother (the only available member of the family). The blood picture in the mother was typical for β-thalassaemia trait and the β:α biosynthetic ratio was consistent with this (Table 1.1). Thus the patient must have inherited the β-thalassaemia gene from her mother and the beta haemoglobin S gene from her father.

For the sake of completeness, the α-globin status was also assessed (see Figure 1.3). Analysis of the α-globin gene cluster revealed the patient to be heterozygous for α^+-thalassaemia (i.e. α-/αα).

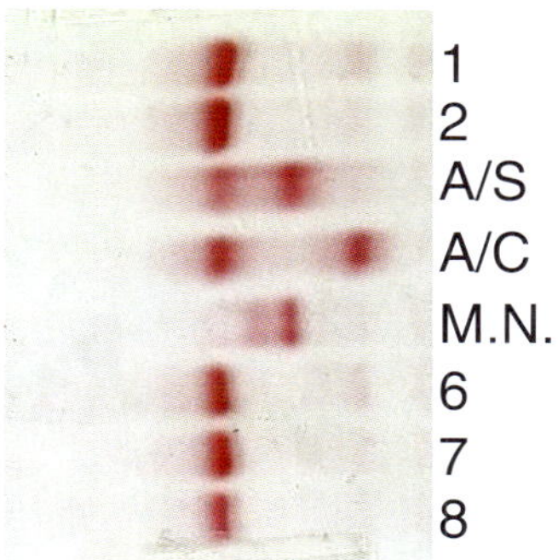

Figure 1.2 Haemoglobin electrophoresis on cellulose acetate membrane; the migration of the haemoglobin fractions is from right to left. An A/S and A/C control are in lanes 3 and 4, respectively. The patient (M.N.) is in lane 5.

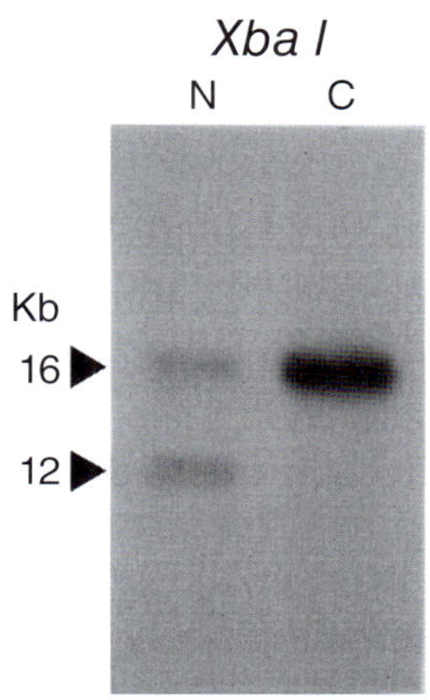

Figure 1.3 Southern blot analysis following an *Xba I* restriction endonuclease digestion of genomic DNA. The normal control DNA (C) yielded a 16 Kb fragment, highlighted by the arrow on the left, when hybridized with an α-globin probe. The patient's DNA (N), in addition to the normal 16 Kb fragment, revealed a smaller size band corresponding to 12 Kb. This is consistent with the patient being heterozygous for deletional α^+-thalassaemia.

Comments

In general, S/β^0 thalassaemia is considerably more severe than S/β^+ thalassaemia [1–3]. However, this patient, a practicing and very active ward sister for most of her working life, although she does suffer recurrent painful episodes especially affecting her limbs, has not had serious complications from her disease: we can designate her S/β^0 thalassaemia as mild. The combination with alpha thalassaemia trait may have ameliorated her sickling disorder; and clearly her erythropoietic system has a high capacity to produce Hb F, which may explain why her Hb A_2 increase is only borderline. Indeed, this patient illustrates the fact that – although S/β^0 thalassaemia is genetically different from S/HPFH – from the clinical point of view the most important determinant of clinical expression is the level of Hb F. At least 3 genetic loci that influence the Hb F level have been identified (*HBS1L-MYB, BCL11A* and the β-globin gene cluster) [4].

Follow-up

Over a 10 year period from the time of presentation, the patient has continued to have a mild clinical course and has never required a blood transfusion.

Conclusion

Sickle cell/β^0 thalassaemia disease with α^+-thalassaemia trait.

Acknowledgements

Referred by Dr. George Moses, Hammersmith Hospital, London, UK.
Dr. Neville, Hanwell Health Centre, London, UK.

References

1. Christakis, J., Vavatsi, N., Hassapopoulou, H. et al. (1991). A comparison of sickle cell syndromes in northern Greece. *Br. J. Haematol.* 77, 386–391.
2. Serjeant, G.R. and Vichinsky, E. (2018). Variability of homozygous sickle cell disease: the role of alpha and beta globin chain variation and other factors. *Blood. Cells. Mol. Dis.* 70, 66–77.
3. Thein, S.L. (2011). Genetic modifiers of sickle cell disease. *Hemoglobin* 35(5–6), 589–606.
4. Menzel, S. and Thein, S.L. (2019). Genetic modifiers of fetal haemoglobin in sickle cell disease. *Mol. Diagn. Ther.* 23(2), 235–244.

Case 2

Plot Twist from Clot Missed

Patient Details

Age: 55 *Sex:* M
Ethnic background: English
Occupation: Retired British Airways engineer

Reason for Referral

Investigation of anaemia.

History and Clinical Findings in Brief

The patient originally presented to his general practitioner in 1973 with flu-like symptoms, abdominal pain and jaundice. He reported passing occasionally dark urine; he was found to be anaemic. A Ham test done as part of his diagnostic work up proved positive, and the patient was referred to the Hammersmith Hospital Haematology department under Sir John Dacie, where the diagnosis of PNH was confirmed and where he was followed up since [1]. In 1977, at the age of 40, the patient developed haematemesis; he had an enlarged spleen and endoscopy revealed bleeding oesophageal varices, deemed to be secondary to portal hypertension caused by portal vein thrombosis. The patient benefited from six sclerosing injections; but by 1980, his splenomegaly had become massive, and it was associated with pancytopenia, which was attributed to hypersplenism. A splenectomy was carried out, and the patient remained reasonably well for some seven years, during which the only treatment was occasional red blood cell transfusion. However, over this length of time his liver functions became progressively more abnormal, and over the last two years he has become symptomatic with recurrent abdominal discomfort and lethargy. His liver edge was palpable and firm; but there was no ascites. After an episode of rectal bleeding, an endoscopy revealed large rectal varices. The patient was noticed to have very red palms, but he said he was no longer passing dark urine.

Laboratory Findings

The patient had a rather severe macrocytic anaemia and a significant reticulocytosis (see Table 2.1). His white cell and platelet counts were within the normal range. On the blood film (see Figure 2.1), we saw anisocytosis, poikilocytosis and many acanthocytes, some of which had large horn-like projections.

Table 2.1 Haematology Data (January 1992)

Hb (g/dl)	7.3
RBC ($\times 10^{12}$/l)	1.99
MCV (fl)	114.6
MCH (pg)	36.7
MCHC (g/dl)	32.0
RDW (S.D.)	94.7
Retic (%)	7.5
Retic ($\times 10^{9}$/l)	149
WBC ($\times 10^{9}$/l)	4.9
Plt ($\times 10^{9}$/l)	298

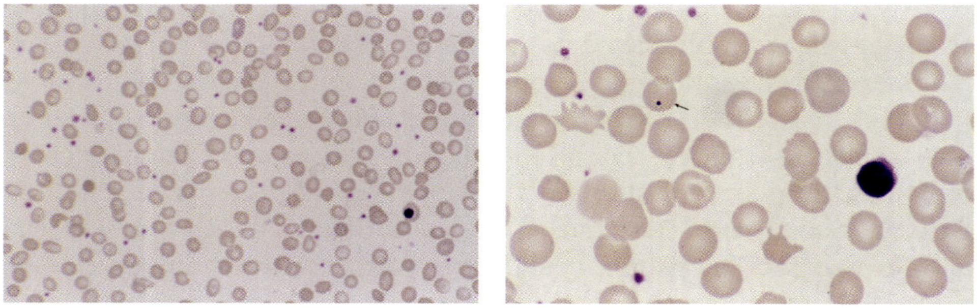

(a) (b)

Figure 2.1 Peripheral blood film: (a) medium power view; (b) high power view (cell with Howell-Jolly body arrowed).

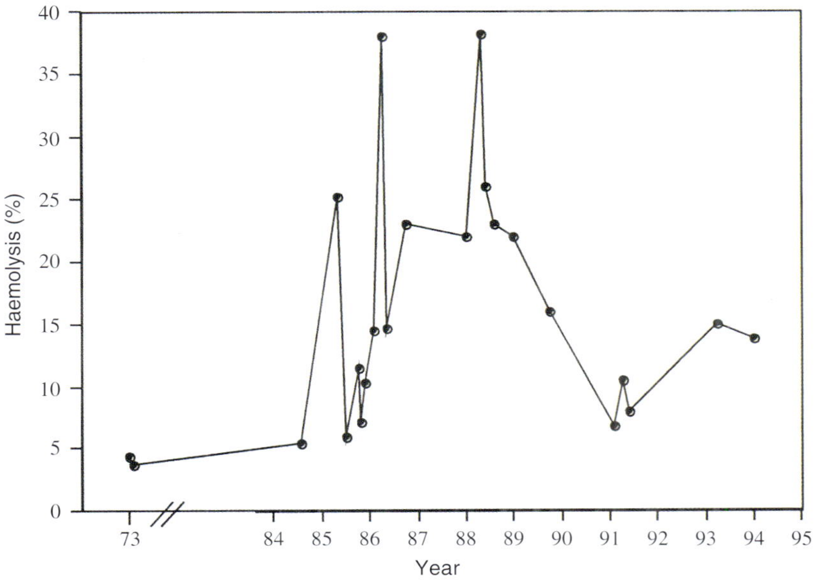

Figure 2.2 Time-course of quantitative Ham tests carried out on this patient from 1973 to 1995. The initial rise may reflect the expansion of the PNH clone, characteristic of this condition [2]; the subsequent considerable fluctuations reflect (i) variable rate of haemolysis of the PNH red cells and (ii) transfusion of non-PNH red cells.

Table 2.2 Additional Studies

Bilirubin (μmol/l)	75
AST (IU/l)	162
GGT (IU/l)	266
Alk. Phos. (IU/l)	141
Ferritin (μg/l)	1668

Target cells, nucleated red cells, polychromatic cells and occasional cells containing a single Howell-Jolly body were also present: overall in keeping with a post-splenectomy status. A direct antiglobulin test was negative.

The Ham test remained always positive (see Figure 2.2). Bilirubin, ferritin and liver enzyme levels were significantly elevated (see Table 2.2).

Initial Assessment

This patient has had PNH for more than 20 years. He now presents with worsening of his clinical condition, which needs reassessment, particularly with respect to anaemia and liver disease.

Further Investigations

First of all, in order to assess the relative roles of haemolysis and of bone marrow failure in the pathogenesis of this patient's anaemia we wanted to establish whether intravascular haemolysis was still a significant factor. For this purpose, we resorted to a low-tech approach, and with the patient's cooperation, we obtained serial urine samples collected at home by the patient himself (see Figure 2.3): obviously, he still had paroxysmal haemoglobinuria in the literal sense of the word. A urinary deposit was positive for haemosiderin. We also obtained a bone marrow aspirate, which showed erythroid hyperplasia. These findings, together with the relatively good white cell and platelet counts indicate that the marrow activity is conserved and that the anaemia is largely haemolytic.

With respect to liver disease, we excluded chronic viral hepatitis by appropriate serological tests, and we knew from history that he had had for a long time portal hypertension sufficiently severe to cause bleeding from oesophageal and rectal varices; we suspected he might have had also hepatic vein thrombosis, but this was never documented. In addition, the high ferritin pointed to iron overload: most unusual in PNH, where so much iron is lost through the urine. Desferal was started (2 G three times a week, as an overnight subcutaneous infusion): it took some time to convince the patient that the urine discoloration from desferal was not more haemoglobinuria, and he became more compliant, but his ferritin remained high (see Figure 2.4).

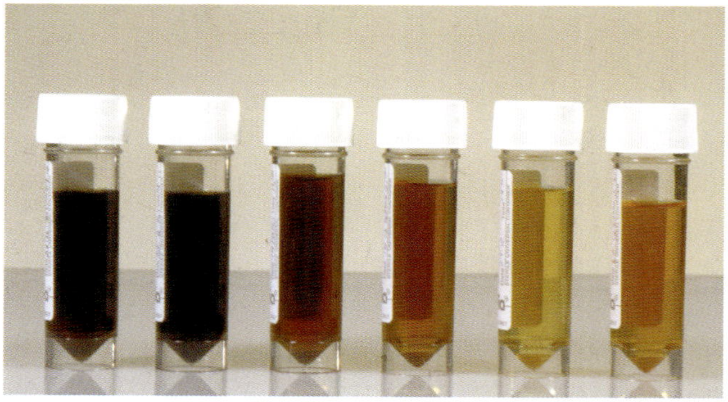

Figure 2.3 Sequential urine samples showing haemoglobinuria, with considerable variation in intensity over a 24 hour period.

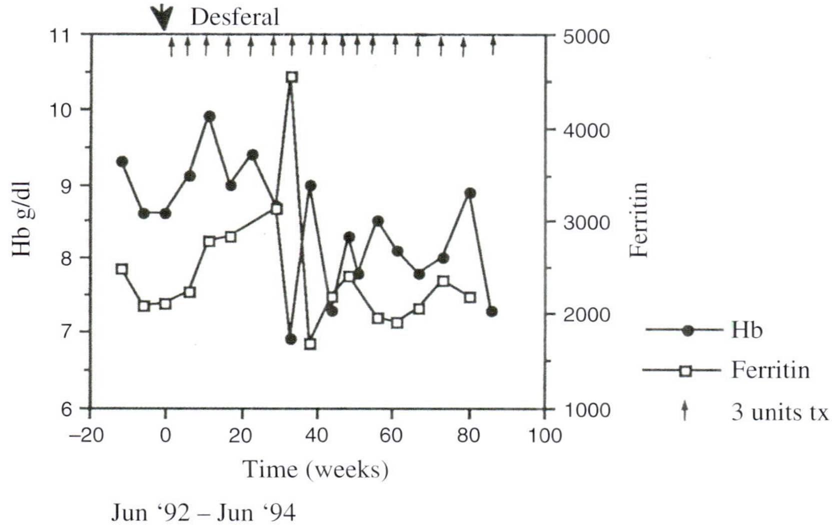

Figure 2.4 Response to desferal infusion.

In the meantime, although we had no doubt about the diagnosis of PNH, this was further confirmed by flow cytometry (see Figure 2.5).[1] This enabled us to measure the PNH cell population not only in red cells but also in white cells (see Table 2.3).

Comments

This patient is an example, from the pre-eculizumab era, of PNH with a stormy course. The patient was diagnosed early and looked after by a unit that had considerable experience of this condition [4]; yet he suffered considerable trials and tribulations. At the same time, even with supportive treatment only, the patient was able to live, since diagnosis, for over 20 years, for many of which he was able to hold on to his profession, even though the burden on his health was significant.

[1] Nowadays, the Ham test has been in practice abandoned in most labs. At the cost of abundantly betraying our age, we wish to register the claim that (unlike the "sugar water test" that is correctly discredited), the Ham test, if executed with all the appropriate controls, is still highly reliable for the diagnosis of PNH: the only "false positive" is in the extremely rare disease CDA type II (see Case 27); and this is easy to exclude. The Ham test is also quantitative (see Figure 2.2); in fact, the % lysis shows a linear correlation with flow cytometry [3]. The main limitation is that it can be applied only to red cells, and not to white cells.

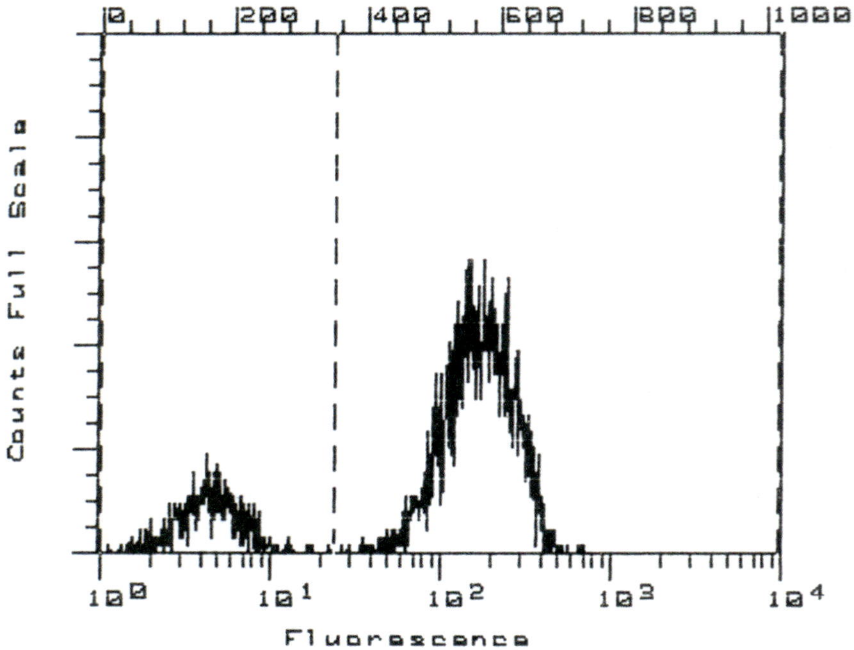

PERCENT	%CV	MEAN	MEDIAN	MODE	PEAK HEIGHT
17.87	46.29	175	165	159	12
82.16	44.59	581	572	552	36

Figure 2.5 Flow cytometry (FACScan) of the patient's red blood cells after staining with anti-CD59 antibody. Two separate populations can be seen; the smaller population (18%) of cells appear to be totally lacking in CD59, while the larger population (82%) show normal expression of CD59.

Table 2.3 Percentage of CD59-negative Cells

Red cells	Granulocytes	Lymphocytes
18[a]	88[b]	73[c]

[a] Same result with CD55.
[b] Same result with CD16.
[c] This high proportion of "PNH lymphocytes" is rather unusual.

The most threatening complication of PNH suffered by this patient has been, characteristically, thrombosis [5], that occurred in his portal vein and caused him to bear life-long portal hypertension, with serious sequelae: massive splenomegaly is not otherwise part of the clinical picture of PNH, and whenever in a PNH patient the spleen is enlarged, splenic or portal vein thrombosis must be suspected. There is no indication at all for splenectomy in most patients with PNH, but in this case, it seemed necessary and it proved beneficial.

It was the very observation of the long-term consequences of abdominal thrombosis in this patient that prompted us to take action, in other PNH patients, when thrombosis is fresh: as we first did at the Hammersmith in 1987 by using the fibrinolytic agent tissue plasminogen activator (tPA) in a young woman who had developed acute Budd-Chiari syndrome. tPA proved successful in re-establishing flow in all three hepatic veins that had been obstructed, and it was subsequently used in more PNH patients [6]. With complement inhibitor therapy, the incidence of thrombosis is drastically reduced [7], but it can still occur [8].

In spite of over 20 years of haemoglobinuria, this patient's renal function has remained normal. This is worth noting because haemoglobinuria is often blamed for renal failure: in fact, when acute renal failure develops in concomitance with massive haemoglobinuria, the likely mechanism is hypovolaemic shock, and it is often reversible. The fact is that, in spite of chronic haemoglobinuria and haemosiderinuria associated with PNH, less than 15% of patients with large PNH blood cell populations develop eGFR below 60 [9].

In contrast, and in spite of chronic iron loss though haemoglobinuria and haemosiderinuria, in this patient, iron overload has been prominent, and it may have made his liver disease worse; although he received many blood transfusions, we doubt this is the explanation. In a somewhat similar case (whose ferritin peaked at 2400 μg/l), a HFE^{H63D} mutation was found [10]; we should have tested this patient with a full haemochromatosis panel.

Follow-up

The patient remained in reasonably good general condition for some time; however, he developed dysphagia and he required recurrent blood transfusion. In spite of desferal, his ferritin continued to increase. Sadly, at the age of 59, the patient passed away.

Conclusion

Portal hypertension and iron overload in a patient with PNH.

Acknowledgements

A. Karadimitris (for Table 2.3), Department of Human Genetics, Memorial Sloan Kettering Cancer Center, New York, USA.

Monica Bessler MD, Haematology Department, Hammersmith Hospital, London, UK.

Professor Ted Gordon-Smith, Haematology Department, Hammersmith Hospital, London, UK.

References

1. Dacie, J.V. (1999). Paroxysmal nocturnal haemoglobinuria. *The Haemolytic Anaemias*. Vol. 5, 3 ed. London: Churchill Livingston. pp. 139–330.
2. Luzzatto, L. and Nakao, S. (2025). Pathogenesis of paroxysmal nocturnal hemoglobinuria. *Blood* 145(26), 3077–3088.
3. Dacie, J.V. and Lewis, S.M. (1995). *Practical Haematology*. London: Churchill Livingstone.
4. Hillmen, P., Lewis, S.M., Bessler, M. et al. (1995). Natural history of paroxysmal nocturnal hemoglobinuria. *N. Engl. J. Med*. 333, 1253–1258.
5. Hill, A., DeZern, A.E., Kinoshita, T. et al. (2017). Paroxysmal nocturnal haemoglobinuria. *Nat. Rev. Dis. Primers*. 3, 17028.
6. Araten, D.J., Notaro, R., Thaler, H.T. et al. (2012). Thrombolytic therapy is effective in paroxysmal nocturnal hemoglobinuria: a series of nine patients and a review of the literature. *Haematologica* 97(3), 344–352.
7. Hillmen, P., Muus, P., Duhrsen, U. et al. (2007). Effect of the complement inhibitor eculizumab on thromboembolism in patients with paroxysmal nocturnal hemoglobinuria. *Blood* 110(12), 4123–4128.
8. Fishman, J., Kuranz, S., Yeh, M.M. et al. (2023). Changes in hematologic lab measures observed in patients with paroxysmal nocturnal hemoglobinuria treated with C5 inhibitors, ravulizumab and eculizumab: real-world evidence from a US based EMR network. *Hematol. Rep*. 15(2), 266–282.
9. Schrezenmeier, H., Roth, A., Araten, D.J. et al. (2020). Baseline clinical characteristics and disease burden in patients with paroxysmal nocturnal hemoglobinuria (PNH): updated analysis from the International PNH Registry. *Ann. Hematol*. 99(7), 1505–1514.
10. Gooneratne, L., Giorgini, A., Elebute, D. et al. (2012). Aplastic anaemia and PNH transformation with deposition of liver iron. *Br. J. Haematol*. 157(5), 518.

Case 3

Unstable: But Stable

Patient Details

Age: 13 *Sex:* F
Ethnic background: Pakistan

Reason for Referral

Investigation of anaemia and jaundice.

History and Clinical Findings in Brief

This young girl from parents who are first cousins had been generally well since birth; the mother informed us that there had been no medical problem up until nine months previously, when she developed dizzy spells with fainting attacks. She presented at her local hospital as an emergency case with an upper respiratory infection and severe anaemia (Hb 3.8 g/dl). Because of impending heart failure, she was transfused three units of blood over a period of 48 hours. Subsequently, the patient was referred to the Hammersmith Hospital, where her immediate complaint was that for the past two weeks, she has had spots all over her body, which tend to erupt on her skin and are quite itchy. She has also had fever on and off, and a non-productive cough. On examination, her general condition was fair, although she looked rather thin, pale and slightly jaundiced. Her spleen was palpable to 5 cm below the costal margin. She had a skin rash on both trunk and extremities. The individual lesions were 3–9 mm in size at different stages. Most of them were crusting, but some looked like vesicles rapidly turning into pustules with little or no surrounding erythema. A dermatologist colleague gave a diagnosis of pityriasis lichenoides and varicelliformis acuta (PLEVA); this was treated with erythromycin.

Laboratory Findings

The patient had a moderate normochromic normocytic anaemia with marked reticulocytosis (see Table 3.1; Subject III-2). The (steady state) blood film (see Figure 3.1) showed cells with punctate basophilia, ranging from fine to very coarse stippling. Also, occasional dense cells, bite cells and crenated cells could be seen.

Additional baseline studies (see Table 3.2) revealed a slightly elevated bilirubin, normal vitamin B12, folate, iron studies and G6PD activity.

Table 3.1 Haematology Data

	Subject								
	I-3	II-1	II-2	II-3	II-4	III-1	III-2	III-3	III-4
Age (yr)/Sex	66/M	37/F	40/M	34/F	36/M	18/M	**13/F**	12/M	8/F
Hb (g/dl)	14.3	13.0	15.5	11.8	16.3	14.0	**10.1**	15.2	10.5
RBC ($\times 10^{12}$/l)	4.78	4.31	5.36	4.14	5.75	4.84	**3.53**	5.36	3.72
MCV (fl)	92.7	91.6	91.0	94.2	81.0	90.9	**95.5**	79.9	86.0
MCH (pg)	29.9	30.2	28.9	28.5	28.3	28.9	**28.6**	28.4	28.2
MCHC (g/dl)	32.3	32.9	31.8	30.3	35.0	31.8	**30.0**	35.5	32.8
RDW (S.D.)	41.7	46.4	45.2	45.0	39.3	43.7	**51.7**	36.6	41.2
Retic (%)	2.3	4.9	4.4	5.0	1.3	6.1	**16.3**	1.5	4.7
Retic ($\times 10^9$/l)	110	215	236	207	74	295	**575**	80	175
Hb A_2 (%)[a]	4.1	4.4	4.4	4.0	3.0	4.6	**5.0**	2.9	4.6
Hb F (%)	0.8	1.8	0.5	0.7	0.5	1.6	**1.7**	2.0	2.2
β-globin-genotype[b]	β^A/β^B	β^A/β^B	β^A/β^B	β^A/β^B	β^A/β^A	β^A/β^B	$\boldsymbol{\beta^B/\beta^B}$	β^A/β^A	β^A/β^B

Subject III-2 is our patient.
[a] Increased levels are artefactual.
[b] $\beta^B = \beta^{Bushwick}$.

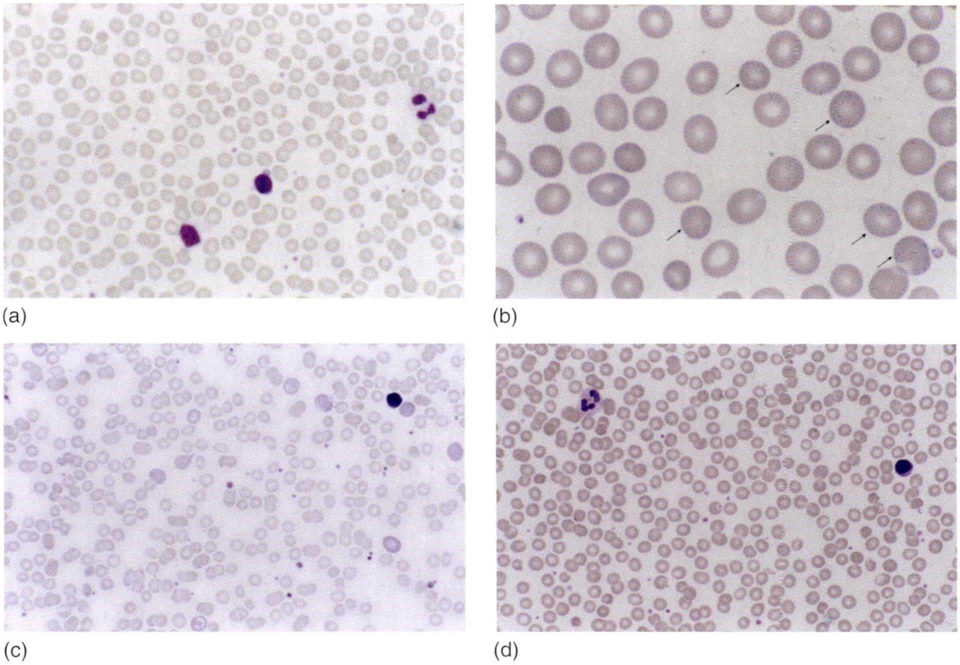

Figure 3.1 Peripheral blood films: (a) patient at presentation (medium power); (b) high power to show basophilic stippling (arrowed); (c) during episode of severe anaemia (Hb 3.8 g/dl); (d) patient's mother.

Table 3.2 Additional Studies

Bilirubin (μmol/l)	28
B12 (ng/l)	719
Serum folate (μg/l)	6.4
Serum iron (μmol/l)[a]	14.3
Ferritin (μg/l)	11
G6PD (IU/gHb)	11.7

[a] Range for age = 9–21 (μmol/l).

Seven of the nine members of the family we were able to test (all except II-4 and III-3) had significant reticulocytosis; but they had normal or nearly normal haemoglobin levels, normal RBC indices and minimal morphological abnormalities (see Table 3.1 and Figure 3.2).

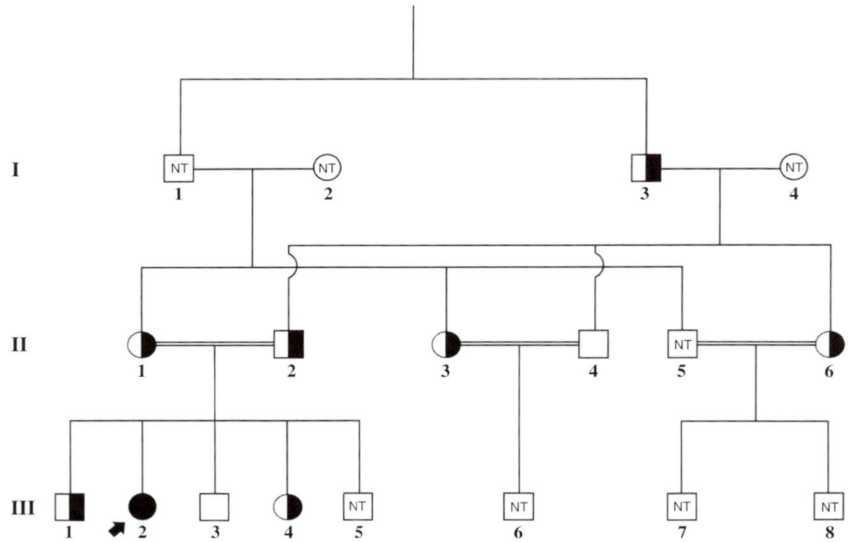

Figure 3.2 Pedigree of family. The three second-generation marriages (II-1 and II-2; II-3 and II-4 also II-5 and II-6) are marriages between first cousins. Because II-1 and II-3 are heterozygous, we presume that I-1 is also heterozygous, like his brother (I-3).

Initial Assessment

The patient had evidence of haemolysis; we thought the basophilic stippling was a significant feature on her blood film. In spite of the elevated Hb A_2, the blood count and red cell morphology were not suggestive of β-thalassaemia trait; however, in view of the significant findings in the family, we focused on a possible genetic abnormality.

Further Investigations

Haemoglobin electrophoresis revealed normal Hb A and Hb A_2, plus a minor band in a position midway between them. This abnormal minor component quantitated to 3.4%, whereas the Hb A_2 was 1.6%; thus, the previously reported Hb A_2 of 5% was clearly the sum total of the true A_2 with the other component. When an electrophoretic strip was stained in Ponceau S (see Figure 3.3), a diffuse smear could be seen between Hb A_2 and Hb A. We inferred that the same artefactual over-estimation of Hb A_2 accounted for the apparent increase in Hb A_2 in other family members. On a fresh blood sample from the patient, processed immediately, the smear between Hb A_2 and Hb A was not seen. This suggested an unstable haemoglobin,

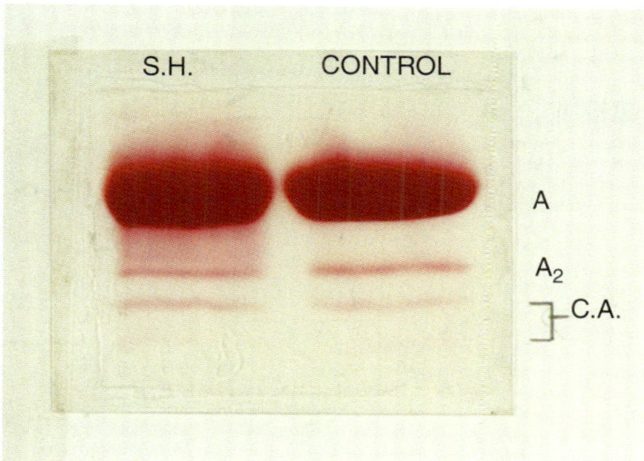

Figure 3.3 Haemoglobin electrophoresis on cellulose acetate membrane. A normal control was electrophoresed on the same strip. The haemolysates were deliberately overloaded to demonstrate the smeary band between the Hb A_2 and Hb A, which explains the artefactually increased Hb A_2 levels. The major and minor bands of carbonic anhydrase (C.A.) are also seen.

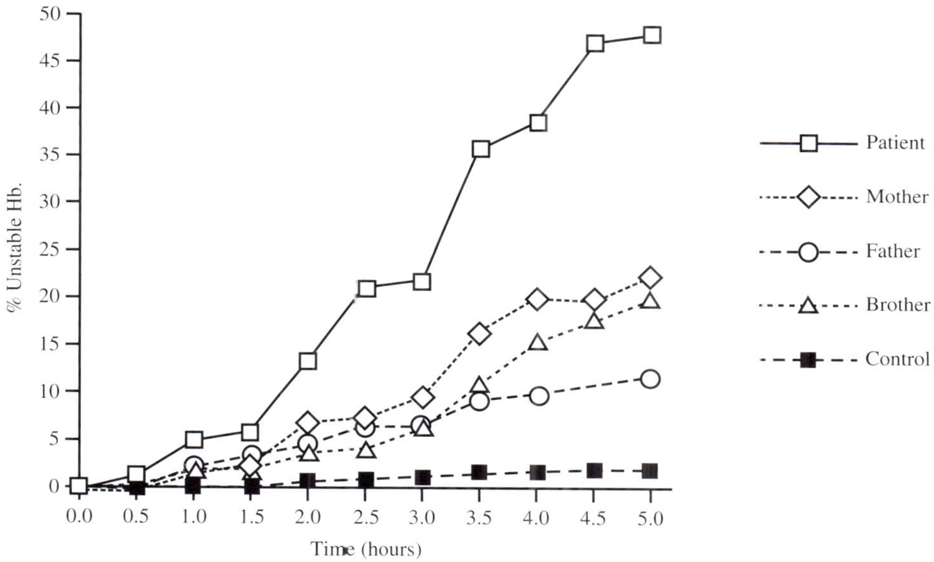

Figure 3.4 Heat denaturation studies. Blood samples were heated in Tris buffer (pH 7.4) at 50 °C. After five hours, the heat-denatured Hb was 50% in the patient's sample, 12–20% in samples from heterozygotes and less than 2% in the normal control. Learning from this case, in our testing for unstable Hb, we have extended the incubation time from the recommended 1–3 hours to 5 hours; we have not yet encountered any false-positive results.

and this was confirmed by the finding of a heat-labile Hb component by both the heat stability and isopropanol precipitation tests.

Heat denaturation studies confirmed the presence of an unstable haemoglobin, far more abundant in the patient than in other members of the family (see Figure 3.4), We surmised that the patient, from parents who were first cousins, was homozygous for an unstable haemoglobin and that other family members were heterozygous.

The patient's biosynthetic globin chain analysis showed two globin peaks eluting at the normal positions of β and α-globin. Because we believed the patient to be homozygous, we inferred that the variant globin chain eluted from the column at the same position as the normal globin chain. From quantitation of the radioactivity incorporated, a progressive deficit of β-globin chains was observed with increasing incubation time (see Table 3.3). This result must be due to rapid degradation of abnormal β-chains.

Sequencing of the β-globin gene (see Figure 3.5) showed a G to T base substitution within codon β^{74} (i.e. GGC to GTC), with the patient being

Table 3.3 Globin Chain Biosynthesis in Patient Homozygous for Hb Bushwick

	Incubation Time (min)	Ratio β:α
Normal	90	1.00 (±0.05)
Mother	90	0.88
Patient	5	0.84
Patient	20	0.71
Patient	30	0.51
Patient	90	0.54

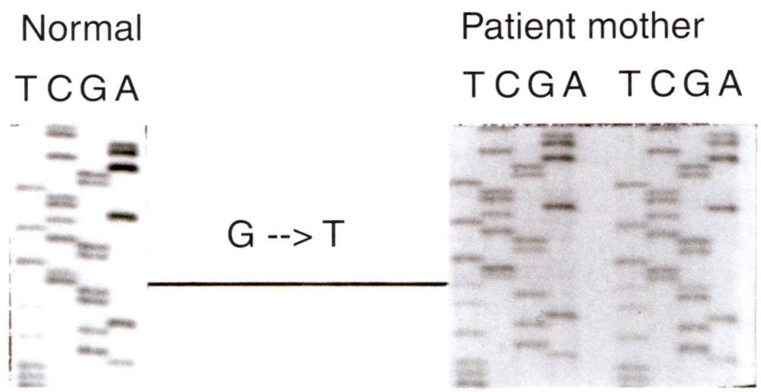

Figure 3.5 Sequencing of the β-globin gene. The normal coding strand sequence of exon 2 of the β-globin gene is shown on the left reading 5′ to 3′ from the bottom. On the right is the patient's and the mother's sequence data. The patient's sequence revealed a substitution in codon β^{74} of G by T (highlighted in bold), predicting the replacement of glycine by valine, previously reported as Hb Bushwick; since only the mutant base T is detectable, the patient must be homozygous for this abnormal Hb. The mother's sequence revealed both G and T within codon β^{74}, showing her to be heterozygous for Hb Bushwick.

homozygous for this mutation; p.Gly74Val, previously reported in an unstable haemoglobin called Haemoglobin Bushwick [1]. The G to T base change causes the loss of an *Hae III* restriction enzyme site, and by taking advantage of this, we confirmed that both parents, two siblings, the grandmother and two aunts of the patient were heterozygous for the Hb Bushwick mutation (see Figure 3.2).

Comments

Unstable haemoglobin disease due to a β-chain abnormality has an autosomal dominant pattern of inheritance (OMIM entry 141900); this is understandable, as in heterozygotes approximately one-half unstable haemoglobin will be enough to cause intra-erythrocytic precipitation of denatured protein, with consequently shortened red life span. Since Hb Bushwick was first discovered as an unstable haemoglobin causing chronic haemolytic anaemia, isolated cases have been reported from various countries (Table 3.4). The severity of clinical manifestations caused by different unstable haemoglobins varies, with Hb Bushwick (OMIM entry 141900.0037) being towards the milder end of the spectrum.

Our family conforms with autosomal dominant inheritance; but the surprise was that one member, our patient, is a homozygote for this mutation. At the time we studied our patient, she was the first example of homozygosity not just for Hb Bushwick, but for any unstable haemoglobin. One might have thought that having red cells with nearly 100% unstable haemoglobin may be incompatible with life, but our patient shows that this is not the case, at least with this mutation. To the best of our knowledge, there has been no further report of homozygosity for an unstable haemoglobin with a β-globin mutation. However, since the discovery of the very unstable α-chain variant haemoglobin Agrinio (*HBA2*:c.89T>C;

Table 3.4 Reported Cases of Hb Bushwick

Ethnic origin	Age (yr)/Sex	β-globin genotype	Hb (g/dl)	Retics (%)	Reference
Italy	–/F	β^A/β^B	11.1	4.1	[1]
Japan	71/F	β^A/β^B	10.0	–	[2]
Yugoslavia	20/M	β^A/β^B	14.0	–	[3]
Pakistan	37/F	β^A/β^B	13.0	5.0	[4]
Pakistan	13/F	β^B/β^B	10.1	16.3	[4]
Japan	10/M	β^A/β^B	7.6[a]	<0.1	[5]

[a] During aplastic crisis.

p.Leu29Pro) [6], several patients who are homozygotes for this mutation have been reported. Since the α-globin gene is duplicated, there are still two normal α genes present, and the phenotype is that of α-thalassaemia, reminiscent of Hb H disease [7].

Our patient certainly has a chronic haemolytic anaemia, with jaundice and persistent reticulocytosis, and her weight and height were below the 10th centile, yet her significant clinical condition had gone undiagnosed until 13 years of age. Her condition was obviously far more serious than that of heterozygotes in her family, demonstrating a dosage effect that is not surprising. Homozygosity for Hb Bushwick is compatible with life, probably because it is less unstable than some other Hbs (homozygosity for e.g. Hb Köln would be probably impossible).

The instability of Hb Bushwick increases once the haeme group is oxidized; when it drops out of the haeme pocket, the protein rapidly denatures. One might visualize the molecule as being in a precarious balance that is tipped when an infection or a drug causes oxidative damage, leading to severe haemolysis, as illustrated by our patient's presenting episode and in other reported cases. Based on our globin chain biosynthetic studies showing unstable β-chains, we suspect that the anaemia may have a component of ineffective erythropoiesis.

Follow-up

Over the following three years, the patient has continued to be only moderately anaemic, maintaining a haemoglobin level of between 10 and 11 g/dl (see Figure 3.6). Her chronic haemolysis persists, but she has not had any further episode of acute exacerbation.

Conclusion

Chronic haemolytic anaemia caused by Hb Bushwick, homozygous state.

This case has been previously published [4].

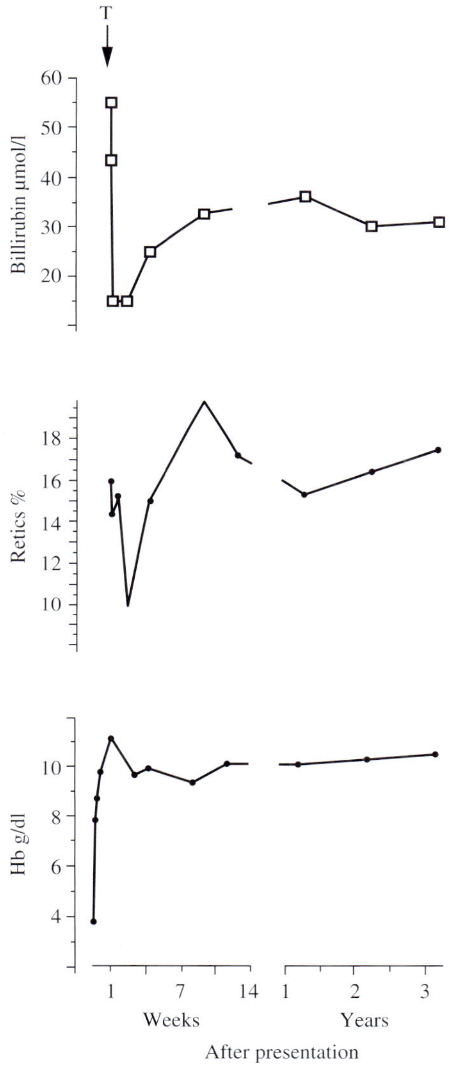

Figure 3.6 Long-term follow-up. The patient's clinical course over a period of three years shows mild chronic haemolytic anaemia after an episode of acute exacerbation, which required blood transfusion (T).

Acknowledgements

Referred by Dr. P. Srivastava, Department of Haematology, Burton District Hospital Centre, Staffordshire, UK.

Margaret Buckley, Department of Haematology, Burton District Hospital Centre, Staffordshire, UK.

References

1. Rieder, R.W., Wolf, D.J., Clegg, J.B. et al. (1975). Rapid postsynthetic destruction of unstable hemoglobin Bushwick. *Nature* 254, 725.
2. Ohba, Y., Miyaji, T., and Shibata, A. (1985). Hb Bushwick, an unstable hemoglobin with a tendancy to lose haem. *Hemoglobin* 9, 517.
3. Efremov, G.D., Jankovic, L., Juricic, D. et al. (1987). Hb Bushwick [beta 74 (E18) Gly→Val] heterozygotes in a Yugoslavian family have 35 to 40% of the unstable variant. *Hemoglobin* 11, 557–562.
4. Srivastava, P., Kaeda, J.S., Roper, D. et al. (1995). Severe hemolytic anemia associated with the homozygous state for an unstable hemoglobin variant (Hb Bushwick). *Blood* 86, 1977–1982.
5. Kitazawa, J., Tono, C., Terui, K. et al. (2000). Sporadic case of hemoglobin Bushwick detected by chance in aplastic crisis. *Pediatr. Int.* 42, 160–163.
6. Hall, G.W., Thein, S.L., Newland, A.C. et al. (1993). A base substitution (T–>C) in codon 29 of the alpha 2-globin gene causes alpha thalassaemia. *Br. J. Haematol.* 85(3), 546–552.
7. Szepetowski, S., Berger, C., Joly, P. et al. (2022). Homozygosity for the hyperunstable hemoglobin variant Hb Agrinio (HBA2:c.89T>C) leads to severe antenatal anemia: eight new cases in three families. *Am. J. Hematol.* 97(11), E393–E395.

See related Cases 9 and 31.

Case 4

Nurture and Nature

Patient Details

Age: 82 *Sex:* F
Ethnic background: Indian

Reason for Referral

Abnormal blood count.

History and Clinical Findings in Brief

This patient had been admitted to the Acute Elderly Unit at the Hammersmith Hospital since falling over in her own home, where she lived alone. She had a complex medical history of osteomalacia, mild chronic renal failure, cardiac failure and mental illness. On examination, she appeared frail and wasted, but there were no specific physical findings.

Laboratory Findings

The patient had a rather severe anaemia with borderline low red cell indices (see Table 4.1). On the blood film (see Figure 4.1), there was marked anisocytosis and poikilocytosis; large oval cells were made very conspicuous by being adjacent to tiny hypochromic cells; some of the cells were

Table 4.1 Haematology Data

Hb (g/dl)	7.2
RBC (×10^{12}/l)	2.95
MCV (fl)	80.0
MCH (pg)	24.4
MCHC (g/dl)	30.5
RDW (S.D.)	59.1

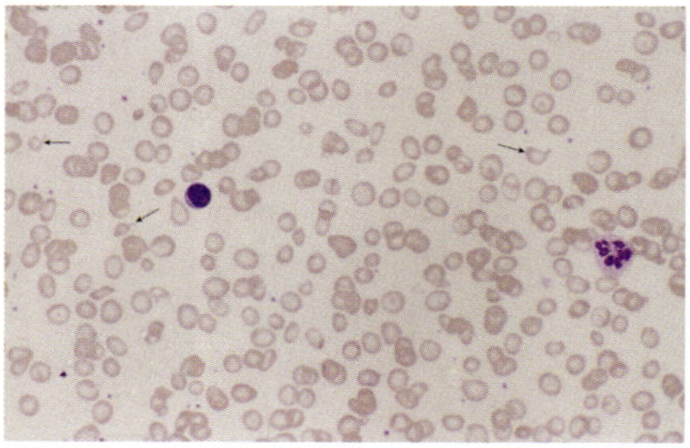
(a)

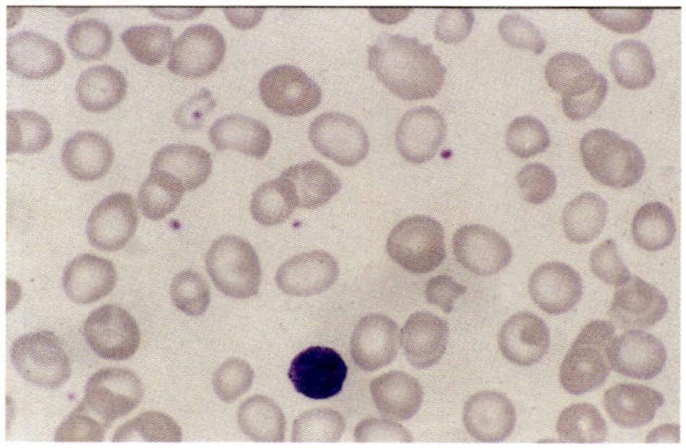
(b)

Figure 4.1 Peripheral blood film: (a) medium power view "malakocytes" arrowed; (b) high power view.

elliptocytes, others were target cells, and a few had one or more horn-like projections ("malakocytes"; *after snail*). Some dense cells were also seen. Several large neutrophils contained as many as 10 nuclear lobes.

The MCH (<27) triggered our computer to calculate discriminant function (DF) values [1, 2] (see Case 42), aiming to tell us whether this patient had iron deficiency anaemia (IDA) or β-thalassaemia trait. The computer favoured IDA.

Initial Assessment

Based on her medical history, this patient seemed *a priori* a good candidate for a multifactorial aetiology of anaemia. The patient probably had iron deficiency and this could well explain some of the changes observed on the blood film. There was no evidence of chronic blood loss and therefore, insufficient dietary iron intake seemed the likely problem. However, the red cell indices, with the MCHC only moderately decreased and the MCV almost normal, did not fit with straightforward iron deficiency. In view of this, and in view of the presence of ovalocytic macrocytes and hypersegmented neutrophils, we thought there was probably a combination of iron and folate deficiency; this combination would explain well the very high RDW. In addition, chronic renal failure may have contributed to the anaemia.

Further Investigations

First of all, in view of the low MCV and MCH, we needed to rule out iron deficiency (this is a frequent problem in the diagnostic laboratory, and to assist us, we refer to an algorithm – see Figure 4.2; Courtesy of David Savage).

Additional studies related to the patient's nutritional status confirmed that she had both iron and folate deficiencies; vitamin B12 was instead normal (see Table 4.2).

The patient was started on iron and folate therapy. Three months later, her haemoglobin level had risen by over 2 grams; ironically, her red cell indices had fallen (see Table 4.3). The blood film was still abnormal, but the morphology was less florid than on first presentation; specifically, there was less anisocytosis (reflected in the RDW value, now in the normal range). The red cells were hypochromic with the exception of an occasional very dense cell. A few cigar-shaped cells and cells with a single projection were still seen (see Figure 4.3).

The patient was still anaemic and obviously not fully iron replete. Her red cell count had risen to normal, with a concomitant sharp drop in her MCV; this could be attributed to folate administration, since hyper-segmented neutrophils could no longer be seen. Upon repeat DF calculation, the computer now favoured, rather than IDA, thalassaemia trait; this was indeed confirmed by an elevated Hb A_2 level (Table 4.3).

Comments

It is well known that heterozygous thalassaemia (both alpha [3, 4] and beta [4–6]) can mask megaloblastic anaemia by preventing the MCV from rising into the typical macrocytic range (see also Case 13). This did occur in our patient; at the same time, we also observed the reverse: namely, folate deficiency masked the beta thalassaemia (that one would hardly suspect with an MCV of 80). Having initially missed the β-thalassaemia trait did not have consequences in this case; however, it would have to be regarded as a serious failure, if it had occurred in a person of child-bearing age.

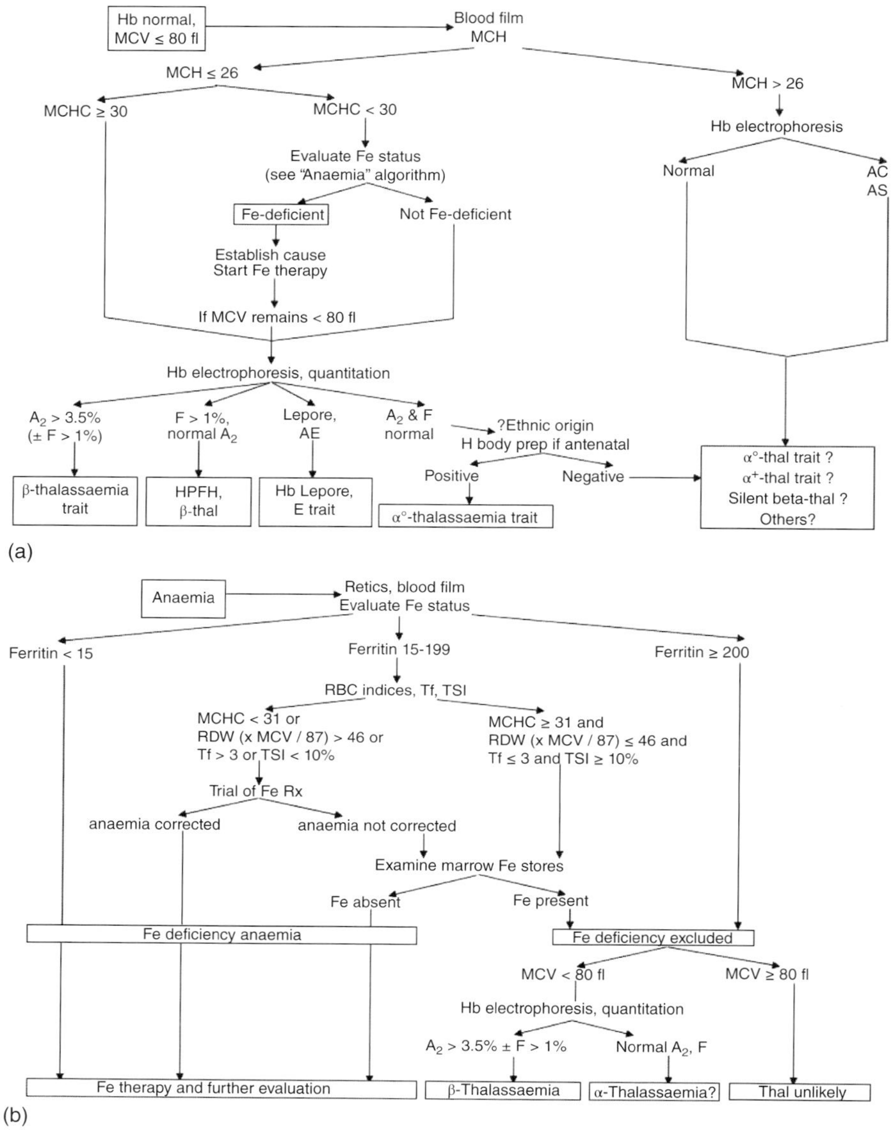

Figure 4.2 Laboratory algorithm used to investigate patients presenting with microcytosis; (a) associated with normal Hb; (b) associated with anaemia.

Thus, the patient's anaemia was indeed multifactorial, since she had: (i) iron deficiency anaemia; (ii) folate deficiency; (iii) β-thalassaemia trait; (iv) chronic renal failure. That must be why her anaemia was not fully corrected by iron and folic acid. It is noteworthy that, in spite of folate deficiency, the MCV not only failed to be increased, but it was actually

Table 4.2 Additional Baseline Studies

Serum B12 (ng/l)	378
Red cell Folate (µg/l)	79
Iron (µmol/l)	7.7
Transferrin (g/l)	1.84
Tfn. saturation (%)	16

Table 4.3 Blood Counts After Three Months Fe + Folate Therapy

Hb (g/dl)	9.5
RBC ($\times 10^{12}$/l)	5.53
MCV (fl)	59.9
MCH (pg)	17.2
MCHC (g/dl)	28.7
RDW (S.D.)	41.9
Hb A_2 (%)	4.4
Hb F (%)	0.8

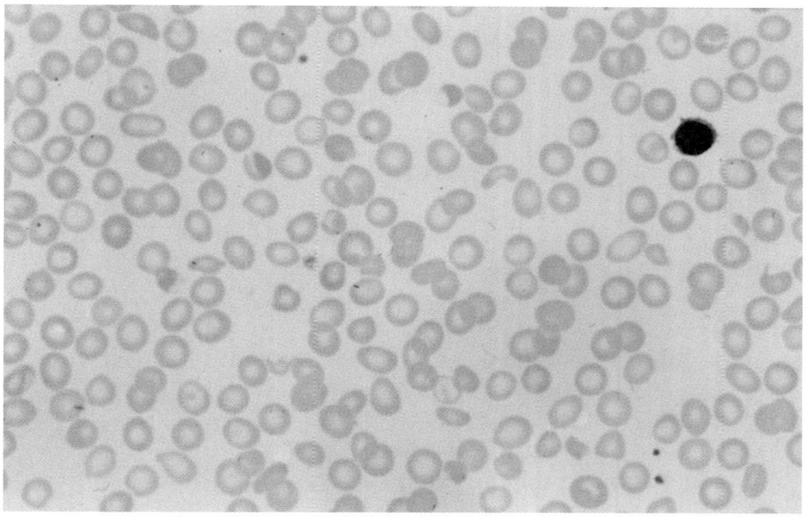

Figure 4.3 Follow-up blood film.

decreased, presumably thanks to the added effects of iron deficiency and thalassaemia. Even in retrospect, it would have been difficult to spot the β-thalassaemia trait on presentation, and certainly the DF failed us in this respect (not for the first time). Nowadays, there are more sophisticated algorithms based on neural networks [7]; one wonders whether their power of discrimination is superior.

Follow-up

Upon subsequent visits, the patient still had moderate anaemia. From repeat assays, folate deficiency was clearly corrected, but iron deficiency was not. Optimal management of IDA in the elderly is not much evidence-based [8]; however, when the iron status is not corrected by oral iron, whether due to intolerance or to sub-optimal adherence, expert opinion supports parenteral iron treatment [9], that at this point, this patient deserved.

Conclusion

Nutritional deficiency of folate and iron in a patient with β-thalassaemia trait and chronic renal failure.

Acknowledgements

Professor Bulpitt, Acute Elderly Unit, Hammersmith Hospital, London, UK.
Dr. D. Savage (for Figure 4.2), Division of Medical Oncology, Columbia-Presbyterian Medical Center, New York, USA.

References

1. England, J.M. and Fraser, P.M. (1973). Differentiation of iron deficiency from thalassaemia trait by routine blood-count. *Lancet* 1, 449–452.
2. Shine, I. and Lal, S. (1977). A strategy to detect beta-thalassaemia minor. *Lancet* 1, 692–694.
3. Green, R., Kuhl, W., Jacobson, R. et al. (1982). Masking of macrocytosis by alpha-thalassemia in blacks with pernicious anemia. *N. Engl. J. Med.* 307, 1322–1325.
4. Mazzone, A., Vezzoli, M., and Ottini, E. (2001). Masked deficit of B(12) and folic acid in thalassemia. *Am J Hematol.* 67(4), 274.
5. Lee, C.A. and Fielding, J. (1975). Letter: combined dietary vitamin B12 deficiency and beta-thalassaemia trait. *Lancet* 2, 127–128.
6. Das Gupta, A. (2002). Abrogation of macrocytosis in pernicious anemia by beta-thalassemia does not mask the diagnosis of vitamin B12 deficiency. *Am. J. Hematol.* 71(1), 61–62.
7. Mo, D., Zheng, Q., Xiao, B. et al. (2023). Predicting thalassemia using deep neural network based on red blood cell indices. *Clin. Chim. Acta.* 543, 117329.
8. Soiza, R.L., Donaldson, A.I.C., and Myint, P.K. (2018). The pale evidence for treatment of iron-deficiency anaemia in older people. *Ther. Adv. Drug. Saf.* 9(6), 259–261.
9. Camaschella, C. (2015). Iron-deficiency anemia. *N. Engl. J. Med.* 373(5), 485–486.

Case 5

Patient Knows Best

Patient Details

Age: 48 *Sex:* F
Ethnic background: Sierra Leone
Occupation: Teacher

Reason for Referral

Acute sickle cell crisis.

History and Clinical Findings in Brief

The patient's past medical history revealed relatively infrequent admissions to hospital due to sickle cell pain crises. She also reported having had laser therapy because of retinopathy; but no other significant complications. A mother of two teenage children, for the past three years she had noticed heavy periods. A gynaecological examination had revealed fibroids, with the largest being about 6 cm, and a small ovarian cyst. She had also suffered occasionally from a burning pain in her left hip; she does not do specific exercise, but she enjoys long walks. This time she developed severe pain in her lower extremities, affecting especially her knees and ankles, and she also had chest pain. On examination in the casualty department of Hammersmith Hospital, the main findings were pallor, dehydration and a spleen of 3 cm which was not tender. She was rehydrated by intravenous fluids; in the evening, she developed a temperature of 38.8 °C and she was started on erythromycin.

Laboratory Findings

The blood count revealed a moderate to severe, microcytic-hypochromic anaemia (see Table 5.1). On the blood film (see Figure 5.1), a striking feature was the degree of anisocytosis; some red cells were smaller than platelets, while others were larger than some of the lymphocytes; in a few of the macrocytic cells, the area of central pallor appeared like a large pool. Tear-drop and other poikilocytes were present, including cells with a tail-like appendage ("icthiocytes"). Of the numerous target cells, some had

Table 5.1 Haematology Data

Hb (g/dl)	7.8
RBC ($\times10^{12}$/l)	3.76
MCV (fl)	68.9
MCH (pg)	20.7
MCHC (g/dl)	30.1
RDW (S.D.)	62.8
Retic (%)	2.1
Retic ($\times10^{9}$/l)	79
Hb A_2 (%)	6.9
Hb F (%)	6.8

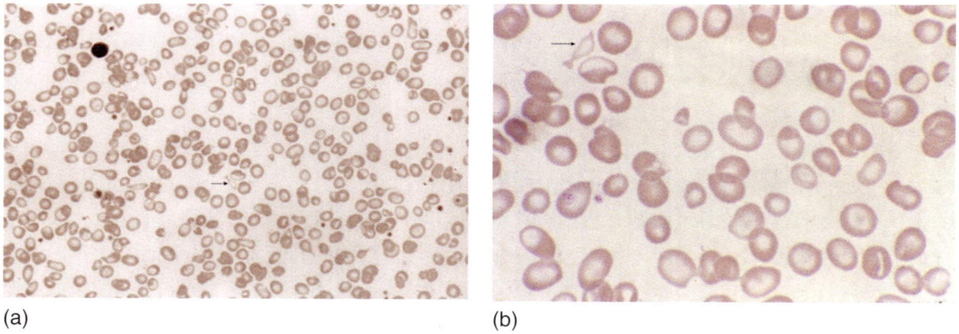

Figure 5.1 Peripheral blood film: (a) medium power view ("icthiocyte" arrowed); (b) high power view ("icthiocyte" arrowed).

the classic appearance; in others, the central area, instead of being round and isolated, formed either a band across the diameter of the cell, or gave the appearance of haemoglobinization across one entire half of the cell. An occasional polychromatic cell could also be seen.

Initial Assessment

The patient was fully aware of her sickle cell disease, but she has had relatively few clinical manifestations. Her level of anaemia would be in keeping with homozygous haemoglobin S disease: however, her red cells are very microcytic and we could not find any irreversibly sickled cells on the blood film. Thus, the obvious alternative possibility was a form of sickle cell disease other than homozygous sickle cell anaemia.

Further Investigations

Haemoglobin electrophoresis (see Figure 5.2) showed absence of Hb A with a slight increase in Hb F and an elevated Hb A_2. These were quantitated at 6.8 and 6.9% respectively. This is consistent with S/β^0 thalassaemia.

Additional baseline studies (see Table 5.2) indicated borderline iron deficiency, with a marginally elevated bilirubin and moderately elevated urea and creatinine.

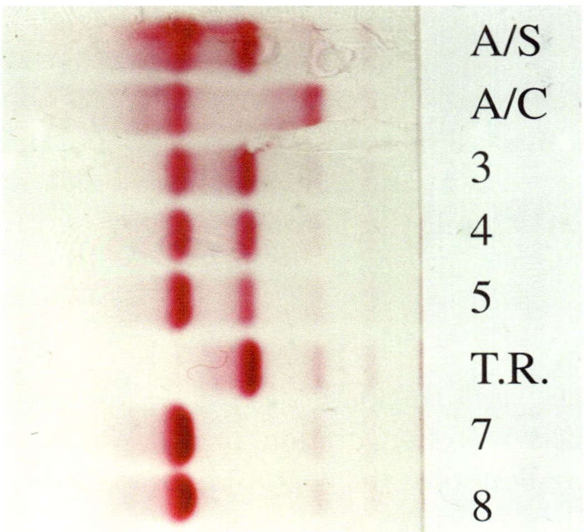

Figure 5.2 Haemoglobin electrophoresis on cellulose acetate membrane; the migration of the haemoglobin fractions is from right to left. An A/S control and A/C control are in lanes 1 and 2 respectively. The patient (T.R.) is in lane 6.

Table 5.2 Additional Baseline Studies

Serum iron (μmol/l)	10.5
Transferrin (g/l)	3.02
Tfn. Saturation (%)	13
Ferritin (μg/l)	46
Urea (mmol/l)	10.6
Creatinine (μmol/l)	164
Bilirubin (μmol/l)	22

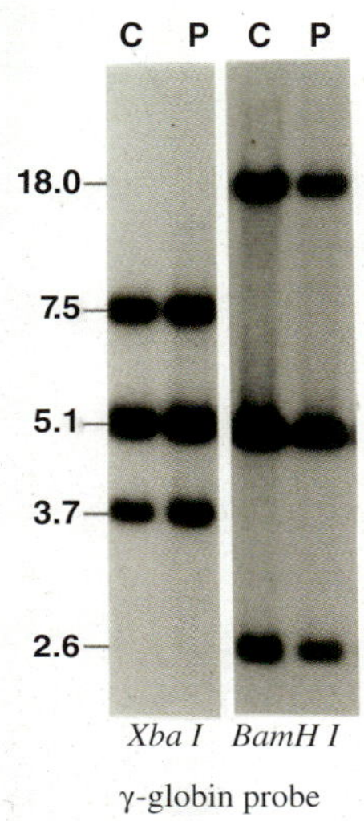

Figure 5.3 DNA from patient (P) and from a control subject (C) was digested with *Xba I* and *BamH I* restriction enzymes.

Southern blot analysis (Figure 5.3) revealed normal gamma globin genes, thus ruling out a deletional type of hereditary persistence of foetal haemoglobin. Analysis of the patient's β-globin gene revealed a 1393 bp deletion, a β^0 mutation previously observed in African patients [1]. For the sake of completeness, the α-globin status was also assessed: the patient was found to be heterozygous for α^+ thalassaemia (i.e. α–/αα).

Comments

It seems likely that the crisis that brought this patient to our hospital on this occasion was triggered by infection, or dehydration, or both. Sickle/β thalassaemia varies in its severity and outlook; the degree of anaemia may be as marked as in homozygous Hb S, as was the case here, or the haemoglobin concentration may be nearly normal (see Case 1). S/β^0 thalassaemia tends to be more severe than S/β^+ thalassaemia: the anaemia is worse; there are usually more irreversibly sickled cells (although we did not find any on this patient's blood film); and patients have more frequent vaso-occlusive problems. The coexistence of alpha thalassaemia may contribute to our patient's relatively mild phenotype.

From the diagnostic point of view, the differentiation between S/S and S/β thal can be helped, as in this case, by the Hb A_2 level and red cell indices (MCH and MCV). Abnormalities of both of these parameters could be masked as a result of blood transfusion (which was not the case with our patient). In such cases, DNA analysis is the most direct approach to this differential diagnosis.

Elevated Hb A_2 is of course the classic diagnostic landmark of heterozygous beta thalassaemia, but we still do not know exactly why the range of increased A_2 level is so variable (from 4 to 7%). It is generally accepted that in normal people, transcription of the δ-globin gene, compared to that of the β-globin gene is so low because of the δ gene promoter being "largely disabled." The deletion found in this patient removes part of the β-globin promoter altogether, and it has been suggested that lack of competition by this promoter would enhance δ-globin gene transcription [2, 3]. This might explain the high A_2 level in this patient.

Follow-up

The patient was managed conservatively and did generally well. After nearly two years, because she continued to be iron deficient and her MCH had dropped further, she was started on iron treatment. This was followed by a sharp increase in Hb and MCH, but also by three severe crises in rapid succession (see Figure 5.4). One crisis was assessed as being due to a spleno-hepatic sequestration; there was a precipitous fall in her haemoglobin (from 6.8 to 3.6 g/dl in 48 hours). This was associated with an increase in spleen size (from her usual 2 cm to 6 cm below the coastal border), and also a palpable liver. She received blood transfusion and made a prompt recovery.

The patient is a very articulate person with considerable insight into her condition. She observed that she feels better when her haemoglobin is in the 6.5–8.0 g/dl range, than when it is higher. She is aware that iron and folic acid can be rate-limiting for erythropoiesis, and was concerned that her "high" haemoglobin might be a trigger for painful crises. On one occasion, with Hb at 10.5 g/dl, she persuaded us to do a venesection of about 350 ml, which was followed by clinical improvement. At this point, we agreed that her iron treatment would be interrupted, while she was to continue taking folic acid.

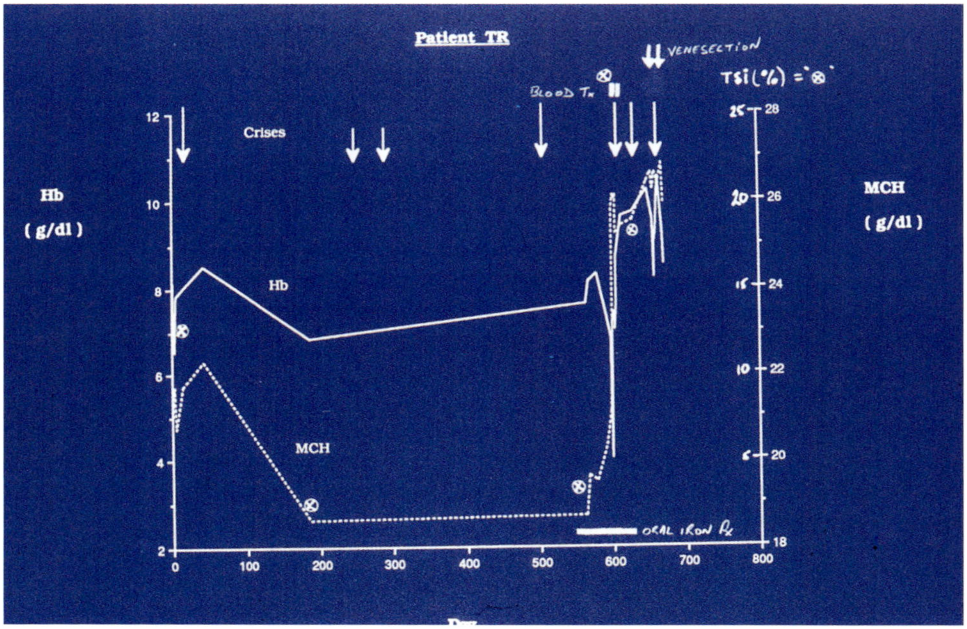

Figure 5.4 Progress chart indicating periods of sickle cell crises with haemoglobin and MCH measurements.

In the subsequent one year, the patient has had several episodes of pain, some of which were quite severe (for example during a harsh winter in Nova Scotia): however, she has not required further hospital admission. The possibility of hysterectomy was debated for some time because of her bleeding, but in the end, we took the "expectant attitude" and fortunately with the menopause, her bleeding stopped.

Currently, the patient, aged 74, is doing well, except for reduced vision due to her retinopathy complicated by lenticular cataracts and glaucoma. She does regular physical exercise. Regarding her haemoglobin level, here in an excerpt from a recent email. "I need my Hb to be in the region of 70 gm/l or slightly less: sticking to that level has served me well for the past 30 years .... On my last visit to Haematology (11 April 2022), my haemoglobin was 71 gm/l, so I did not get phlebotomized."

We have learned several lessons from this patient; (i) splenic sequestration, often regarded mainly as a threat in children, can occur in adults as late as in their 5th decade; (ii) chronic blood loss from fibroids may have been a blessing in disguise in this patient (many years ago, induction of iron deficiency has been advocated, for the treatment of sickling disorders) [4]; (iii) we should be humble enough to admit that the same patient may justifiably ask us to receive blood at one time and to remove it at another time.

Conclusion

Sickle cell/β^0 thalassaemia disease, possibly ameliorated by α^+ thalassaemia; and mild iron deficiency.

Acknowledgements

Referred by Dr. Konetey-Ahulu, Harley Street, London, UK.

References

1. Padanilam, B.J., Felice, A.E., and Huisman, T.H.J. (1984). Partial deletion of the 5' beta-globin gene region causes beta zero-thalassaemia in members of an American black family. *Blood* 64, 941–944.
2. Thein, S.L., Hesketh, C., Brown, J.M. et al. (1989). Molecular characterisation of a high Hb A2 beta thalassaemia by direct sequencing of single stranded enriched amplified genomic DNA. *Blood* 73, 924–930.
3. Serjeant, G.R. (1985). *Sickle Cell Disease*. Oxford University Press, Oxford.
4. Castro, O., Poillon, W.N., Finke, H. et al. (1994). Improvement of sickle cell anaemia by iron-limited erythropoeisis. *Am J Haematol*. 47, 74–81.

See also related Cases 1 and 12.

Case 6

Not Only Males Are Affected

Patient Details

Age: 2 *Sex:* F
Ethnic background: Egyptian (Cairo)

Reason for Referral

History of severe neonatal jaundice.

History and Clinical Findings in Brief

This patient was the second child born of healthy, unrelated parents. Like her older sister, she was born prematurely at 31 weeks gestation by vaginal delivery in a hospital in Cairo. She was noticed to be jaundiced from the third day, and by the fifth day her bilirubin had risen to a level of 290 µmol/l, at which point she was given an exchange blood transfusion. Unfortunately, on the sixth day, the bilirubin level had risen to 330 µmol/l, and on the seventh day another exchange transfusion was performed. On examination, the patient appeared to be developmentally delayed, with all body measurements below the third centile; she had a high arched palate, funnel-shaped chest and hyper-extensibility of joints. There was no splenomegaly or hepatomegaly. The patient had multiple neurological abnormalities i.e. severe sensorineural hearing loss, spastic paraparesis, ataxia and involuntary movements; a formal assessment of her mental state was not carried out, but she was said to be mentally retarded. Her multiple neurological defects were regarded as consistent with kernicterus.

Laboratory Findings

We did not draw blood from the patient because we wished to spare her an invasive procedure at a time when there was no acute clinical problem. However, a blood count done elsewhere, had yielded a haemoglobin level of 11.6 g/dl (see Figure 6.2), with normal red cell indices, normal blood film morphology and normal reticulocytes. The parents had normal blood counts with the exception of slightly raised reticulocyte counts. There were no obvious abnormalities on their blood films (see Figure 6.1), except for an occasional polychromatic red cell on the mother's film.

Initial Assessment

The patient had the full-blown picture of neurological damage from kernicterus. The question was why this severe complication of neonatal jaundice (NNJ) had developed. Of course, prematurity is a known risk factor; however, this was not likely to account for the severity of the damage the patient suffered. Extensive serological investigations had ruled out iso-immune haemolytic disease of the newborn.

Further Investigations

Haemoglobin electrophoresis and autohaemolysis tests performed on the parents were normal. A G6PD assay on the mother was also normal but a level of 1.1 IU/g Hb in the father indicated he was G6PD deficient, which of

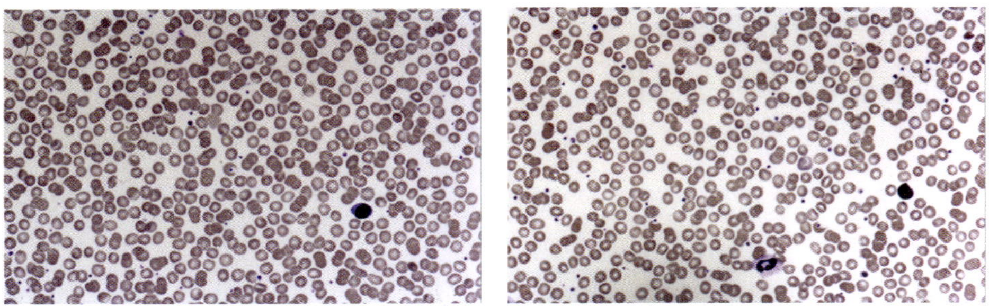

(a) (b)

Figure 6.1 Parents' peripheral blood films: (a) father; (b) mother.

Figure 6.2 Family pedigree.

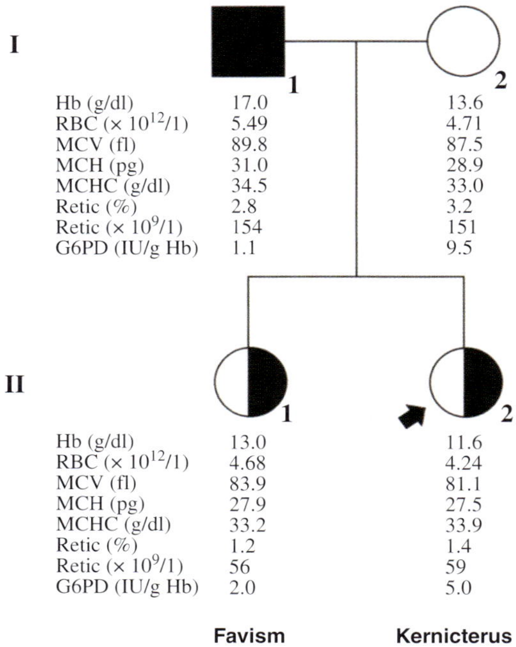

course predicts that both daughters must be heterozygotes. In fact, a G6PD assay carried out elsewhere on the girl with kernicterus gave a value in the heterozygous range (see Figure 6.2).

We next proceeded to molecular analysis and, having excluded G6PD A – and G6PD Mediterranean, the entire coding region of the G6PD gene was systematically screened for mutations using single strand conformation polymorphism (SSCP) analysis [1].[1] This revealed a mutation in exon V, that was confirmed by sequence analysis (see Figure 6.3). The A→C substitution within codon 135 implies the substitution in that position of Asn by Thr; at the time, this was a novel mutation.

Another, no-less-important further investigation was supplementary family history. We learned that the patient's sister, now five years old, had also had NNJ and had been treated with phototherapy. The sister developed normally, but at the age of six months, she had a severe attack of haemoglobinuria. Questions on dietary habits revealed that the whole family had an elevated (almost daily) consumption of fava beans – a very popular food

[1] This analysis is based on the principle that the mobility of single stranded DNA electrophoresed through non-denaturing polyacrylamide gels is determined by its fragment length and the secondary structure; the latter is sequence dependent. Therefore, a PCR product amplified from a mutant allele will have a different mobility to the PCR fragment with wild type sequence.

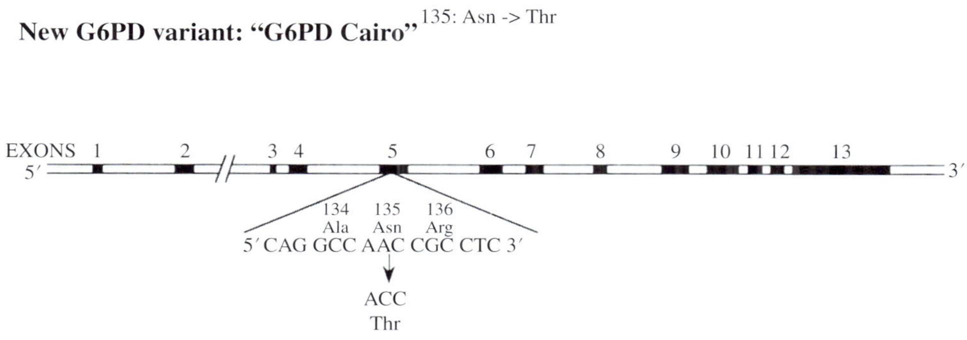

Figure 6.3 A schematic representation of the G6PD gene is shown. The exons and the introns are represented by black and white boxes respectively. The SSCP analysis revealed a putative mutation in exon V; direct sequence analysis of this exon revealed an A→C substitution within codon 135. This mutation predicts a replacement of Asn by Thr.

item in Egypt. The mother was able to recall that she had fava beans more than once in the days immediately preceding her second daughter's birth.

Comments

Since the discovery of G6PD deficiency, susceptibility to NNJ of G6PD deficient newborns, including the risk of kernicterus, was recognized early on [2, 3]. There is by now a vast literature on this subject [4–6]; in spite of this, it is still not clear why some but not all G6PD deficient babies develop NNJ, although it is known that one factor is the coexistence of the *UGT1A* mutation characteristic of Gilbert's syndrome [7]. It is also not clear whether and in what cases hyperbilirubinaemia results mainly from haemolysis or through other mechanisms. It has been suggested [8] that there may be two types of NNJ associated with G6PD deficiency: (i) a more common type, like an exaggerated form of "physiological jaundice of the newborn," generally benign and requiring phototherapy, if any therapy; (ii) a more rare type, with frank haemolysis, probably due to some environmental agent interacting with the genetic abnormality of G6PD, requiring active therapy including exchange transfusion in order to prevent kernicterus. One of the worst possible scenarios is a baby being exposed to fava beans that cause haemolysis before birth, or in the neonatal period through mother's milk; this is probably what happened in this case, and it is not unprecedented [9, 10]. Although placental transfer of the damaging components of the fava bean (divicine and isouramil, aglycones of pyrimidine glycosides) has not been documented, other glycosides are known to be transferred.

Although, since the G6PD gene is X-linked, both favism and NNJ are more common in males, they are well-documented also in heterozygous females [11, 12]. That the patient's father was used to eating fava beans with impunity is not surprising for several reasons. (i) Haemolysis is strongly dose-related; hence the much greater risk for children. (ii) From talking to the family, they normally consume dried and cooked (rather than fresh and raw) fava beans, and these are less dangerous [13].

While finding G6PD deficiency in Egypt is not surprising, because the prevalence in males is about 6% [14], we did not expect to find, rather than G6PD Mediterranean (probably the commonest variant in that country), a new variant that we called G6PD Cairo. Interestingly, it was found subsequently that G6PD Cairo is one of the commonest G6PD variants in Gaza, and it is frequently associated with favism [15]. Asparagine 135 is a highly conserved amino acid residue [16]; therefore, it is not surprising that when it is replaced by threonine it results in G6PD deficiency, probably through decreased *in vivo* stability of the enzyme protein.

In summary, this unfortunate girl heterozygous for G6PD deficiency suffered severe NNJ, associated with haemolytic anaemia, probably from maternal ingestion of fava beans; although as a baby she received treatment including exchange transfusion, she developed kernicterus. For a heterozygote, her G6PD level was in the middle range, i.e. about 50% of normal; her serious sequelae are a stark reminder of the fact that this level means that, consequent on X-chromosome inactivation, about 50% of her red cells are G6PD deficient, as severely deficient as in a hemizygous male.

Conclusion

Kernicterus in a girl heterozygous for G6PD deficiency: G6PD Cairo.

Acknowledgements

Referred by Dr. I. Hann, Department of Haematology, Great Ormond Street Hospital for Children, London, UK.
Dr. J. Wilson, Department of Neurology, Great Ormond Street Hospital for Children, London, UK.

References

1. Orita, M., Iwahana, H., Kanazawa, H. et al. (1989). Detection of polymorphisms of human DNA by gel electrophoresis as single-strand conformation polymorphisms. *Proc. Natl. Acad. Sci. USA*. 86, 2766–2770.

2. Doxiadis, S.A., Fessas, P.H., and Valaes, T. (1960). Erythrocyte enzyme deficiency in unexplained kernicterus. *Lancet* ii, 44–40.
3. Panizon, F. (1960). Erythrocyte enzyme deficiency in unexplained kernicterus. *Lancet* ii, 1093–1090.
4. Bienzle, U., Effiong, C.E., and Luzzatto, L. (1976). Erythrocyte glucose 6-phosphate dehydrogenase deficiency (G6PD type A−) and neonatal jaundice. *Acta Paediatr. Scand.* 65, 701–703.
5. Kaplan, M., Herschel, M., Hammerman, C. et al. (2004). Hyperbilirubinemia among African American, glucose-6-phosphate dehydrogenase-deficient neonates. *Pediatrics* 114, e213–e219.
6. Kaplan, M. and Hammerman, C. (2009). The need for neonatal glucose-6-phosphate dehydrogenase screening: a global perspective. *J. Perinatol.* 29(Suppl 1), S46–S52.
7. Kaplan, M., Renbaum, P., Levy-Lahad, E. et al. (1997). Gilbert syndrome and glucose-6-phosphate dehydrogenase deficiency: a dose-dependent genetic interaction crucial to neonatal hyperbilirubinemia. *Proc. Natl. Acad. Sci. USA*. 94, 12128–12132.
8. Luzzatto, L. and Poggi, V.E. (2015). Glucose-6-phosphate dehydrogenase deficiency. In: Orkin, S.H., Fisher, D.E., Ginsburg, D. et al. editor. *Nathan and Oski's Hematology and Oncology of Infancy and Childhood*. Vol. 1. Elsevier Saunders. pp. 609–629.
9. Corchia, C., Balata, A., Meloni, G.F. et al. (1995). Favism in a female newborn infant whose mother ingested fava beans before delivery. (Review) *J. Pediatrics* 127, 807–808.
10. Mentzer, J.W.C. and Collier, E. (1975). Hydrops fetalis associated with erythrocyte G6PD deficiency and maternal ingestion of fava beans and ascorbic acid. *J. Pediatrics* 86, 565–567.
11. Meloni, T., Forteleoni, G., and Meloni, G.F. (1992). Marked decline of favism after neonatal glucose 6-phosphate dehydrogenase screening and health education: the northern Sardinian experience. *Acta. Haematologica*. 87, 29–31.
12. Pamba, A., Richardson, N.D., Carter, N. et al. (2012). Clinical spectrum and severity of hemolytic anemia in glucose 6-phosphate dehydrogenase-deficient children receiving dapsone. *Blood* 120, 4123–4133.
13. Luzzatto, L. and Arese, P. (2018). Favism and glucose-6-phosphate dehydrogenase deficiency. *N. Engl. J. Med.* 378, 1068–1069.
14. Luzzatto, L., Ally, M., and Notaro, R. (2020). Glucose-6-phosphate dehydrogenase deficiency. *Blood* 136, 1225–1240.
15. Reading, N.S., Sirdah, M.M., Shubair, M.E. et al. (2016). Favism, the commonest form of severe hemolytic anemia in Palestinian children, varies in severity with three different variants of G6PD deficiency within the same community. *Blood. Cells. Mol. Dis.* 60, 58–64.
16. Notaro, R., Afolayan, A, and Luzzatto, L. (2000). Human mutations in glucose 6-phosphate dehydrogenase reflect evolutionary history. *FASEB J.* 14, 485–494.

Case 7

A Levels Without Haemoglobin A

Patient Details

Age: 5 *Sex:* F
Ethnic background: Parents from Iraq

Reason for Referral

Second opinion on a patient with beta thalassaemia.

History and Clinical Findings in Brief

The patient, who grew up in Bahrain, was well until the age of four, when she was admitted to hospital with fever and anaemia. She subsequently received a single blood transfusion. Her family recently moved to the United Kingdom; it was confirmed that she had moderate anaemia, with haemoglobin levels fluctuating between 9 and 10 g/dl, but she was clinically well and had required no further blood transfusions. On examination she had no icterus, but marked splenomegaly (8 cm below the costal margin), and the liver was also palpable. Malocclusion was noted on the left, consistent with some facial skeletal changes.

Laboratory Findings

The patient had a moderate microcytic anaemia (see Table 7.1). The blood film confirmed a microcytic picture (see Figure 7.1). In addition, it showed hypochromia and a very marked anisocytosis and poikilocytosis. We also saw dense cells, not quite spherical (we are tempted to call them pseudo-spherocytes); target cells, large polychromatic cells and an occasional nucleated red blood cell.

Initial Assessment

The clinical and haematological features immediately suggested a thalassaemic condition, and beta thalassaemia is relatively common in Iraq. The patient fits with the clinical picture of what has been known for a long time as thalassaemia intermedia, which we now prefer to call non-transfusion-dependent thalassaemia (NTDT).

Table 7.1 Haematology Data

Hb (g/dl)	10.7
RBC ($\times 10^{12}$/l)	4.87
MCV (fl)	69.6
MCH (pg)	22.0
MCHC (g/dl)	31.8
RDW (S.D.)	82.1
Retic (%)	5.7
Retic ($\times 10^{9}$/l)	278
Hb A_2 (%)	2.0
Hb F (%)	98
Non-α : α ratio[a]	0.32

[a] Globin chain biosynthetic ratio.

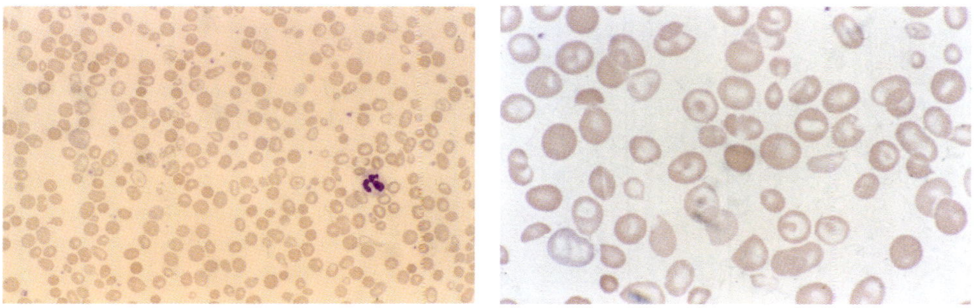

(a) (b)

Figure 7.1 Peripheral blood film: (a) medium power view; (b) high power view.

Further Investigations

Haemoglobin electrophoresis revealed Hb F and Hb A_2 only (see Figure 7.2). This would be compatible with homozygous hereditary persistence of foetal haemoglobin (HPFH) or homozygous beta thalassaemia. HPFH was immediately ruled out by the fact that Hb F was normal in both parents (Figure 7.5), and the globin chain biosynthetic ratio (non-α/α) was markedly abnormal at 0.32 (see Figure 7.3). A Southern blot β-globin gene analysis ruled out a major deletion, as would be seen in most cases of HPFH; on the other hand, PCR amplification of the β-globin gene after *Hph I* digestion, followed by sequencing, revealed an IVS II nt 1 (G→A) mutation without a normal base in this position, indicating that the patient is homozygous for this mutation (see Figure 7.4). Both of the patient's parents were heterozygous for this mutation. In addition, analysis of the alpha globin gene cluster (not shown) revealed that the patient and the family members tested were all heterozygous for α^+ thalassaemia (i.e. α–/αα) (see Figure 7.5).

Comments

Genotype–phenotype correlations have been extensively explored in β-thalassaemia [1]. The IVS II nt 1 (G→A) mutation prevents splicing; therefore, it is in the β^0 class and, not surprisingly, in general, β^0 is more severe than β^+ [2] However, there are exceptions, and this patient, homozygous for this mutation, is one of them. IVS II nt 1 (G→A) was in fact classified as "mild" by Cao et al. [3]; and three homozygotes for this mutation were classified as mild or moderate by Ho et al [4]. Since the excess of α chains not finding a partner is the main agent of ineffective erythropoiesis in β-thalassaemia [5], a high rate of γ chain production is beneficial in β-thalassaemia; another homozygote for the IVS II nt 1 (G→A) mutation had, like our patient, >98% Hb F and was classified as "moderate" by Diaz-Chico et al. [6], who attributed this to the mutation being in a haplotype context

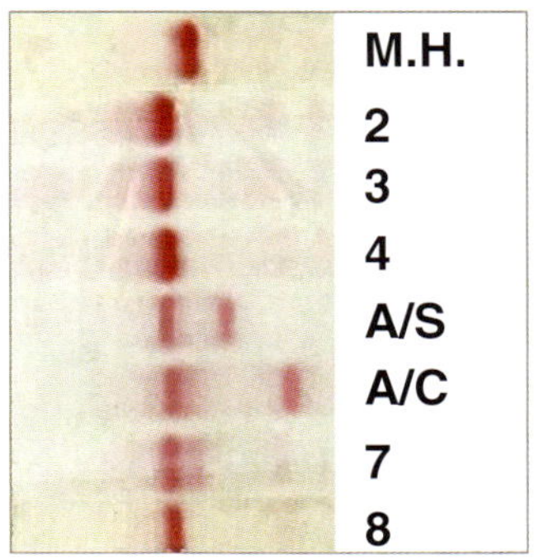

Figure 7.2 Haemoglobin electrophoresis on cellulose acetate membrane; the migration of the haemoglobin fractions is from right to left. An A/S control and A/C control are in lanes 5 and 6, respectively. The patient (M.H.) is in lane 1.

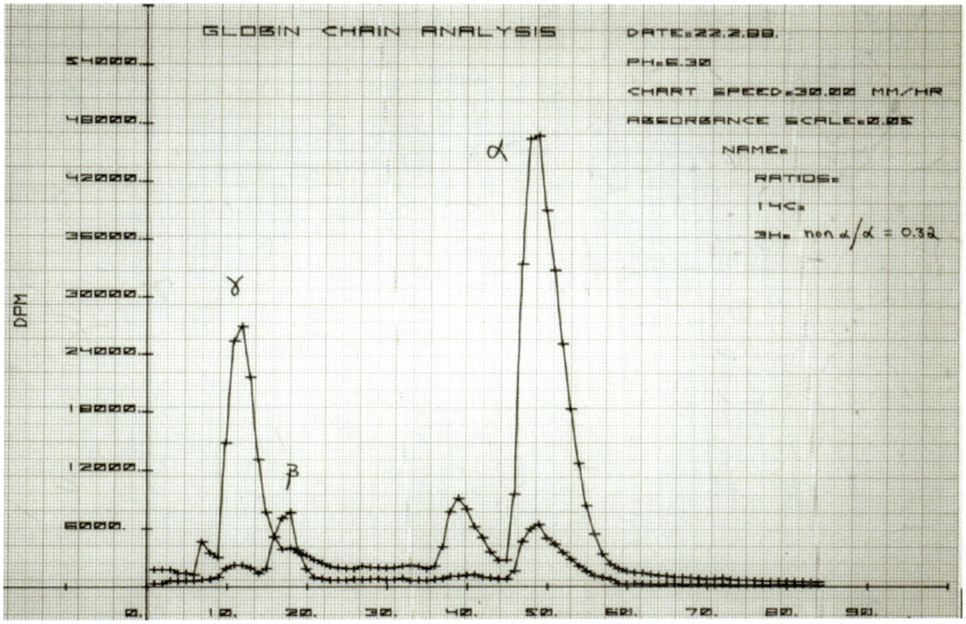

Figure 7.3 *In vitro* globin chain synthesis. The Y-axis represents the radioactivity incorporated; the X-axis is the tube number (or elution time). The incorporation of labelled leucine by newly synthesized globin chains is represented graphically following ion-exchange column chromatography. The two curves are the normal control labelled with ^{14}C-leucine (curve close to the X-axis) and the patient's globin chains labelled with ^{3}H-leucine. The two small peaks eluting at points 18 and 48 mark the normal β and α globin chains positions, respectively. The control α : β globin chain ratio was determined to be 0.96 (normal range 0.95–1.05). The patient's curve revealed two major peaks corresponding to γ and α globin chains, the virtual absence of β-globin chains, peaking at tube 18, is characteristic of a β^0-phenotype. The non-α: ratio α ratio was 0.32, in the range of thalassaemia intermedia.

favourable to a high rate of γ chain synthesis. In addition, in our patient the α chain excess was decreased by the coexistent α-thalassaemia gene.

Follow-up

This patient has continued to do remarkably well. As a young girl, she reports "never missing a day off school," studying for her "A"-levels. However, her spleen remains moderately enlarged (7 cm below the costal margin), and NTDT is highly heterogeneous from both the genetic and the clinical point of view [7]; in adults there is often iron overload that may need correction. This patient may also be a candidate for luspatercept, the first medicine, recently approved, that can ameliorate ineffective erythropoiesis [8].

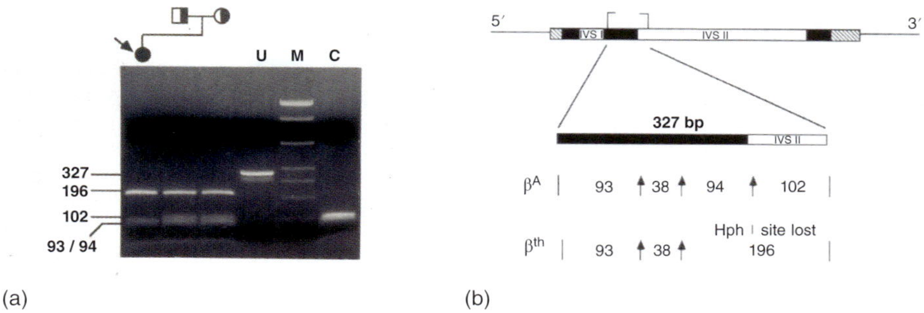

Figure 7.4 (a) Ethidium bromide stained mini-agarose gel, showing the fragments generated by *Hph I* digestion of the PCR products from: normal control (C), the patient and her parents (see pedigree above); U: undigested fragment; M: molecular size marker. (b) Schematic representation of the β-globin gene; also illustrated is the region of the gene amplified using PCR; the location of the primers; the restriction sites for the enzyme *HpH I*, with expected fragment sizes (bp) in both the normal (β^A) and the thalassaemic (β^{th}) allele.

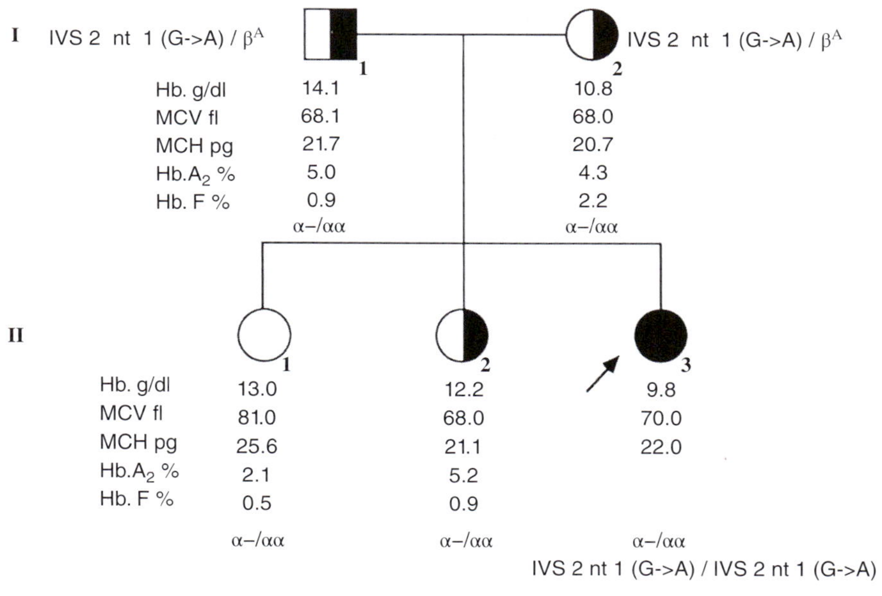

Figure 7.5 Family pedigree.

Conclusion

β-thalassaemia (homozygous for IVS II nt 1 mutation), heterozygous for α-thalassaemia, resulting in NTDT (thalassaemia intermedia phenotype).

Acknowledgements

Professor Antonio Cao, University of Cagliari, Cagliari, Italy.
Dr. Irene Roberts, Department of Haematology, Hammersmith Hospital, London. UK.

References

1. Taher, A.T., Musallam, K.M., and Cappellini, M.D. (2021). β-thalassemias. *N. Engl. J. Med*. 384(8), 727–743.
2. Weatherall, D.J. and Clegg, J.B. (2001). *The Thalassaemia Syndromes* 4 ed. Copyright © 2001 Blackwell Science Ltd.
3. Cao, A., Galanello, R., and Rosatelli, M.C. (1994). Genotype-phenotype correlations in beta-thalassemias. *Blood. Rev*. 8(1), 1–12.
4. Ho, P.J., Hall, G.W., Luo, L.Y. et al. (1998). Beta-thalassaemia intermedia: is it possible consistently to predict phenotype from genotype? *Br. J. Haematol*. 100, 70–78.
5. Kihm, A.J., Kong, Y., Hong, W. et al. (2002). An abundant erythroid protein that stabilizes free alpha-haemoglobin. *Nature* 417(6890), 758–763.
6. Diaz-Chico, J.C., Yang, K.G., Stoming, T.A. et al. (1988). Mild and severe beta-thalassemia among homozygotes from Turkey: identification of the types by hybridization of amplified DNA with synthetic probes. *Blood* 71, 248–251.
7. Musallam, K.M., Rivella, S., Vichinsky, E. et al. (2013). Non-transfusion-dependent thalassemias. *Haematologica* 98(6), 833–844.
8. Piga, A., Perrotta, S., Gamberini, M.R. et al. (2019). Luspatercept improves hemoglobin levels and blood transfusion requirements in a study of patients with β-thalassemia. *Blood* 133(12), 1279–1289.

See also related Cases 11, 12, and 17.

Case 8
A Hot Blood Smear

Patient Details

Age: 6 *Sex:* F
Ethnic background: Turkish-Cypriot

Reason for Referral

Chronic haemolytic anaemia.

History and Clinical Findings in Brief

The patient was first found to be anaemic when she was 6 months old. Since then, her anaemia has persisted and she has required several blood transfusions; intermittently she has been clinically jaundiced. On examination, the patient's height and weight were at the 25th centile. There were no "thalassaemia-like" changes in her facial appearance; but she had splenomegaly.

Laboratory Findings

There was a moderate normocytic normochromic anaemia (see Table 8.1). The red cell morphology was striking (see Figure 8.1), partly because of the wide range of cell sizes (reflected in the high RDW); but especially

Table 8.1 Haematology Data

	Patient	Mother	Father	Sister	Brother
Hb (g/dl)	9.3	12.9	15.5	13.6	15.6
RBC ($\times 10^{12}$/l)	3.52	4.51	4.98	4.96	5.72
MCV (fl)	77.0	85.8	93.0	87.7	79.2
MCH (pg)	26.4	28.6	31.1	27.4	27.3
MCHC (g/dl)	34.3	33.3	33.5	31.3	34.4
RDW (S.D.)	78.1	38.9	41.7	43.8	37.2

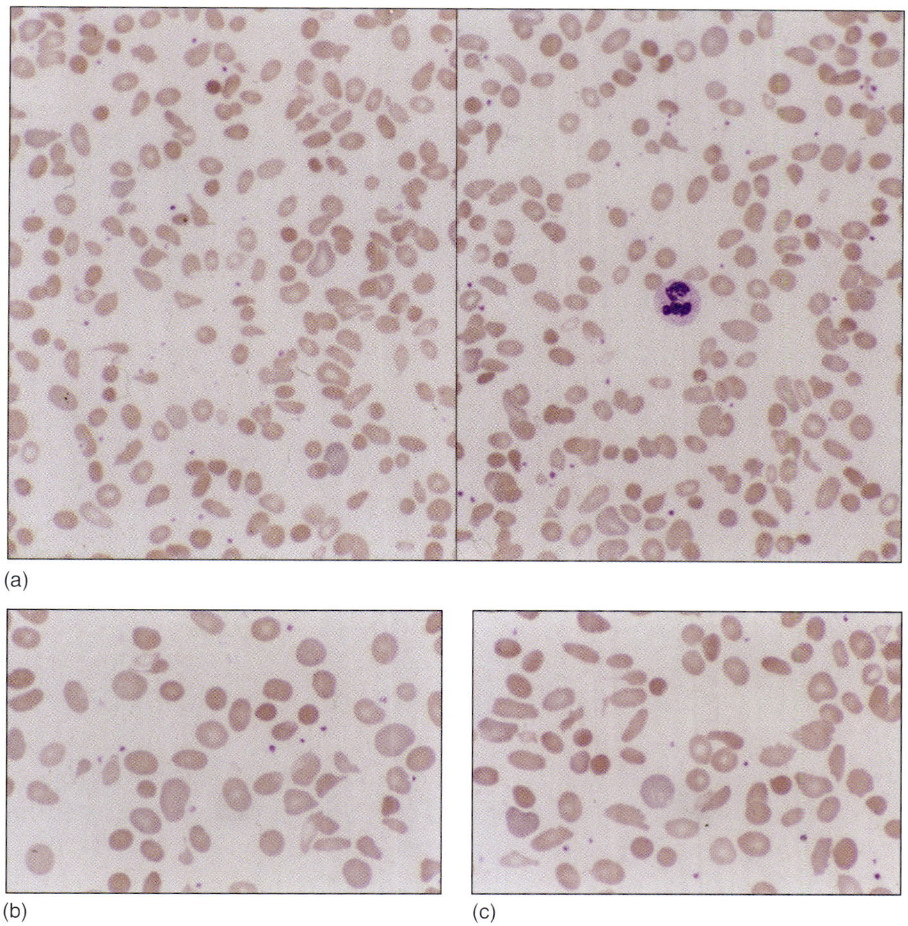

Figure 8.1 Peripheral blood film; (a) medium power view (composite); (b) and (c) high power view.

because we saw an extraordinary range of morphology, from compact micro-spherocytes to very large polychromatic macrocytes (which must have been 120 fl or more; see Figure 8.2). Many of the red cells were very

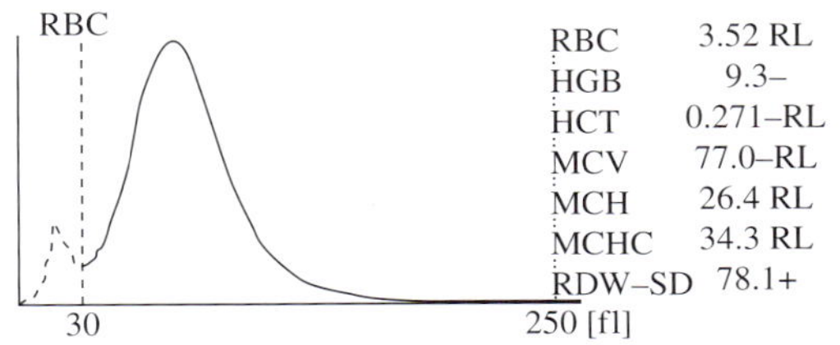

Figure 8.2 Red cell size distribution profile showing increased RDW.

dense and some of these were true spherocytes. Whether they had central pallor or not, a high proportion of the red cells had one axis longer the other, which gave an overall ovalocytic/elliptocytic appearance. Many poikilocytes were seen; some with very irregular contours and fimbriated edges; some tear-drop-shaped with long "tails," which made them look like tadpoles; a few smaller cells were either angular in appearance ("trigonocytes") and well haemoglobinized, or oval-shaped but very hypochromic. We even saw shapes that were a reasonable imitation of a sickle cell! Polychromatic cells were abundant (retic count 22.3%).

Initial Assessment

The patient had a history compatible with chronic haemolytic anaemia and a blood picture highly suggestive of the severe form of elliptocytosis known as hereditary pyropoikilocytosis (HPP) [1].

Further Investigations

The osmotic fragility curve (see Figure 8.3) was markedly right shifted (MCF 4.6 g/l), with a large tail that reflected hyper-fragile cells. After preincubation for 24 hours at 37 °C, the curve was so abnormal that it nearly lost its typical sigmoidal shape and became linear (MCF 6.3 g/l). The autohaemolysis test was also markedly abnormal, with correction by glucose of only about 50% (see Table 8.2).

A family study showed normal blood counts in parents and two siblings (Table 8.1).

A G6PD assay on the patient gave a level of 6.4 IU/g Hb, just below our normal range, and very significantly low when one considers her high reticulocytosis. The assay on the mother was normal (see Table 8.3), but the father proved to be a hemizygote deficient, with an enzyme level of only 0.1 IU/g Hb; thus, the child was an obligate heterozygote. Molecular analysis revealed the G6PD Mediterranean mutation.

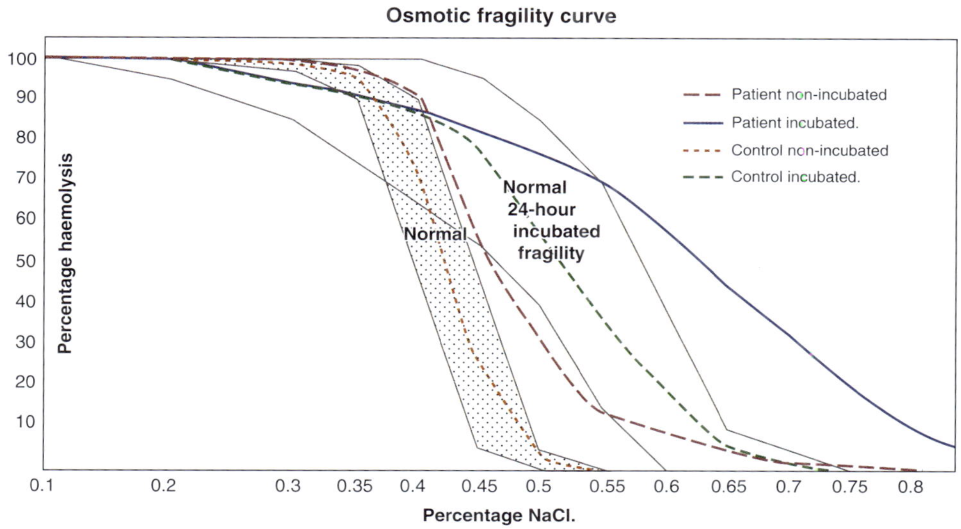

Figure 8.3 Osmotic fragility curves of the patient's sample before incubation (red line) and after 24 hours of incubation at 37 °C, together with the normal ranges. A normal control is shown also, before (orange line) and after (green line) incubation. Normal ranges are indicated by the shaded area (for freshly tested sample) and by the black unbroken lines (post 24-hour incubated sample).

Table 8.2 Results of Autohaemolysis Test

	% Lysis at 48 hours	
	Without glucose	Addition of glucose
Control	1.7	0.2
Patient	28.7	14.9
Mother	2.4	0.4
Father	1.7	0.4

Table 8.3 G6PD Activity (IU/g Hb)

Control	8.9
Patient	6.4
Mother	10.3
Father	0.1
Sister	3.7
Brother	10.2

Overall, we felt confident about the diagnosis of pyropoikilocytosis, with the added finding that the patient was also heterozygote for G6PD deficiency.

Follow-up

The following year a splenectomy was performed: there were no post-operative problems.

Further Follow-up and Subsequent Investigations

Many years later, Dr. G Bozkurt, who had originally referred this patient, kindly provided an update. The patient, now 38 years old, has been doing well; she is leading a normal life and she works full-time in her office. Her haemoglobin level is near-normal (see Table 8.4), and she has not required any more blood transfusions after her splenectomy; however, her blood film (see Figure 8.4, courtesy of Dr. Bozkurt) still shows marked anisopoikilocytosis, elliptocytosis, spherocytes and red cell fragments, much like before. Platelet counts are elevated, and she has been advised to take 100 mg aspirin daily. She also receives an annual preventive pneumococcal vaccine.

Achille Iolascon and Immacolata Andolfo have carried out further tests on blood samples from the patient and her family. On the patient's sample,

Table 8.4 Haematology Data (Age 36)

Hb (g/dl)	11.7
RBC ($\times 10^{12}$/l)	4.27
MCV (fl)	79.6
MCH (pg)	27.4
MCHC (g/dl)	34.4
WBC ($\times 10^{9}$/l)	10.4
Plt ($\times 10^{9}$/l)	820

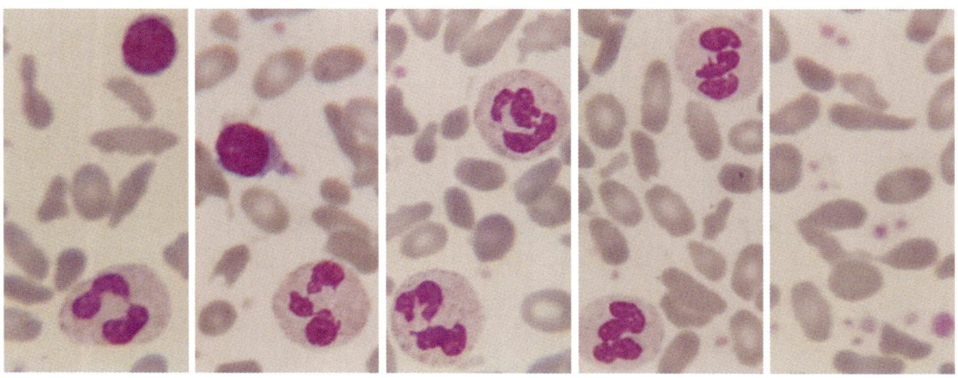

Figure 8.4 Follow-up peripheral blood film (courtesy of Dr. Gulsen Bozkurt).

in the eosin-5′-maleimide (EMA) binding test, fluorescence was reduced by 40%. The ektacytometry profile [2] showed an impressive "flattening" in the patient and a shift to the right in both parents (Figure 8.5). DNA analysis of 30 genes that can underlie haemolytic anaemia – currently referred to as an "appropriate NGS panel" [3] – yielded interesting results (see Figure 8.6).

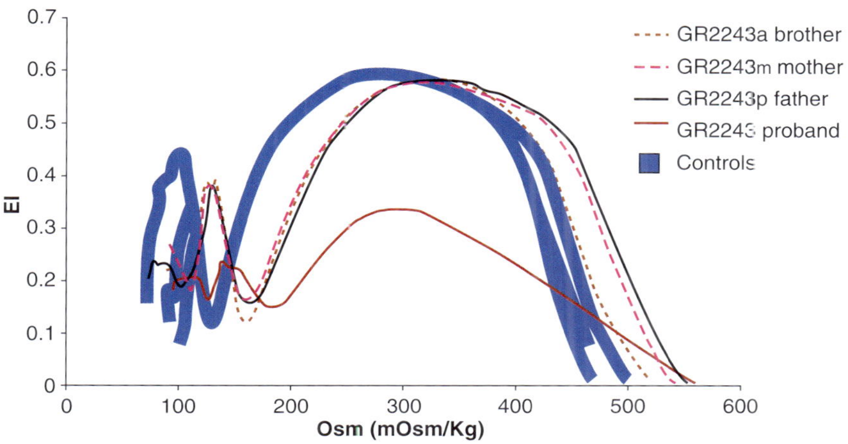

Figure 8.5 Ektacytometry profiles of patient and family members. Osm, osmolarity; EI, erythrocyte deformability index.

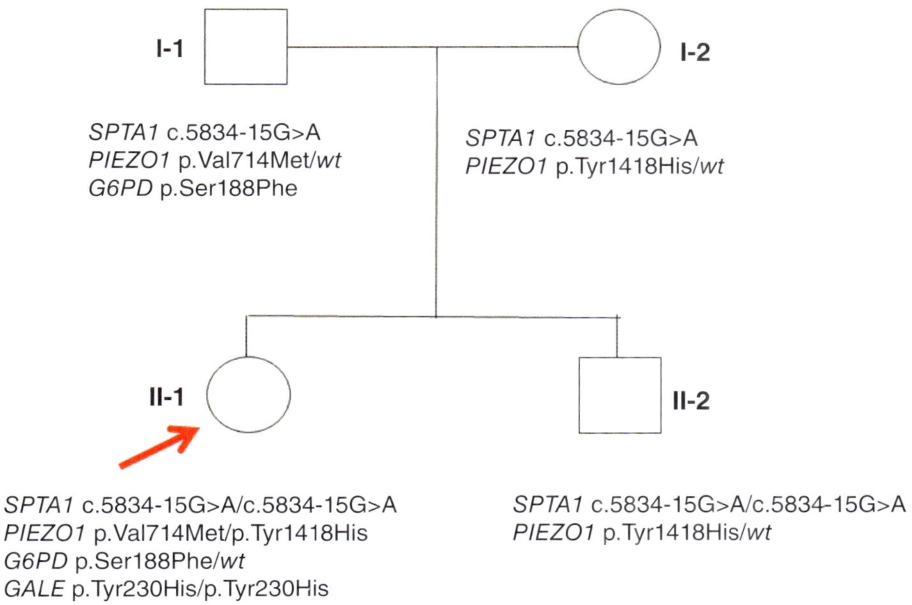

Figure 8.6 Genetic studies on the family and of patient (red arrow). The genotypes detected by DNA analysis are shown; wt, wild type.

First, not surprisingly, G6PD deficiency was confirmed. Second, both parents are heterozygous for a mutation in the gene encoding α-spectrin, *SPTA1,* and both the patient and her brother are homozygous for this mutation; however, it is an intronic mutation, 15 nucleotides upstream of the intron-exon boundary, and it has almost certainly no clinical significance. Third, the patient's mother is heterozygous for a missense mutation in exon 33 of *PIEZO1*, and the patient's father as well as the patient's brother are heterozygous for a missense mutation in exon 16 of this same gene; notably, the patient herself has inherited both *PIEZO1* mutations. Then, whole exon sequence (WES) analysis uncovered a surprise: the patient is also homozygous for a missense mutation (p.Tyr230His) of the galactose-4-epimerase gene *GALE*.

Comments

From the point of view of traditional haematology, in this patient HPP was a spot diagnosis from just looking at the blood film.[1] The rather spectacular results of old-fashioned tests such as osmotic fragility and auto-haemolysis were in keeping with this diagnosis; and so was the good clinical response to splenectomy.

Coming to aetiology, whereas the genotype-phenotype relationship is straightforward with hemoglobinopathies, as they are caused by mutations of either the α-globin genes (*HBA1, HBA2*), or the β-globin genes (*HBB*); and whereas each enzymopathy is due to mutations of the respective structural gene, with the membrane-cytoskeleton group of red cell disorders [4] the situation has proven more complex. The same phenotype, e.g. spherocytosis, can be due to mutations of one of several genes: the spectrin genes (*SPTA1, SPTB*), the ankyrin gene (*ANK*), the band 3 gene (*SLC4A1*), and possibly others. Conversely, other *SPTA1* or *SPTB* mutations will give elliptocytosis rather than spherocytosis [5]. For this reason, in this group of disorders, NGS on an appropriate gene panel is particularly valuable [6, 7].

HPP has occurred with homozygous or bi-allelic *SPTA1* or *SPTB* mutations, each one of which would cause, in a heterozygote, the milder disease hereditary elliptocytosis (HE). In many cases of HPP [3, 8], one mutation in *SPTA1* interferes with self-association, whereas the other causes a quantitative decrease in α-spectrin [9]; and some HPP patients have one *SPTA1* mutation and one *SPTB* mutation (each one inherited from one of the

[1] The term pyropoikilocytosis originates from the fact that similarly highly abnormal red cell morphology can be seen in patients with severe burns, or by deliberately exposing red cells to heat. Therefore, the use of this term for a severe form of HE has been criticized, but it is by now entrenched in the literature.

parents). In our case, although the red cells morphology was not that of HE in either parent, the mother had a slightly abnormal osmotic fragility curve, and both parents had a slightly abnormal ektacytometry profile (very marginally also the brother).

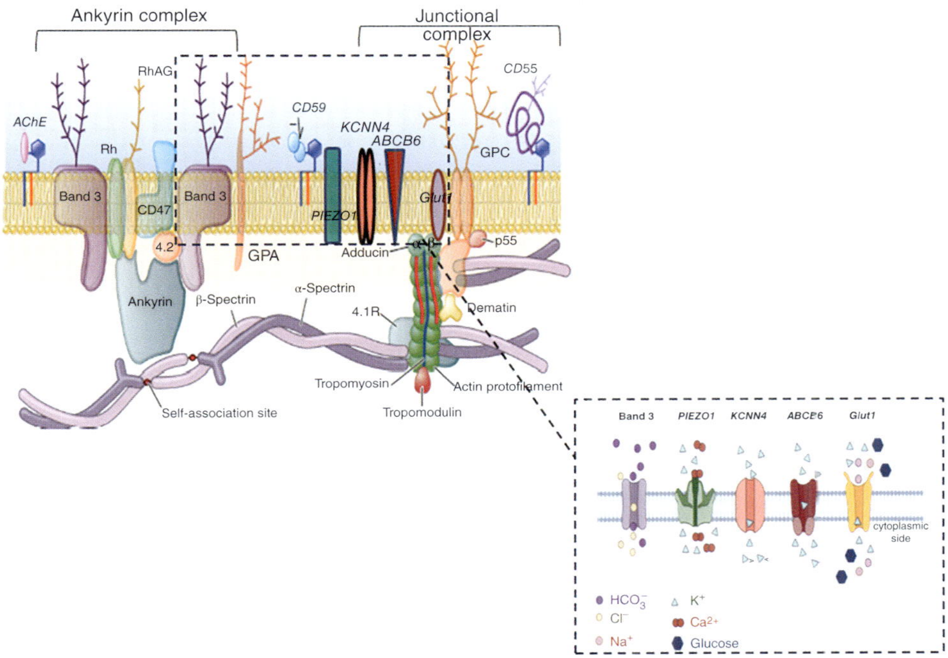

Figure 8.7 The red cell membrane and cytoskeleton. Within the lipid bilayer several proteins are integral to the membrane; other proteins, e.g. acetylcholinesterase (*AChE*) and the two complement-regulatory proteins CD59 and CD55, are tethered to the membrane through the glycosylphosphatidylinositol (GPI) anchor, whereby the entire polypeptide chain is extracellular. Many of the membrane proteins bear polypeptide and/or carbohydrate red cell antigens. Underneath the membrane, the α-β spectrin dimers, which associate head-to-head into tetramers, together with actin and other proteins, form most of the cytoskeleton. The ankyrin complex, which provides mainly radial (vertical) connections, and the junctional complex, that provides mainly tangential (horizontal) connections, link the membrane to the cytoskeleton. The inset is a schematic diagram of membrane transporters, abnormalities of which underlie channelopathies. Band 3 (anion exchanger 1 [AE1]) is the most abundant, and mutations of *SLC4A1* (encoding band 3) can inactivate anion exchange, thus causing cation leak; *PIEZO1*, a homotrimer with a three-bladed, propeller-shaped structure, is a mechano-sensitive cation channel that regulates red blood cell volume; *KCNN4* encodes a Ca^{2+} activated K^+ channel, also known as the Gardos channel; *ABCB6* encodes a mitochondrial porphyrin transporter, and some mutations can cause increase K^+ efflux from red cells and stomatocytosis; *Glut1* facilitates glucose transport [12]/with permission of McGraw Hill.

Our patient illustrates that even NGS and even WES may not always give a straightforward answer. The phenotype of *GALE*-related disease ranges from severe galactosemia to thrombocytopenia with neurological abnormalities: although the WES report classified the *GALE*Y230H mutation as "deleterious," our patient had none of the above and we feel this finding is not relevant to her HPP.

Of course, we were expecting to find mutations in one of the HE/HPP genes mentioned above. Instead, two *PIEZO1* mutations turned up: the maternal one is classified as "of uncertain significance," and the paternal one, shared also by the patient's unaffected brother, is novel; the only member of the family with two *PIEZO1* mutations is the patient. The best-known red cell morphology of *PIEZO1* mutations is stomatocytes [10], not elliptocytes; however, considering the very close solid-state arrangement of proteins in the membrane–cytoskeleton complex of the red cell (see Figure 8.7), it seems not impossible that some *PIEZO1* mutations, when bi-allelic, may cause HPP. We must also note that in patients with stomatocytosis, particularly in dehydrated xerocytosis, splenectomy is contraindicated, because it is often complicated by life-threatening thrombosis [11]: fortunately, it was not the case in our patient.

Deficiency of G6PD has been reported before in families with HE, and in most instances there has been no evidence of the former enhancing chronic haemolysis associated with the latter [13, 14]. However, infection, or a drug, may be a trigger of acute on chronic haemolytic anaemia; and we did advise our patient to avoid fava beans absolutely.

Conclusion

Pyropoikilocytosis with bi-allelic *PIEZO1* mutation in a heterozygote for G6PD deficiency.

Acknowledgements

Referred by Dr. Gulsen Bozkurt, Hematological Diagnosis and Treatment Centre, Nicosia, Cyprus.

Prof. Achille Iolascon, Department of Molecular Medicine and Biotechnology, University of Naples Federico II, Naples, Italy.

Dr. Immacolata Andolfo, Department of Molecular Medicine and Biotechnology, University of Naples Federico II, Naples, Italy.

Dr. Irene Roberts, Department of Haematology, Hammersmith Hospital, London, UK.

Dr. Marion Reid, International Blood Group Reference Laboratory (IBGRL), Bristol, UK.

References

1. Dacie, J.V. (1954). *The Haemolytic Anaemias, Congenital and Acquired*. London Churchill.
2. Llaudet-Planas, E., Vives-Corrons, J.L., Rizzuto, V. et al. (2018). Osmotic gradient ektacytometry: a valuable screening test for hereditary spherocytosis and other red blood cell membrane disorders. *Int. J. Lab. Hematol.* 40(1), 94–102.
3. Niss, O., Chonat, S., Dagaonkar, N. et al. (2016). Genotype-phenotype correlations in hereditary elliptocytosis and hereditary pyropoikilocytosis. *Blood. Cells. Mol. Dis.* 61, 4–9.
4. Lux, S.E. (2014). Red cell membrane. In: Orkin, S.H., Fisher, D.E., Ginsburg, D. et al. editor. *Nathan and Oski's Hematology and Oncology of Infancy and Childhood*. Vol. 1, Philadelphia: Elsevier Saunders. pp. 455–514.
5. Lux, S.E. (2014). Disorders of the red cell membrane. In: Orkin, S.H., Fisher, D.E., Ginsburg, D. et al. editor. *Nathan and Oski's Hematology and Oncology of Infancy and Childhood*. Vol. 1, Philadelphia: Elsevier Saunders. pp. 515–579.
6. Vives-Corrons, J.L., Krishnevskaya, E., Rodriguez, I.H. et al. (2021). Characterization of hereditary red blood cell membranopathies using combined targeted next-generation sequencing and osmotic gradient ektacytometry. *Int. J. Hematol.* 113(2), 163–174.
7. Russo, R., Andolfo, I., Manna, F. et al. (2018). Multi-gene panel testing improves diagnosis and management of patients with hereditary anemias. *Am. J. Hematol.* 93(5), 672–682.
8. Lawler, J., Palek, J., Liu, S.C. et al. (1983). Molecular heterogeneity of hereditary poikylocytosis: identification of a second variant of the spectrin alpha-subunit. *Blood* 62, 1182–1189.
9. Iolascon, A., Andolfo, I., and Russo, R. (2019). Advances in understanding the pathogenesis of red cell membrane disorders. *Br. J. Haematol.* 187(1), 13–24.
10. Andolfo, I., Iolascon, A., and Russo, R. (2025). The evolving landscape of hereditary stomatocytosis. *Blood* 145(26), 3089–3100.
11. Stewart, G.W., Amess, J.A.L., Eber, S.W. et al. (1996). Thrombo-embolic disease after splenectomy for hereditary stomatocytosis. *Br. J. Haematol.* 93, 303–310.
12. Luzzatto, L. and De Franceschi, L. (2025). Hemolytic anemias. In: Jameson, J.L., Fauci, A.S., Kasper, D.L. et al. editor. *Harrison's Principles of Internal Medicine*. Vol. 1, 22 ed. New York: Access Medicine. pp. 791–807.
13. Pryor, D.S. and Pitney, W.R. (1967). Hereditary elliptocytosis: a report of two families from New Guinea. *Br. J. Haematol.* 13, 126–134.
14. Pearson, H.A. (1968). The genetic basis of hereditary elliptocytosis with hemolysis. *Blood* 32, 972–978.

Case 9
More Yellow Than Sick

Patient Details

Age: 37 *Sex:* M
Ethnic background: English

Reason for Referral

Long-standing jaundice.

History and Clinical Findings in Brief

The patient had suffered from neonatal jaundice. In recent years, he complained of intermittent tiredness. His sister was reported to have had anaemia, for which she had been splenectomized. On examination the patient was mildly icteric but not anaemic. There was no hepatosplenomegaly.

Laboratory Findings

The patient had a moderate macrocytosis but did not have anaemia (see Table 9.1). His reticulocyte percentage and absolute count were slightly elevated. On the blood film (see Figure 9.1), the majority of the red cells

Table 9.1 Laboratory Findings

Hb (g/dl)	13.3
RBC ($\times 10^{12}$/l)	4.57
MCV (fl)	106
MCH (pg)	29.1
MCHC (g/dl)	29.5
Retic (%)	2.4
Retic ($\times 10^{9}$/l)	110
WBC ($\times 10^{9}$/l)	4.6
PLT ($\times 10^{9}$/l)	92
Hb A_2 (%)	2.5
Hb F (%)	1.4
Bilirubin (μmol/l)	44

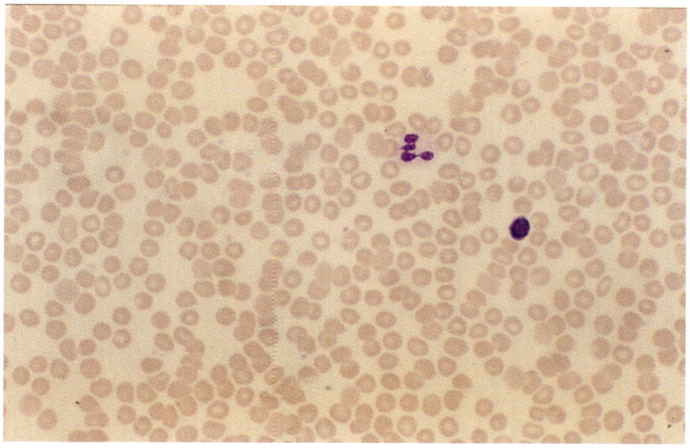

Figure 9.1 Peripheral blood film.

looked normal, but a few cells showed uneven distribution of haemoglobin and some appeared rather dense.

The urinary sediment revealed the presence of haemosiderin. The autohaemolysis test was normal. The osmotic fragility test performed on a fresh sample was normal. However, on the post-incubated aliquot, a left-shifted curve was obtained (not shown). This did not reflect a susceptibly fragile population of red cells, but rather, cells with an increased *resistance* to osmotic lysis; this was quite compatible with his low MCHC.

Initial Assessment

The blood findings are consistent with a well-compensated haemolytic disorder; the modest increase in bilirubin and the positive urinary haemosiderin indicate intravascular haemolysis. The normal autohaemolysis test did not support a membrane defect or enzymopathy; therefore, we focused on the possibility of an abnormal haemoglobin.

Further Investigations

Haemoglobin electrophoresis on cellulose acetate membrane revealed, in addition to the normal bands of Hb A and Hb A_2 (2.5%), a diffuse band anodal to A_2, which was quantitated at 6.8% (see Figure 9.2). Hb F level was 1.4% (see Table 9.1). Globin chain (alkaline) electrophoresis revealed an α- and a β-globin band in their respective normal positions (not shown). The globin chain biosynthetic ratio ($\beta : \alpha$) gave a normal value of 0.94. In view of the abnormal electrophoretic pattern, tests for unstable haemoglobins were performed. After supravital staining with methyl violet, no Heinz bodies were seen. However, the heat stability test was positive, and the unstable Hb was quantitated to be 8.4% (control 3.4%); the isopropanol precipitation test was also positive. Molecular analysis of the patient's β-globin gene revealed that he was heterozygous for a base substitution at codon 98 (Val→Met) (see Figure 9.3), which predicts Hb Köln [1]. We were fortunate enough to have available a blood sample from the patient's sister. Her blood film (see Figure 9.4) showed

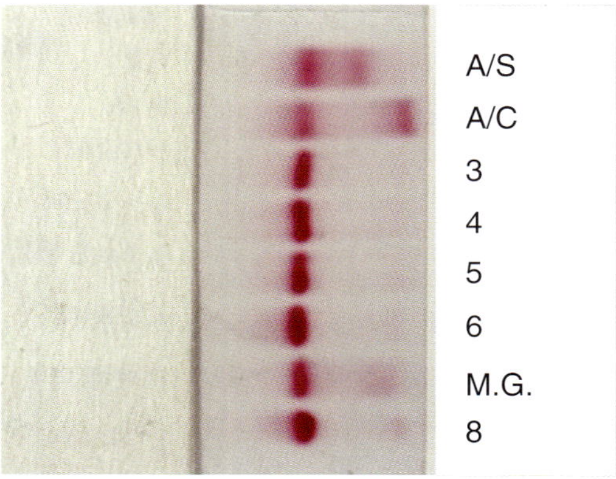

Figure 9.2 Haemoglobin electrophoresis on cellulose acetate membrane; the migration of the haemoglobin fractions is from right to left. An A/S and A/C control are in lanes 1 and 2, respectively. The patient (M.G.) is in lane 7.

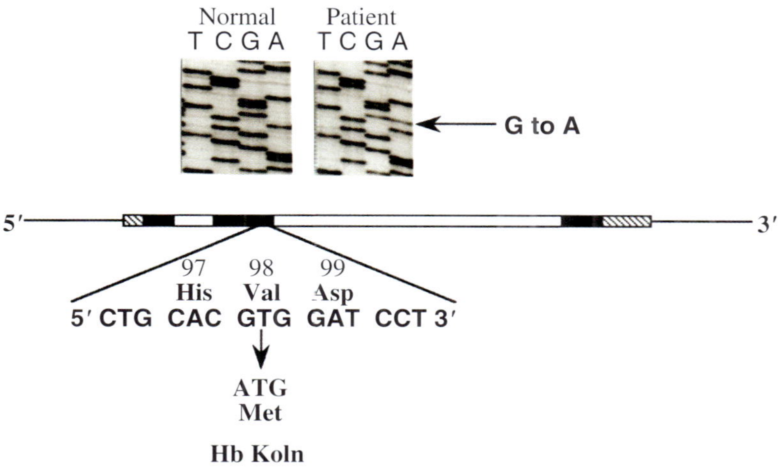

Figure 9.3 Sequence analysis identifies Hb Köln. In a schematic of the β-globin gene, exons and introns are indicated by black and white boxes, respectively. The shaded areas represent the 5′ and 3′ untranslated regions. Above the diagram, the results of direct sequence analysis of PCR products are shown. Within codon β98 a band in both G and A tracks is seen in the patient's DNA (highlighted by the arrow on the right), showing the patient to be heterozygous for a mutation in codon β98. The (G→A) mutation in codon β98 predicts the substitution of Val by Met, known as that of Hb Köln.

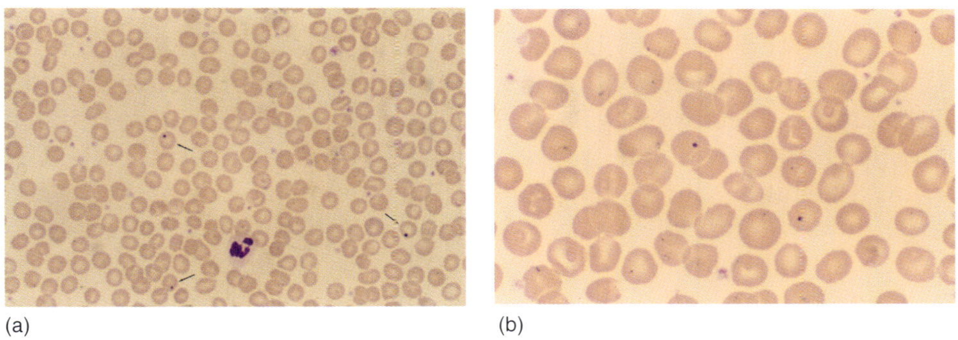

Figure 9.4 Peripheral blood film of the patient's sister: (a) low power view: Howell–Jolly bodies indicated by arrows; (b) high power view.

similar red cell morphology to the brother's, and in addition, some "burr cells," Howell–Jolly bodies (consistent with the fact that she had been splenectomized), and an occasional target cell. After methyl violet staining, approximately 50% of the erythrocytes displayed a single well-stained Heinz body (see Figure 9.5).

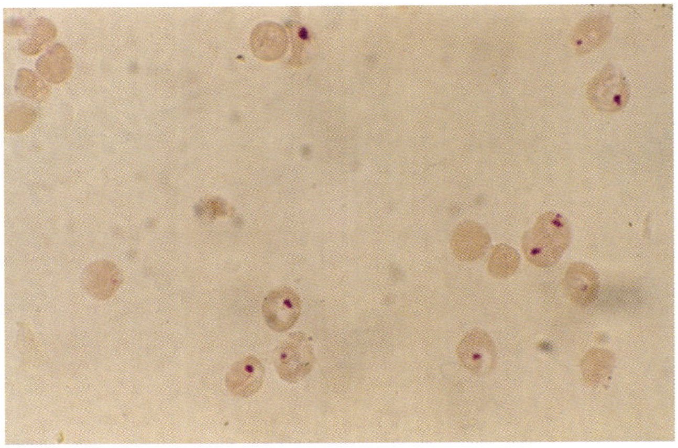

Figure 9.5 Heinz body film of the sister.

Comments

The amino acid substitution in Hb Köln affects haeme binding, because it is situated within the haeme pocket (see Figure 9.6); as a result, haeme may dissociate from the abnormal chain, resulting in a partially haeme-deficient molecule that may become a partially denatured hemichrome, followed by irreversible denaturation. Precipitates of denatured Hb constitute the so-called Heinz bodies, which become attached to the red cell membrane by hydrophobic bonding [2], thus limiting cellular deformability and increasing membrane permeability. Heinz bodies are removed selectively by the spleen, a phenomenon that contributes directly to the haemolytic process and also leaves damaged cells with reduced viability. Our patient (unlike his sister), because he has a normally functioning spleen, had no demonstrable Heinz bodies, even though undoubtedly they are formed. We should have thought of an unstable haemoglobin earlier, because this is one of the few conditions in which, with normal or high MCV and MCH, the MCHC is low, due to the loss of haeme.

Hb Köln is the commonest among the unstable haemoglobins. It is often the result of a *de novo* mutation (absent in the patient's parents); consistent with this, it has been reported in persons from various ethnic groups. The fact that the mutation is recurrent may be due at least in part to the fact that the mutated residue on the non-coding strand is a C in a CpG dinucleotide: in this position, if the C is methylated, it is known to

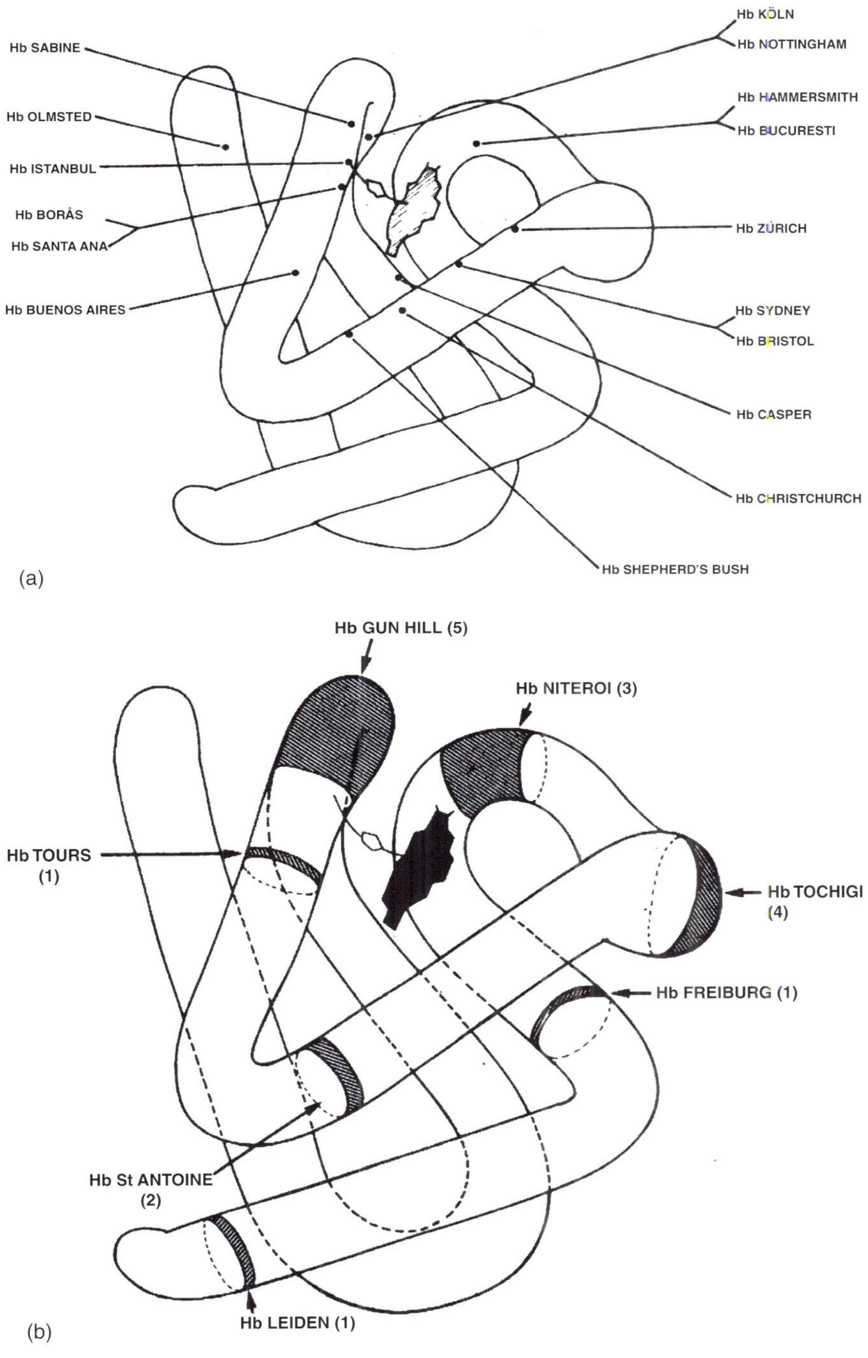

Figure 9.6 Diagram of the β-globin polypeptide chain. (a) Sites of amino acid replacements causing unstable haemoglobins: note that some of them, including that of Hb Köln, are part of the haeme pocket; (b) Sites of single or multiple amino-acid deletions, that also result in unstable haemoglobins (from [3]: used with permission).

be prone to become a T through deamination. Interestingly, at position 98 three other unstable, haemoglobins are known: namely, Hb Nottingham, Hb Djelfa and Hb Mainz.

The haemolytic disorder associated with Hb Köln varies from compensated haemolysis without anaemia, like in this case, to moderate chronic haemolytic anaemia (like in his sister). We noticed in this patient and in two others with an unstable haemoglobin (one is Case 31) that the platelet count was moderately decreased, and there is some precedent for this in the literature [4, 5]. Pedersen et al. suggested the decrease in platelet count in their patient was most likely due to splenic sequestration of platelets, as the count returned to normal after splenectomy [6].

Follow-up

Only after writing these notes, did we discover that a large study of this patient's family had been carried out already many years earlier [3] (Figure 9.7).

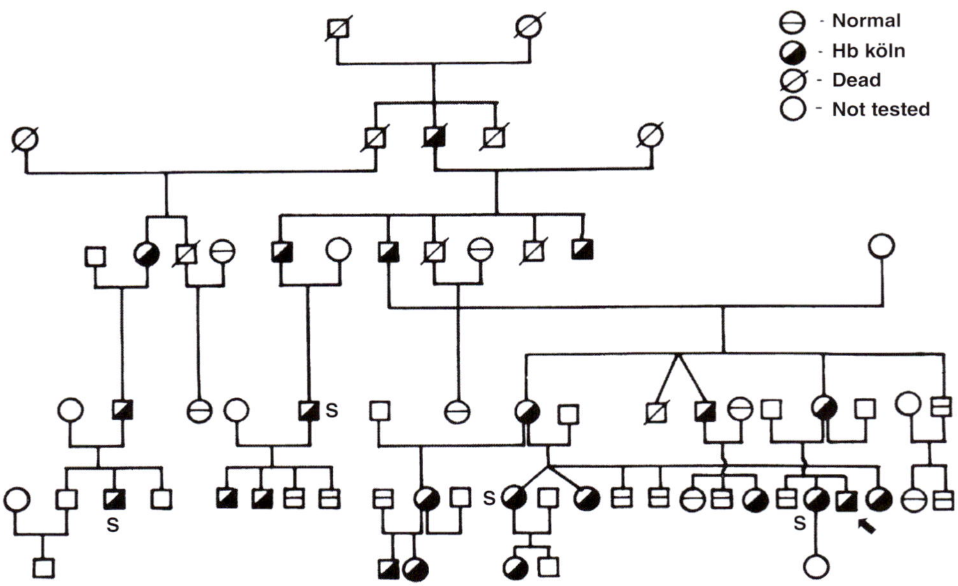

Figure 9.7 Family pedigree. The family tree over five generations of individuals heterozygous for Hb Köln; four members have been splenectomized (S). (From [3]: used with permission.) The diagram has been edited to illustrate our patient.

Conclusion

Chronic low grade haemolytic disorder due to heterozygous state for haemoglobin Köln.

Acknowledgements

Professor Ted Gordon-Smith, Department of Haematology, Hammersmith Hospital, London, UK.
Dr. Amin Rahemtulla, Department of Haematology, Hammersmith Hospital, London, UK.

References

1. Carrell, R.W., Lehmann, H., and Hutchison, H.E. (1966). Haemoglobin Koln (β-98) Valine→Methionine): an unstable protein causing inclusion-body anaemia. *Nature* 210, 915–916.
2. Winterbourn, C.C. and Carrell, R.W. (1973). The attachment of Heinz bodies to the red cell membrane. *Br. J. Haematol*. 25, 585–592.
3. White, J.M. (1974). The unstable haemoglobin disorders, In: Weatherall, D.J., editor. *Clinics in Haematology*. Vol 3, No 2. W.B. Saunders Company.
4. Hutchison, H.E., Pinkerton, P.H., Waters, P. et al. (1964). Hereditary Heinz body anaemia, thrombocytopenia and haemoglobinopathy (Hb Köln) in a Glasgow family. *Br. Med. J*. 2, 1099–1103.
5. Warang, P., Nair, S., Nadkarni, A, et al. (2014). Hb Koln [β98(FG5) [GTG → ATG, Val → Met]: the first report from India. *Hematology* 19(4), 199–201.
6. Pedersen, P.R., McCurdy, R., Wrightstone, R.N. et al. (1973). Hemoglobin Koln in a Black: pre-and post-splenectomy red cell survival (DF 32P and 51Cr) and the pathogenesis of hemoglobin instability. *Blood* 42, 771–781.

See also related Case 31.

Case 10

A Blue Baby with a Normal Heart

Patient Details

Age: 23 *Sex:* M
Ethnic background: Pakistan

Reason for Referral

Abnormal component detected on haemoglobin electrophoresis (blood sample only).

History and Clinical Findings in Brief

We learnt from referral documents that this young man living in Qatar had, since birth, bluish discoloration of nails on his fingers and toes, as well as of his lips and tongue; this was interpreted as cyanosis. No other family members were affected. As a result of an accident, the patient also had left foot dorsiflexion weakness and stepping gait.

Laboratory Findings

The blood count showed an elevated haemoglobin level and marked erythrocytosis (see Table 10.1). Morphology of red cells was difficult to assess on the regular blood film because of their very high number, and in trying to spread a film more thinly, distortion of the cells resulted (see Figure 10.1a). We centrifuged an aliquot of the blood, and we prepared a "diluted" film by mixing a drop of the patient's whole blood with a drop of his own plasma. On this film (see Figure 10.1b), most of the red cells appeared normal, but with some anisocytosis, and with occasional cigar-shaped cells and polychromatic cells.

As from the referral letter we had received, there was, in addition to the normal bands of Hb A and Hb A_2, an abnormal band on cellulose acetate electrophoresis (see Figure 10.2): it was very close to the position of Hb F, and it quantitated to 40.8%.

Table 10.1 Haematology Data

Hb (g/dl)	19.5
RBC ($\times 10^{12}$/l)	6.32
MCV (fl)[a]	101.3
MCH (pg)	30.9
MCHC (g/dl)	30.5
RDW (S.D.)	53.8
Retic (%)	2.0
Retic ($\times 10^9$/l)	126
Hb A_2 (%)	3.0
Hb F (%)	3.6
Abnormal Hb (%)	40.8

[a] The sample was one day old when analyzed and therefore the true MCV is probably lower and might be within the normal range.

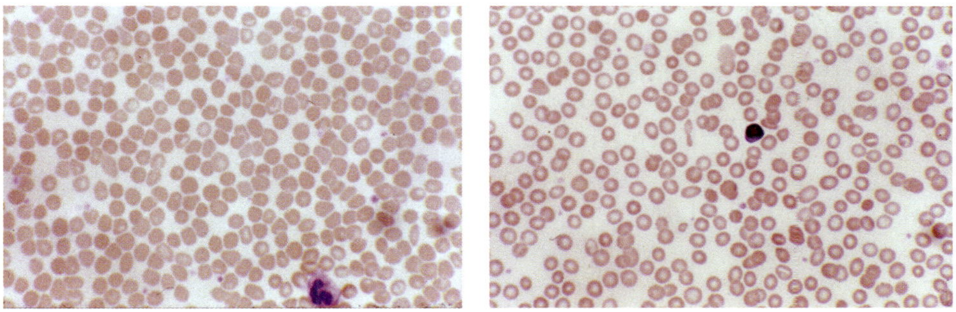

(a) (b)

Figure 10.1 Peripheral blood film: (a) made in the normal way; (b) after 50% dilution with patient's own plasma (we found this approach very useful in order to display red cell morphology whenever the haematocrit is high).

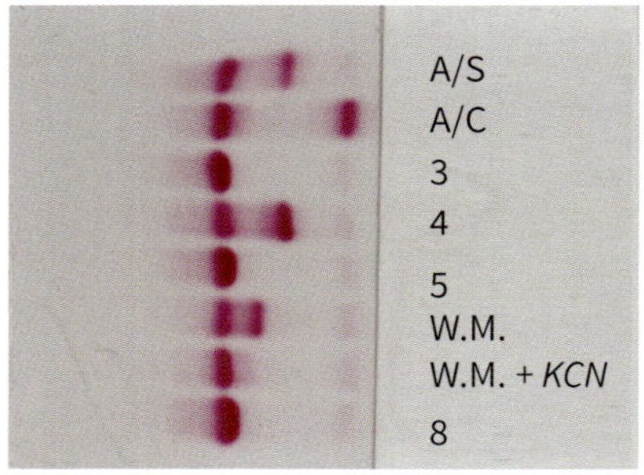

Figure 10.2 Haemoglobin electrophoresis on cellulose acetate membrane; the migration of the haemoglobin fractions is from right to left. An A/S control and A/C control are in lanes 1 and 2, respectively. The patient (W.M.) is in lane 6, and his sample after treatment with potassium cyanide solution is in lane 7.

Initial Assessment

On the clinical side, the most conspicuous sign was "cyanosis"; on the blood count, it was the erythrocytosis; on the electrophoretic pattern, it was the abnormal band. If this band was as a high oxygen affinity Hb, it would explain the erythrocytosis but not the cyanosis. On the other hand, if the abnormal band was a low oxygen affinity Hb, it could explain the cyanosis but not the erythrocytosis.

Further Investigations

When haemoglobin electrophoresis was repeated on Cellogel,[1] we noticed that the abnormal component was of a light mahogany-brown colour (unlike the Hb A band, which was the usual light orange/red colour). The penny dropped (to use an English idiom made obsolete by cell phones) when we repeated electrophoresis after adding potassium cyanide (20 g/l): the abnormal band disappeared (see Figure 10.2). This finding indicated that there was no abnormal Hb; rather, there was a large amount of methaemoglobin (MetHb: that KCN had converted to cyanmethaemoglobin, migrating like normal Hb). MetHb was confirmed by spectrophotometric analysis of the patient's haemolysate (signal at 630 nm in Figure 10.3). By the method of Evelyn and Malloy, MetHb amounted to 37% (in good agreement with the 40% value originally estimated from electrophoresis).

We next performed an assay for cytochrome b_5 reductase: this enzyme activity was undetectable.

[1] Cellogel electrophoresis strips are composed of cellulose acetate membrane combined with a gel matrix. The unique porosity prevents band spreading and provides very sharp separations of proteins, etc.

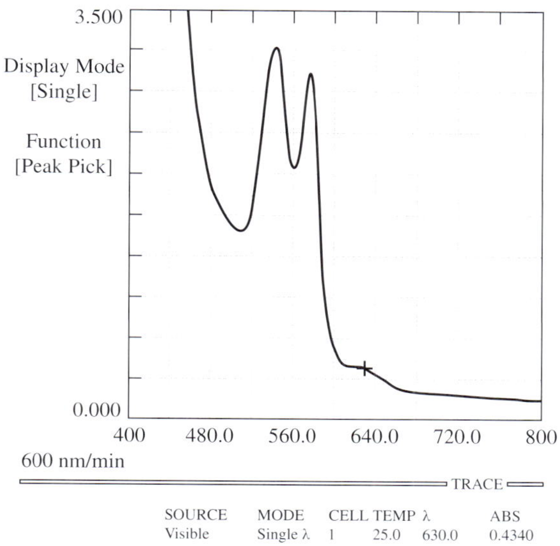

Figure 10.3 Spectral scan of blood sample after haemolysis in water. Analysis revealed the typical haemoglobin peaks at 540 nm and 576 nm; plus, a signal at 630 nm (indicated by a cursor): this is typical of methaemoglobin.

Comments

A small amount of metHb is formed normally as a by-product of the cyclic oxygenation and deoxygenation of haemoglobin: it has been estimated that each day 2–3% of haemoglobin is converted to methaemoglobin [1]. However, the steady-state methaemoglobin level in normal people is only about 0.6%, because in red cells two enzyme systems effectively reduce metHb back to haemoglobin. One is the NADH-requiring cytochrome b_5 reductase (formerly called diaphorase); the other, a flavo-enzyme, relies as electron donor on NADPH, provided by G6PD (see Figure 10.4).

Methaemoglobinaemia can be caused by an α-globin or β-globin mutation (Hb M) that produces amino acid replacements that alter the haeme environment in a manner that stabilizes the oxidized ferric state of iron over the reduced ferrous state. This was suggested when the patient was referred to us; instead, he had the other form of methaemoglobinaemia, caused by enzyme deficiency. The most compelling evidence that cytochrome b_5 reductase, encoded by the *CYB5R3* gene (on chromosome 22q13-qter), is the more important enzyme in the physiological maintenance of haeme in the ferrous state is provided by patients like this one. Many mutations are known [2, 3] in *CYB5R3*: expression of this gene produces, through alternative splicing, a membrane-bound form of the enzyme that in many cells is anchored to the cytoplasmic face of the endoplasmic reticulum, where it is an integral part of the microsomal electron transport system; as well as

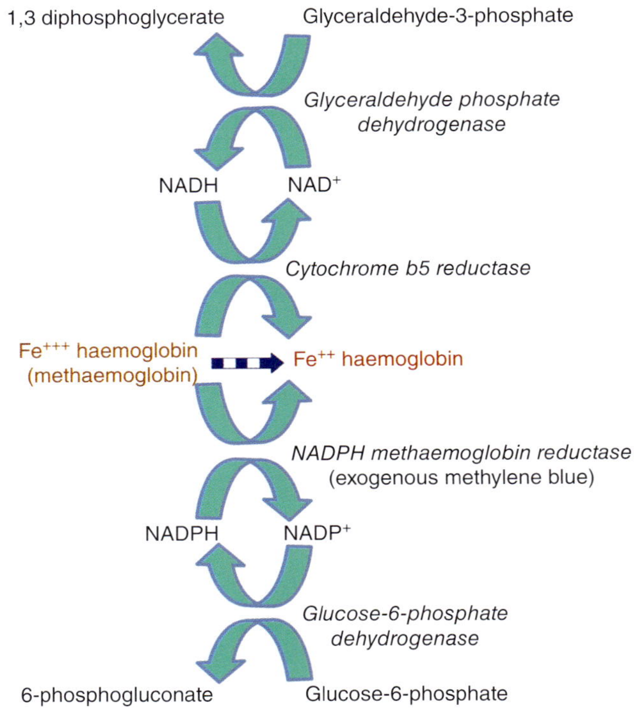

Figure 10.4 Metabolic pathways for the reduction of methaemoglobin. The major pathway for methaemoglobin reduction is the nicotinamide adenine dinucleotide (NADH)-dependent cytochrome b_5 reductase. An alternative pathway is the nicotinamide adenine dinucleotide phosphate (NADPH)-dependent methaemoglobin reductase, a flavo-enzyme that requires an intermediary electron acceptor (e.g. methylene blue) A small amount of methaemoglobin is reduced through a non-enzymatic pathway.

the soluble form present in red cells. Some point mutations, called type I, cause only methaemoglobinaemia; others (either point mutations or *non-sense* mutations causing protein truncation) [4], called type II, cause, in addition, a devastating neurological disorder with early mortality [5].

Like most enzymopathies, methaemoglobinaemia due to cytochrome b_5 reductase deficiency is recessive: although we were unable to test our patient's parents, we assume that they are both asymptomatic heterozygotes. Only homozygotes or patients with bi-allelic mutations have increased methaemoglobin, which lacks any ability to exchange oxygen; hence the clinical cyanosis[2] and tissue hypoxia that triggers erythropoietin-driven erythrocytosis, prominent in our patient.

Methaemoglobinaemia due to cytochrome b_5 reductase deficiency is often higher than with M haemoglobins: the proportion of metHb can be up to 50% in the former, but it is rarely above 20% in the latter.[3] However,

---

[2] Strictly speaking the term cyanosis indicates discoloration due to excess deoxyhaemoglobin, as in pulmonary insufficiency; the discoloration of a patient with methemoglobinemia ought to be called more exactly "pseudo-cyanosis."

[3] We have followed for years one patient with Hb M Hyde Park (β92 His>Tyr), diagnosed at the age of 7 [9]. Currently, aged 44, she is a clinical scientist, and she has had one successful pregnancy.

even a patient homozygous for a *CYB5R3* mutation may present at age 61 with mild symptoms [6]. Thus, patients with this condition may not need treatment. When treatment is desirable, it is similar to that used in acquired methaemoglobinaemia due to toxic causes, such as nitrites. In such cases, there is indication for the oral administration of methylene blue (MB), which serves as electron carrier and brings the NADPH-dependent reductase into operation. Before using this treatment it is recommended to check the G6PD level, because MB can cause acute haemolytic anaemia in G6PD deficient persons [7, 8].

We found that in fact, the patient's G6PD level was only 0.1 IU/g Hb: thus, he was not only cytochrome b_5 reductase deficient but also G6PD deficient. Since it is G6PD that supplies the NADPH required for the activity of the other metHb-reductase, it is possible that the combined deficiency has made the methaemoglobinaemia more severe, although clearly our patient is still to be regarded as having type I disease.

Follow-up

In view of the above, treatment with ascorbic acid was recommended.

Conclusion

Methaemoglobinaemia due to cytochrome b_5 reductase (diaphorase) deficiency; associated with G6PD deficiency.

Acknowledgements

Referred by Dr. Awidi Abbadi, Hamad General Hospital, Doha, Qatar.

References

1. Keise, M. (1974). *Methaemoglobinaemia: A Comprehensive Treatise.* Cleveland: CRC Press.
2. Vieira, L.M., Kaplan, J.C., Kanh, A. et al. (1995). Four new mutations in the NADH-cytochrome b_5 reductase gene from patients with recessive congenital methaemoglobinaemia type II. *Blood* 85, 2254–2262.
3. Manabe, J., Arya, R., Sumimoto, H. et al. (1996). Two novel mutations in the reduced nicotinamide adenine dinucleotide (NADH)-cytochrome b_5 reductase gene of a patient with generalised type, hereditary methemoglobinemia. *Blood* 88, 3208–3215.

4. Percy, M.J. and Lappin, T.R. (2008). Recessive congenital methaemoglobinaemia: cytochrome b(5) reductase deficiency. *Br. J. Haematol.* 141, 298–308.
5. Siendones, E., Ballesteros, M., and Navas, P. (2018). Cellular and molecular mechanisms of recessive hereditary methaemoglobinaemia type II. *J. Clin. Med.* 7, 341.
6. de Geus, K.F., Anas, A.A., Franssen, R. et al. (2018). Congenital methaemoglobinaemia in a 61-year-old patient with normal haemoglobin levels. *Neth. J. Med.* 76, 194–197.
7. Rosen, P.J., Johnson, C., McGehee, W.G. et al. (1971). Failure of methylene blue treatment in toxic methemoglobinemia. Association with glucose-6-phosphate dehydrogenase deficiency. *Ann. Intern. Med.* 75, 83–86.
8. Askerova, T.A., Kichibekov, B.R., and Panakhova, Kh.G. (1995). Familial case of methemoglobinemia associated with glucose-6-phosphate dehydrogenase deficiency. *Klin. Lab. Diagn.* 1, 51–53.
9. Rotoli, B., Camera, A., Fontana, R. et al. (1992). Hb-M "Hyde Park": a *de novo* mutation, identified by mass spectrometry and DNA analysis. *Haematologica* 77(2), 110–118. PMID: 1398295.

Case 11

Detecting and Managing Point Mutations

Patient Details

Age: 14 months *Sex:* M
Ethnic background: Italian (Calabria/Sicily)

Reason for Referral

Investigation of anaemia in a child whose mother had β-thalassaemia trait.

History and Clinical Findings in Brief

This child had been delivered by caesarean section in another hospital after a prolonged labour: at birth, he was a healthy baby, weighing just over 3.7 kg. Over the course of the next 14 months, the child's growth and development were normal. However, the mother reported occasional febrile episodes, which were attributed in turn to a urinary infection, an upper respiratory infection, and an ear infection. On examination the child's general condition was good; his pulse rate and blood pressure were normal, but he did appear pale. Abdominal examination revealed a spleen tip and a barely palpable liver.

Laboratory Findings

The patient had a moderate microcytic hypochromic anaemia (see Table 11.1). On the blood film (see Figure 11.1), the red cells were indeed very small, some of them being no larger than platelets. In addition, the cells showed quite a range of haemoglobinization (anisochromasia): at one extreme there were hypochromic cells and target cells, and at the other extreme, occasional contracted cells and deeply stained polychromatic cells. Teardrop poikilocytes and occasional nucleated red cells were also seen.

A blood test on the mother was consistent with her known β-thalassaemia trait; a blood test on the patient's father revealed low MCV, low MCH and an elevated Hb A_2: he too had β-thalassaemia trait. Globin chain biosynthetic studies (see Table 11.1) were in keeping with this: the β:α ratio in the patient was much lower.

Table 11.1 Haematology Data

	Patient	Mother	Father
Hb (g/dl)	8.3	11.3	14.0
RBC ($\times 10^{12}$/l)	3.98	5.31	6.39
MCV (fl)	64.6	64.1	66.6
MCH (pg)	21.0	21.4	21.8
MCHC (g/dl)	32.3	33.2	32.9
Retic (%)	0.2	–	–
Retic ($\times 10^9$/l)	29	–	–
Hb A_2 (%)	2.5	4.7	4.9
Hb F (%)	31.0	0.9	1.7
β:α ratio[a]	0.27	0.65	0.57

[a] Globin chain biosynthetic ratio.

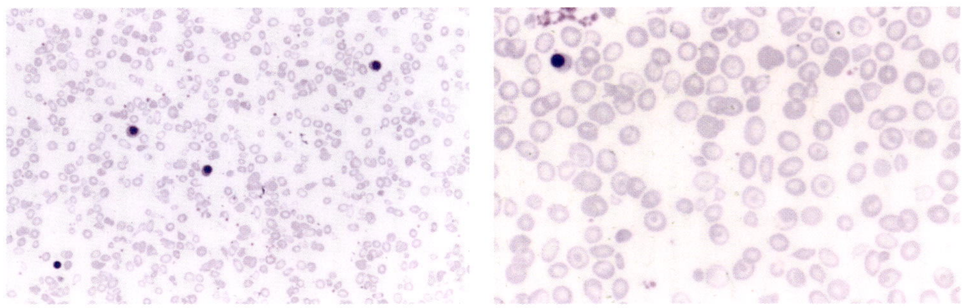

(a) (b)

Figure 11.1 Peripheral blood film: (a) low power view; (b) medium power view.

Initial Assessment

Clearly, this young child has a thalassaemia syndrome more severe than just β-thalassaemia trait. Since both parents are heterozygotes for beta thalassaemia, he might be suffering from thalassaemia major. However, at this time, he has not required any blood transfusion. Because initiating a regular blood transfusion regimen is a major commitment, which usually proves irreversible, this differential diagnosis must be taken very seriously. From the literature and from previous experience [1] with a β:α ratio of 0.27, this child might still have thalassaemia intermedia rather than thalassaemia major.

Further Investigations

At about the time this child was being investigated, a relatively mild form of β-thalassaemia was reported from Northern Portugal and had become known as the "Portuguese" β^+-thalassaemia type [2]. The underlying mutation, IVS 1 nt 6 T→C, affects splicing, but it is associated with significant residual synthesis of β globin: our patient's father was heterozygous for this mutation; the β-thalassaemia mutation in the mother was not yet known. Restriction fragment length polymorphism (RFLP) analysis revealed the mother was homozygous for a haplotype consisting of seven restriction enzyme sites: and therefore at the time we could not tell which one of her chromosomes had her β-thalassaemia mutation (see Figure 11.2).

Follow-up of Family

The parents had very much wanted another baby for some time (the mother's second pregnancy had been terminated for social reasons). In a subsequent pregnancy, globin-chain analysis was performed on a foetal blood sample obtained by fetoscopy at 20 weeks. The β:α ratio was 0.007, which implied that the foetus must have again inherited β-thalassaemia mutations from both parents who, having requested genetic counselling, chose to have the pregnancy terminated. In the fourth pregnancy, at 10 weeks of gestation, DNA analysis was performed on a chorion villus sample: this showed that the foetus had inherited the father's thalassaemic chromosome, and therefore there was a 50% chance of a severely affected baby; the parents opted to have again termination. In a fifth pregnancy, at 13 weeks of gestation, DNA analysis on a chorion villus sample showed that this time the

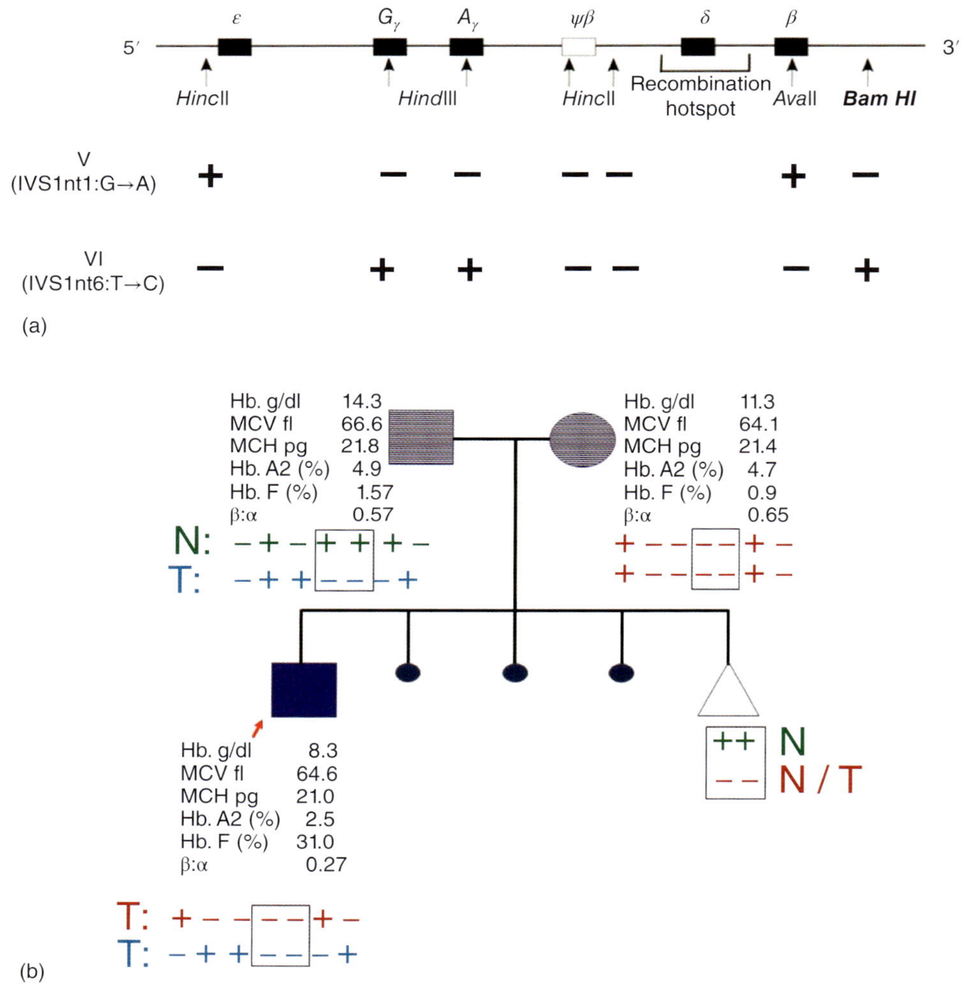

Figure 11.2 Molecular genetics of patient and family. (a) Top: the β-globin gene cluster, with arrows pointing to seven restriction enzyme cleavage sites; underneath: the haplotypes that have the combinations of restriction sites shown (whereby, the sign + indicates the presence, while the sign – indicates the absence of each individual restriction site) are designated as V and VI. (b) The patient's family tree, showing haematological and molecular data. Rows of +/- signs indicate haplotypes as from panel (a). The fact that our patient had inherited from his father haplotype VI and the thalassaemia mutation told us that the paternal thalassaemia mutation was, in this case, within this haplotype (T: shown in blue), whereas the other paternal haplotype (N) does not have a thalassaemia mutation. On the other hand, since the mother was homozygous for haplotype V, from finding this haplotype in an offspring it was impossible to know whether the thalassaemia mutation was there or not (only later did we pinpoint the thalassaemia mutation IVS I nt1 in the mother). In the last pregnancy the foetus had the paternal N haplotype; hence, he must be either normal or heterozygous, but not with severe thalassaemia.

embryo had inherited the normal chromosome from the father. This pregnancy went to term, and a normal baby was delivered. Only subsequently a thalassaemia mutation not uncommon in Southern Italy was identified in the mother, a G→A substitution at IVS 1 nt 1, (see Case 19, Figure 19.3), this mutation also affects splicing, so drastically that it is a β^0 mutation [3].

Follow-up of Child

The child's growth and development continued to be good (see Figure 11.3), but he tended to become very tired towards the end of the day. At about three and a half years of age, his liver had enlarged to 5 cm, his spleen to 11 cm, and his haemoglobin had fallen to 5.3 g/dl. His red cell morphology had become much more abnormal (see Figure 11.4). Furthermore, his β:α biosynthetic ratio was now 0.11. His skull X-ray began to show minimal changes in the diploe. We had to admit the boy had thalassaemia major, currently often referred to as transfusion-dependent thalassaemia (TDT).

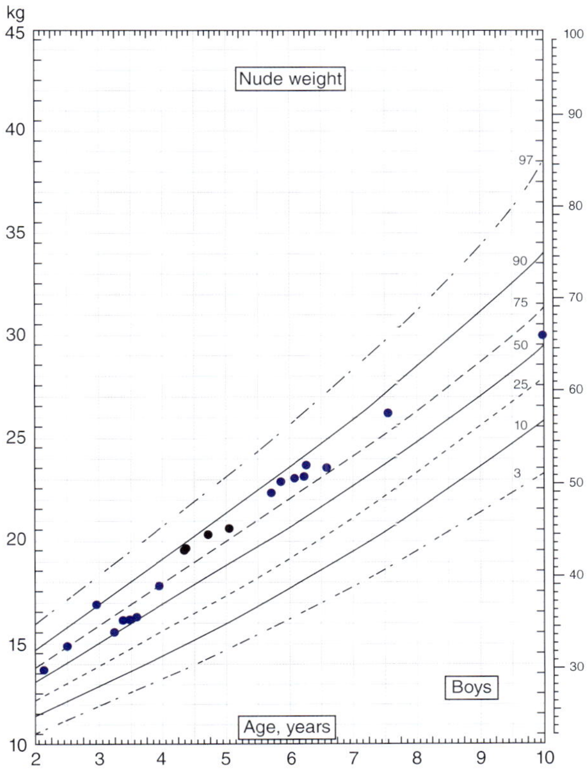

Figure 11.3 Growth curve of patient.

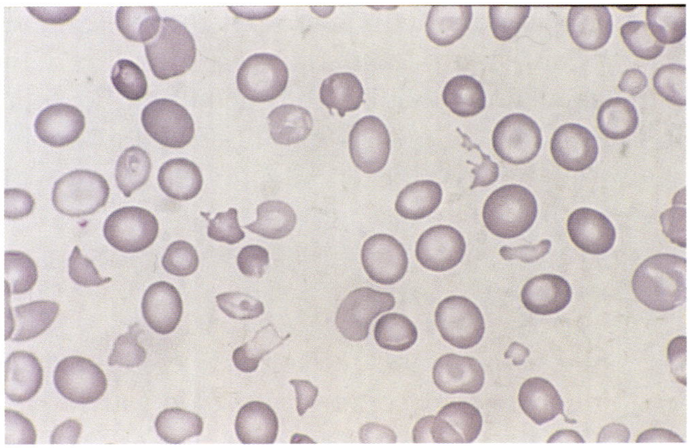

Figure 11.4 Peripheral blood film at 3.5 years of age.

The boy was commenced on a regular blood transfusion regimen, and about a month later he was splenectomized. The child did very well on this regimen, and at age six he was clinically entirely normal, receiving, on average, 20 blood transfusions a year. He was also on nightly desferal by subcutaneous administration using an infusion pump.

Comments

The severity of β-thalassaemia depends, of course, on many factors [4], two of which are prominent: (i) the amount of residual β-globin chain synthesis (which by definition is greater than zero in β^+-thalassaemia); (ii) the amount of γ-chain synthesis, because it can reduce the excess in α chains that are the main culprit of ineffective erythropoiesis. With respect to (i), homozygosity for the IVS 1 nt 6 T→A is associated with a considerable level of β chain synthesis [2], resulting in a "mild" β^+ thalassaemia; but the same mutation, in combination with a β^0 mutation, can give a severe phenotype, i.e. TDT, as it did in this case. With respect to (ii), genetic factors affecting the level of Hb F have been extensively investigated [5]; in addition, although normally most of the switch from Hb F to Hb A occurs during the first 6 months of life, when erythropoiesis is stressed, it may take up to several years for Hb F to decrease to its plateau level [6, 7]. This may justify why we were reluctant to accept that our patient had TDT.

This couple's reproductive history has been trying and painful more than once; at the same time, it illustrates the stepwise progress that molecular medicine has made in the area of genetic counselling and prenatal diagnosis. During the first pregnancy, probably the parents did not realize that there was risk of a severe inherited disorder in their baby; although they both had a trait that is easy to diagnose, no prospective genetic counselling was offered. During the third pregnancy, we were only able to offer late prenatal diagnosis, entailing a rather distressing termination of pregnancy. During the last two pregnancies, early prenatal testing was made available, but at the cost of risking unnecessary termination (which may indeed have been the case in the fourth pregnancy). In the event, both parents were adamant they would not want the risk of the birth of another child with thalassaemia disease. We were greatly relieved when, at the next pregnancy, foetal DNA analysis enabled us to rule out homozygous beta thalassaemia.

Prenatal diagnosis of thalassaemia was pioneered in Italy by the late Antonio Cao: one outcome of his efforts was a drop of births with thalassaemia major in Sardinia from about 100 to about 5 per year [8], and all the approaches briefly mentioned here were gradually implemented in most parts of Italy. Today, if a couple like the one reported here requested genetic counselling, one would directly test DNA from chorionic villi for the specific thalassaemia mutations detected in both parents. An alternative that is actively pursued is non-invasive testing of free foetal DNA in maternal blood [9], but this is not yet routine.

The availability of prenatal diagnosis may encourage couples at risk to pursue reproduction; in the end, our patient had a healthy brother.

Further Follow-up

The family returned to Italy and lived in Siracusa (Sicily), where the child continued to be well controlled on a regular blood transfusion regimen. However, he developed bilateral severe valgismus of his knees (see Figure 11.5a), which had to be attributed to desferal toxicity [10]; he was switched to deferiprone, which was well tolerated, and whereby the valgismus was nearly completely reversed (Figure 11.5b). Having been found to be hepatitis C positive early on, he had two courses of α-interferon in 1993 and in 2003, without success; in 2018, he had a course of sofosbuvir, followed by complete resolution.

This young man (Figure 11.6) has been now managed for nearly 30 years by the Thalassemia Unit of the main hospital in Siracusa, strictly adhering to up-to-date guidelines. His blood count is that of a regularly transfused patient with TDT (see Table 11.2: the high white cells and platelets are common in splenectomized patients). He receives, at intervals of 21–23 days, 550 ml of packed red cells (haematocrit 70%); thanks to careful

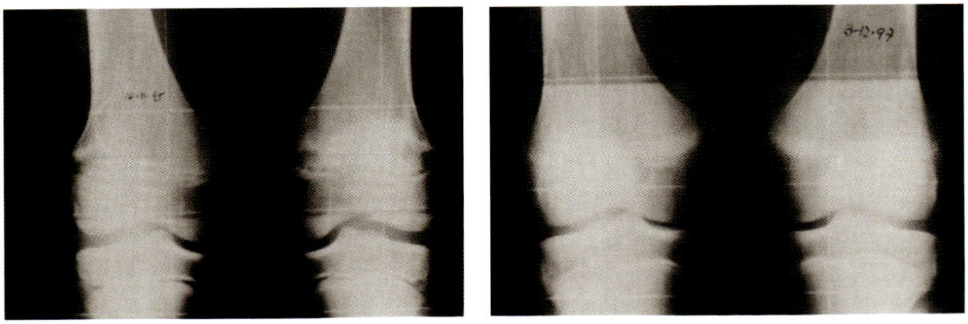

(a) (b)

Figure 11.5 X-ray of knees: (a) age 12: irregularity of metaphyseal edges with deep erosions and sclerotic margins in both knees; (b) age 14: significant improvement two years after switching from deferoxamine to deferiprone. [10]/with permission of Walter de Gruyter GmbH.

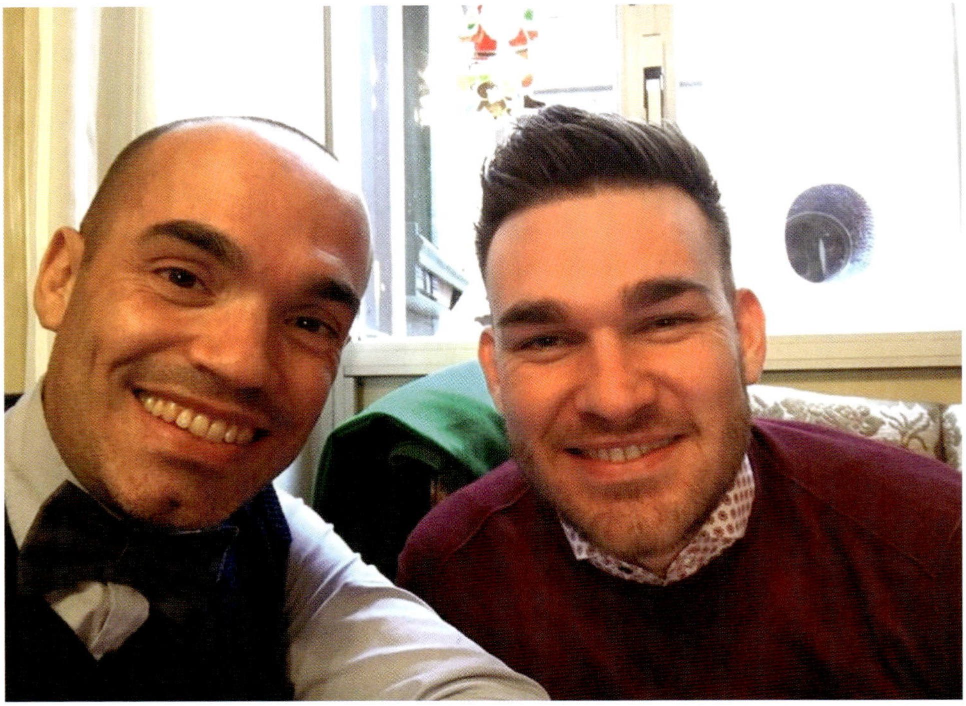

Figure 11.6 Patient's picture: patient at age 39, with his brother, age 36; with permission from both.

red cell matching, he has not developed any alloantibodies; he is still on deferiprone 400 mg/day. MRI studies have not shown evidence of iron overload in the heart, and a full endocrine assessment was normal. Recently the patient has written: "I regard myself as fortunate: I conduct a normal

Table 11.2 Laboratory Data on 04.02.2022

Hb (g/dl)	9.2
RBC ($\times 10^{12}$/l)	3.8
MCV (fl)	80
MCH (pg)	26
MCHC (g/dl)	32
Retic (%)	8.2
Retic ($\times 10^{9}$/l)	312
WBC ($\times 10^{9}$/l)	16.2
Platelets ($\times 10^{9}$/l)	683
Ferritin (ng/ml)	371

life, and I do sports regularly.... I receive professional care, and during the COVID pandemic this has never faltered.... However, I still hope to be able one day to have the long-awaited Gene Therapy."

Conclusion

Thalassaemia major, or transfusion dependent thalassaemia (TDT), resulting from bi-allelic *HBB* mutation: β^0 (IVS 1 nt 1 G→A)/β^+ (IVS 1 nt 6 T→A).

Acknowledgements

Dr. J. Old, Institute of Molecular Medicine, John Radcliffe Hospital, Oxford, UK.
Mr. C. Rodeck, Department of O&G, King's College School of Medicine, London, UK.
Dr. Saveria Campisi, Unit for the Diagnosis and Treatment of Thalassaemia, Umberto I Hospital, Siracusa, Italy.
Dr. A. Whitelaw, Neonatal Unit, Hammersmith Hospital, London, UK.

References

1. Pepe, G., Lupi, L., and Luzzatto, L. (1980). Genetic and biochemical heterogeneity of beta-thalassaemia in Naples. *Br. J. Haematol.* 45(3), 417–429.
2. Tamagnini, G.P., Lopes, M.C., Castanheira, M.E. et al. (1983). Beta+ thalassemia–Portuguese type: clinical, haematological and molecular studies of a newly defined form of beta thalassaemia. *Br. J. Haematol.* 54(2), 189–200.
3. Rosatelli, M.C., Tuveri, T., Scalas, M.T. et al. (1992). Molecular screening and fetal diagnosis of beta-thalassemia in the Italian population. *Hum. Genet.* 89(6), 585–89.
4. Weatherall, D.J. (2000). *The Harvey Lectures Series 94, 1998–1999.* In: Davis MM, Fuchs E, Hunter T et al. editor. ISBN: 978-0-471-40125-4.

5. Weatherall, D.J. and Clegg, J.B. (2001). *The Thalassaemia Syndromes*, 4 ed, Blackwell Science Ltd.
6. Schröter, W. and Nafz, C. (1981). Diagnostic significance of hemoglobin F and A2 levels in homo-and heterozygous beta-thalassemia during infancy. *Helv. Paediatr. Acta* 36(6), 519–25.
7. Mason, K.P., Grandison, Y., Hayes, R.J. et al. (1982). Post-natal decline of fetal haemoglobin in homozygous sickle cell disease: relationship to parenteral Hb F levels. *Br. J. Haematol.* 52(3), 455–63.
8. Cao, A. and Kan, Y.W. (2013). The prevention of thalassemia. *Cold Spring Harb Perspect Med.* 3(2), a011775.
9. Saba, L., Masala, M., Capponi, V. et al. (2017). Non-invasive prenatal diagnosis of beta-thalassemia by semiconductor sequencing: a feasibility study in the Sardinian population. *Eur J Hum Genet.* 25(5), 600–7.
10. De Sanctis, V., Pinamonti, A., Di Palma, A. et al. (1996). Growth and development in thalassaemia major patients with severe bone lesions due to desferrioxamine. *Eur. J. Pediatr.* 155, 368–72.
11. Mangiagli, A., De Sanctis, V., Campisi, S. et al. (2000). Treatment with deferiprone (L1) in a thalassemic patient with bone lesions due to desferrioxamine. *J. Pediatr. Endocrinol. Metab.* 13, 677–80.

Case 12

A Gush of Oxygen for the Baby

Patient Details

Age: 23 *Sex:* F
Ethnic background: Sierra Leone

Reason for Referral

Supervision of first pregnancy.

History and Clinical Findings in Brief

There was no significant medical history except for ritual female circumcision. On a routine ante-natal booking, when the patient was 10 weeks pregnant, she was found to be clinically well and her physical examination was normal.

Lab Findings

The patient was not anaemic, but she had microcytic, hypochromic red cell indices (see Table 12.1). The blood film (see Figure 12.1) confirmed a microcytic picture, with some red cells appearing about the size of large platelets. There was marked anisocytosis and poikilocytosis, with a small number of microspherocytes and pyknocytes. There was a large number of

Table 12.1 Haematology Data

Hb (g/dl)	12.0
RBC ($\times 10^{12}$/l)	5.48
MCV (fl)	64
MCH (pg)	21.9
MCHC (g/dl)	34.2
Hb A_2 (%)	6.0
Hb F (%)	80.0
Non-α:α ratio[a]	0.45

[a] Globin chain biosynthetic ratio.

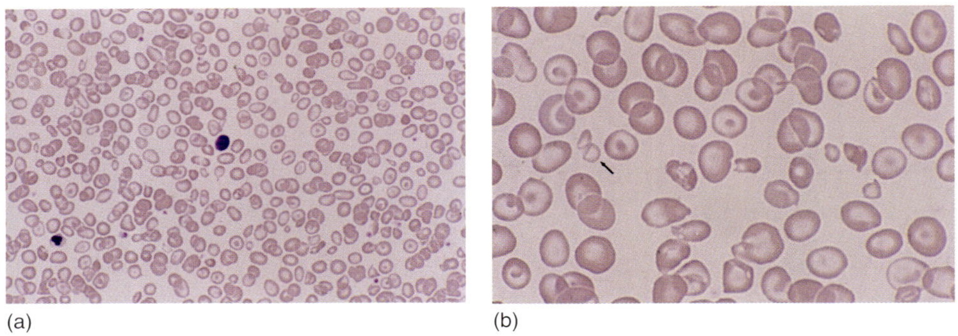

Figure 12.1 Peripheral blood film: (a) medium power view; (b) high power view with "octocyte" arrowed.

target cells, which made the hypochromia especially prominent. In addition, some cells were so thin that they became twisted into a figure-of-8 shape ("octocytes"). An occasional nucleated red cell was also seen.

Haemoglobin electrophoresis on cellulose acetate membrane (part of routine antenatal screening) revealed Hb F to be the major component (80%): the balance consisted of Hb A (14%), and Hb A_2 (6.0%) (not shown).

Initial Assessment

In adults, there are only very few conditions in which haemoglobin F can be 80%. Clearly, the patient does not have thalassaemia major; and she could not be a δβ-thalassaemia homozygote, because her Hb A_2 was elevated. Keeping into account the patient's indices and morphology, we favoured the possibility that she might be heterozygous for β^+-thalassaemia and Hereditary Persistence of Foetal Haemoglobin (HPFH).

Further Investigations and Management

A Kleihauer test performed in order to assess the cellular distribution of foetal haemoglobin, showed that this was homogeneous (so called pancellular Hb F) (see Figure 12.2). An oxygen dissociation study (see Figure 12.3) revealed, not surprisingly, a left-shifted curve (P_{50} of 17.7 mmHg: normal control 20.3 mmHg), with a normal red cell 2,3-BPG level (15.6 mmol/g Hb).

Our first concern was possible foetal hypoxia resulting from the reduced oxygen gradient across the placenta: therefore it was decided to carry out exchange transfusions in this patient. The aim was to reduce the Hb F level to below 50%, while maintaining the total haemoglobin level between 11.0 and 12.0 g/dl. The patient underwent seven exchange transfusions throughout her pregnancy (see Figure 12.4). At 32 weeks gestation, the oxygen dissociation curve was normal (P_{50} of 20.4 mmHg); the patient had a spontaneous uncomplicated premature labour and she delivered a live male infant (weighing 2410 g), who did very well.

We also still needed to explain the very high Hb F level in this patient. A globin chain biosynthesis study revealed a non-α:α ratio of 0.45 (in the range of a β-thalassaemia heterozygote). Analysis of the β-globin genes (see Figure 12.5) revealed on one chromosome a A→G mutation at position −29, in the TATA box of the β-globin gene promoter: a known mild thalassaemia mutation [1]; on the other chromosome, a deletion of 1393 bp, that had been reported already in several persons with African ancestry.

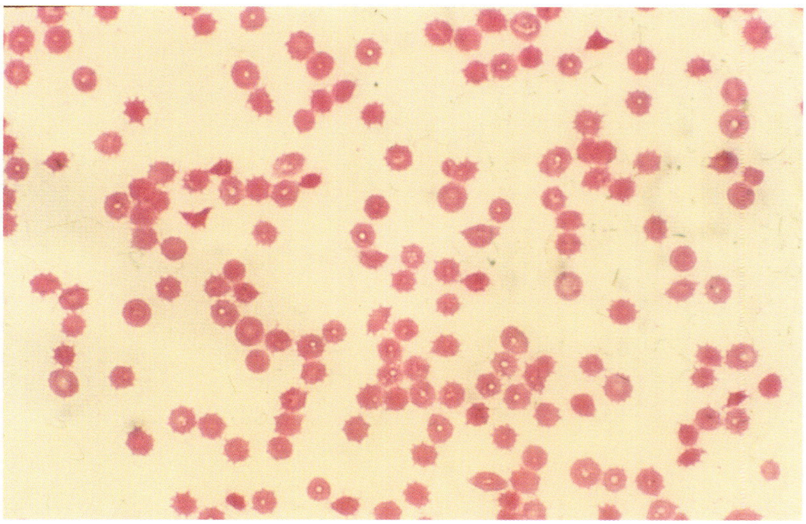

Figure 12.2 Kleihauer film showing pancellular distribution of Hb F (the red cell crenation is an unfortunate artefact).

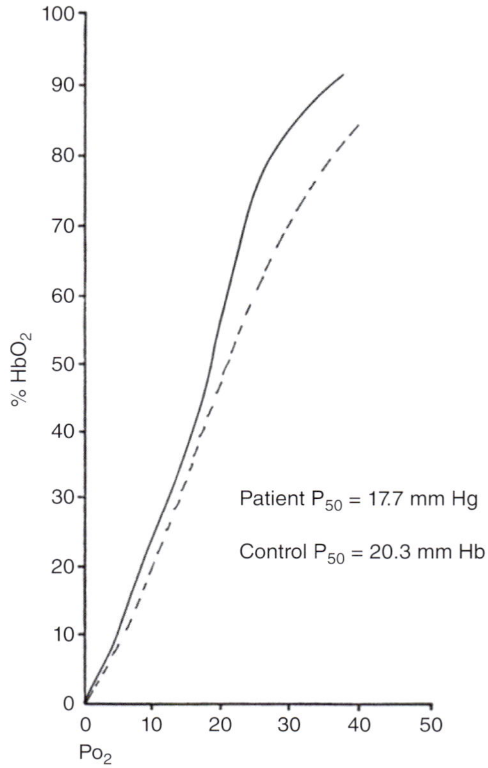

Figure 12.3 Oxygen dissociation curve of the patient's blood (solid line), showing a shift to the left, compared a normal control. The haemoglobin-oxygen dissociation curve is slightly different in whole blood *versus* a free haemoglobin (Hb) solution; it is influenced by pH, temperature, Hb concentration, carbon dioxide, and especially by the concentration of 2,3-bisphosphoglycerate: these factors will therefore affect P50, i.e. the oxygen pressure (in mmHg) at which 50% of haemoglobin is oxygenated. The currently accepted value for P_{50} in normal blood is 26-27; however, under the experimental conditions used at the time in the assays reported here, a normal control had a P_{50} of 20.3: therefore the data in this figure and in figure 12.4 must be seen in that light.

Comments

Our initial assessment, that the patient did not have thalassaemia major, was confirmed: yet, to our surprise, she did have in fact two β-thalassaemia genes. We could not find in the literature any precedent for this particular bi-allelic combination, and therefore, we must try to explain her resulting phenotype, especially with respect to her very high (80%) Hb F level.

To this end, we must consider current understanding of the foetal to adult haemoglobin switch (see Figure 12.6). The locus control region (LCR) can couple with either the promoters of the γ-globin genes *HBG2-HBG1*, or the promoters of the δ and β-globin genes *HBD-HBB*. Between the two alternatives, there is competition, and during foetal life, the balance is in favour of the *HBG2-HBG1* promoters: therefore, Hb F is produced. Around birth, there is an increase in erythroid cells of the transcriptional repressor BCL11A [2], that binds selectively to each one of the *HBG2* and *HBG1* promoters, and thus hinders their coupling to the LCR: as a result, in an adult, the competition turns in favour of the *HBD-HBB* promoters. Comparative analysis of numerous deletions has pinpointed, as critical in this respect,

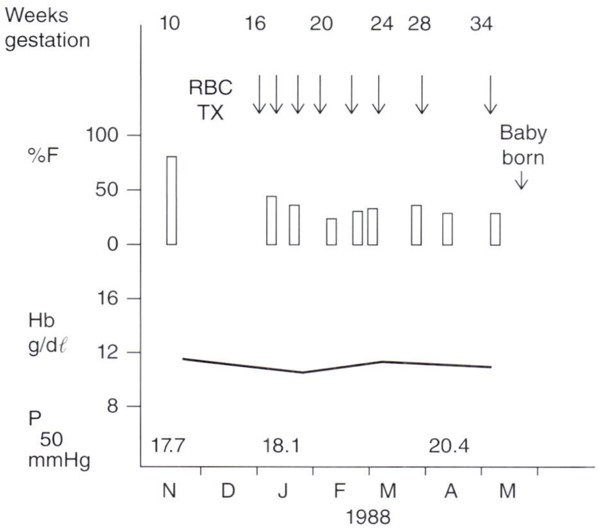

Figure 12.4 Patient's course to delivery.

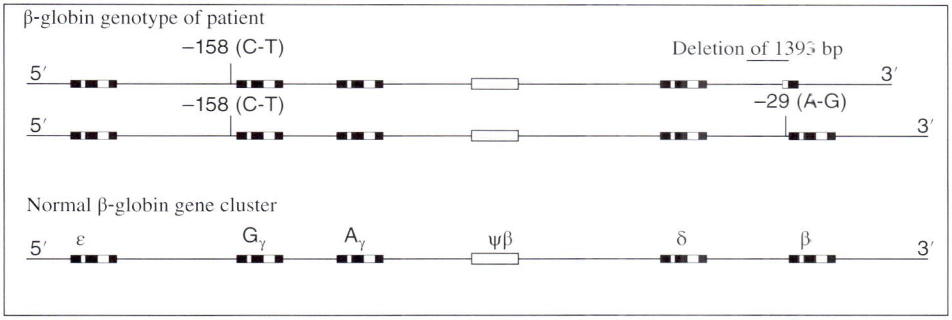

Figure 12.5 The β-globin gene cluster on chromosome 11. Top: the two alleles in this patient. Bottom: normal reference diagram.

the *HBB* promoter [3] that, in our patient has been removed on one chromosome by the 1393 bp deletion [4]: we can infer that, as a consequence, both γ-globin genes in *cis* to the deletion are derepressed, thus explaining the florid production of Hb F; in keeping with this, Hb F is unusually high even in heterozygotes for this deletion, in whom the other allele is normal [5]. The concept that a deletion removing part of the β-globin gene including its promoter would produce changes in the chromatin favouring reactivation of the γ-globin genes was suggested early on in the study of this mutation [6]. In our patient, homozygosity for the −158 T allele at the polymorphic *Xmn* I site upstream of the $^{G}\gamma$ (*HBG2*) globin gene [7], has helped to further increase the output of this gene. Whether the deletion

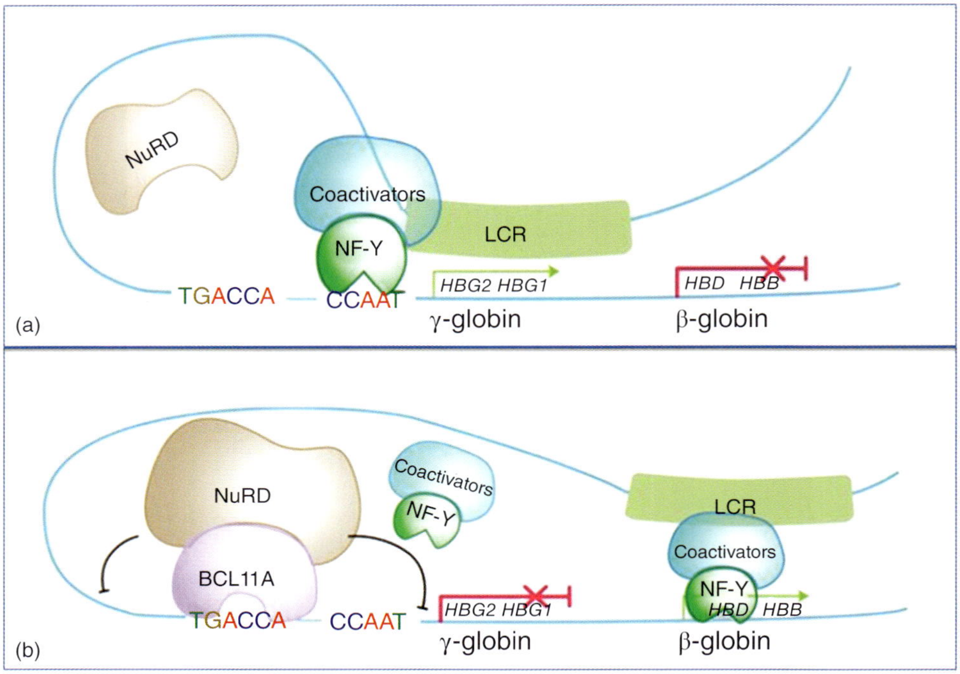

Figure 12.6 Illustration of the foetal to adult haemoglobin switch. In each panel the blue line is the genomic DNA of the β-globin gene cluster; *LCR* (locus control region) is the powerful enhancer located some 40 kb upstream; *NF-Y* (Nuclear Factor Y) is a heterotrimeric transcription factor complex that binds to the highly conserved CCAAT-box sequence found in the promoters of all globin genes; it is able to recruit *coactivators* that favour transcription. *NuRD* is a Nucleosome Remodeling and Deacetylase complex, able to act as a major transcriptional co-repressor. Panel (a) illustrates the situation that prevails during foetal life: the LCR is physically coupled to the foetal haemoglobin genes *HBG2, HBG1*; NF-Y and co-activators provide a high rate of transcription of these genes; the δ gene *HBD* and the β gene *HBB* are not expressed. Panel (b) illustrates the situation that prevails during adult life: the LCR is now physically coupled to the *HBD* and *HBB* genes, whereby NF-Y and co-activators enables their transcription at a high rate; the protein BCL11A, nearly absent during foetal life, together with NuRD, represses almost completely *HBG2* and *HBG1*. Modified from [8].

should be classified as thalassaemia or HPFH is a matter of definition: it cannot make β-globin and it causes mild microcytosis; but a major (beneficial) effect is derepression of the γ-globin genes. In our patient analysis of the α-globin gene cluster (not shown) revealed that she is heterozygous for α^{+}-thalassaemia (i.e. α−/αα), which reduces her α/non-α globin chain imbalance, and must have helped to prevent anaemia. Her clinical phenotype is a mild form of thalassaemia intermedia.

Increased oxygen affinity – compared to Hb A – is not an intrinsic property of Hb F: rather, it is due to its reduced binding of 2,3-bis-phosphoglycerate, the major intra-erythrocytic regulator of the O_2 dissociation curve. In terms of the physiology of pregnancy, the difference between the mother's Hb A and the foetus' Hb F has long been regarded as important in facilitating O_2 transfer across the placenta [9]. Evidence-based guidelines regarding management of pregnancy in thalassaemia patients – not available at the time – recommend "the initiation of transfusion in late pregnancy in some patients with non-transfusion-dependent thalassaemia" [10]; but the guidelines have not yet considered the specific issue of patients with a predominance of Hb F. On this ground, we preferred to be cautious, when we opted for a regular exchange transfusion programme throughout this patient's pregnancy. In retrospect, we may have been over-cautious, and consequently excessively invasive. We did not yet know that a normal baby could be born from a mother who had only Hb F in her blood (see Case 17).

Conclusion

Compound heterozygote for two different β-thalassaemia genes (β^0/β^+), with coexisting heterozygous alpha thalassaemia.

Acknowledgements

Dr. A. B. Mehta, Department of Haematology, The Royal Free Hospital, London, UK. A short report on this patient has been previously published [11].

References

1. Antonarakis, S.E., Orkin, S.H., Cheng, T.C. et al. (1984). β-thalassaemia in American blacks: novel mutations in the TATA box and acceptor splice site. *Proc. Natl. Acad. Sci. USA*., 81, 1154–158.
2. Sankaran, V.G., Menne, T.F., Xu, J. et al. (2008). Human fetal hemoglobin expression is regulated by the developmental stage-specific repressor BCL11A. *Science* 322(5909), 1839–1842.
3. Topfer, S.K., Feng, R., Huang, P. et al. (2022). Disrupting the adult globin promoter alleviates promoter competition and reactivates fetal globin gene expression. *Blood* 139(14), 2107–2118.

4. Padanilam, B.J., Felice, A.E., and Huisman, T.H.J. (1984). Partial deletion of the 5' β-globin gene region causes β^0 thalassaemia in members of an American black family. *Blood* 64, 941–944.
5. Amin, A.B., Pandya, N.L., Diwin, P.P. et al. (1979). A comparison of the homozygous states for G gamma and G gamma A gamma delta beta thalassaemia. *Br. J. Haematol.* 43(4), 537–548.
6. Anand, R., Boehm, C.D., Kazazian Jr., H.H. et al. (1988). Molecular characterization of a beta zero-thalassemia resulting from a 1.4 kilobase deletion. *Blood* 72(2), 636–641.
7. Gilman, J.G. and Huisman, T.H.J. (1985). DNA sequence variation associated with elevated fetal G-gamma globin product. *Blood* 66, 783–87.
8. Liu N, Xu S, Yao Q, et al. Transcription factor competition at the gamma-globin promoters controls hemoglobin switching. Nat Genet. 2021;53(4):511–20.
9. Bunn, H.F., Forget, B.G., and Ranney, H.M. (1977). Hemoglobinopathies. *Major. Probl. Intern. Med.* 12, 1–291. PMID: 323584.
10. Shah, F.T., Nicolle, S., Garg, M. et al. (2024). Guideline for the management of conception and pregnancy in thalassaemia syndromes: a British Society for Haematology Guideline. *Br. J. Haematol.* 204(6), 2194–2209.
11. Kaeda, J.S., Prasad, K., Howard, R.J., Mehta, A., Vulliamy, T.J., Luzzatto, L. Management of pregnancy when maternal blood has a very high level of fetal haemoglobin. Br. J. Haematol 88, 432-434 (1994).

See also related Case 17.

Case 13

PA: Not a Power-Act

Patient Details

Age: 34 *Sex:* F
Ethnic background: Ugandan

Reason for Referral

Investigation of "autoimmune haemolytic anaemia."

History and Clinical Findings in Brief

The patient had enjoyed mostly good health, except that since the age of 20 she has had heavy menses; this problem improved since, after having two children, she began taking the contraceptive pill. At the age of 34, in April 1991, she developed palpitations upon minor exercise, which became increasingly worse, and she was referred to her local hospital in Uganda for investigation. At that time, the patient appeared pale and mildly jaundiced; her haemoglobin level was 5 g/dl. She received several medicines, in both injection form and tablet form, including steroids. By September 1991, the patient's haemoglobin had risen to 13.5 g/dl.

Over the next year and a half, the patient was hospitalized four times, because of malarial infection, a chest infection, anaemia, and severe pain in her left calf. On this last occasion, the patient had emergency treatment because of severe anaemia and was then transferred to a hospital in Nairobi, where a diagnosis of deep vein thrombosis (DVT) was made. The contraceptive pill was stopped and the patient was anticoagulated with warfarin. A blood count confirmed that the patient was severely anaemic (see Table 13.1). It also revealed a reticulocytosis of 45%, and 58 nucleated red cells per 100 white cells. A diagnosis of autoimmune haemolytic anaemia (AIHA) was made and the patient was placed on prednisolone (40 mg/d) and azathioprine (100 mg/d). During the next month, her condition improved, and she was subsequently referred to the Hammersmith Hospital.

On examination, the patient was overweight and frankly cushingoid; her general condition was otherwise good. There were no other significant clinical findings. Upon questioning, the patient reported that during bouts of her illness, she had noticed her urine became darker; but not red or brown. Family history revealed that the patient's father had suffered, sadly, a fatal road traffic accident recently; whereas, her mother had suffered a stroke eight years previously.

Laboratory Findings

The patient had a normal haemoglobin level (see Table 13.1); however, her red cell indices were decreased. On the blood film (see Figure 13.1), the red cells were small; most of them looked hypochromic, but some appeared fully haemoglobinized. Target cells and poikilocytes, some of which were shaped like goldfish ("icthiocytes"), were also seen. We could not find

Table 13.1 Haematology Data

	April '91	Sept '92	Nov '92	Dec '94
	(Uganda)	(Nairobi)	(London)	(London)
Hb (g/dl)	5.8	4.4	12.3	12.2
RBC ($\times10^{12}$/l)	–	1.30	5.59	5.02
MCV (fl)	–	114	74.1	76.3
MCH (pg)	–	33.8	22.0	24.3
MCHC (g/dl)	–	29.7	29.6	31.9
RDW (S.D.)	–	–	58.1	46.3
Retic (%)	4.5	45	0.5	1.6
Retic ($\times10^9$/l)	–	585	28	80
WBC ($\times10^9$/l)	4.1	6.2	15.7	7.9
Plt ($\times10^9$/l)	–	112	422	328

spherocytes or fragmented cells that one might have expected in a patient with AIHA; but we knew of course that she had received treatment.

The patient had had two previous bone marrow aspirates: one had been reported as normoblastic, and one as suspicious of megaloblastosis. In a bone marrow aspirate done now (see Figure 13.2), we found somewhat hypocellular fragments, with normocellular trails. Both erythropoiesis and leucopoiesis were normal (see Figure 13.2). Iron stores were reduced.

A biochemistry profile was normal. The patient's DAGT was negative by the standard technique and by Polybrene[1] also. A red cell antibody screen was negative. The patient's serum folate level was normal, but her levels of vitamin B12, iron and ferritin were low (see Table 13.2).

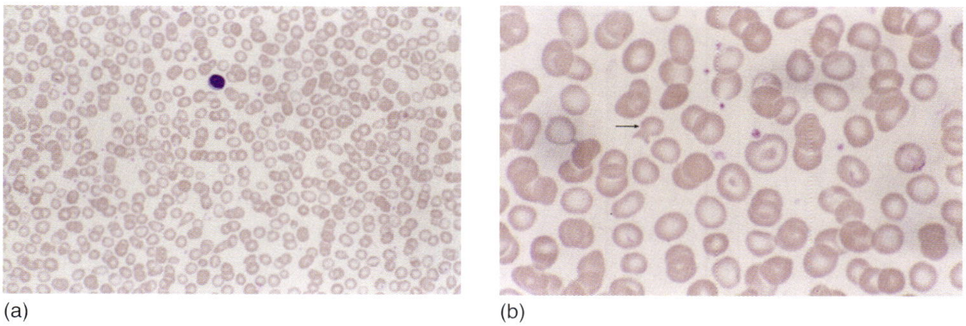

Figure 13.1 Peripheral blood film: (a) medium power view; (b) high power view, with "icthiocyte" arrowed.

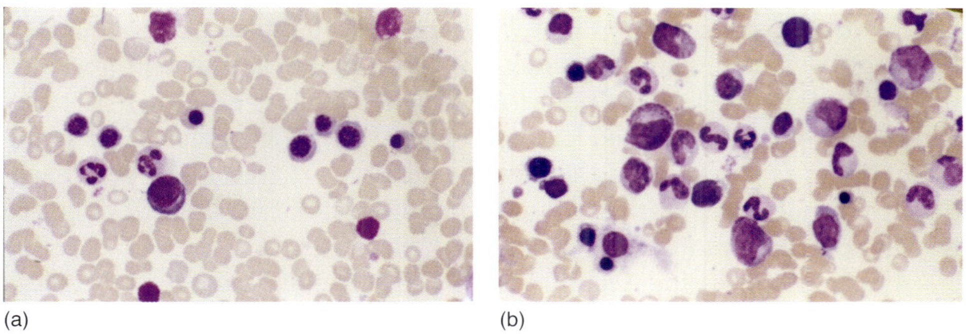

Figure 13.2 Bone marrow aspirate: (a) and (b) are two medium power fields.

[1] Polybrene (hexadimethrine bromide) was introduced into serological practice to increase the sensitivity of detection of antibody-coated red cells [1]: it is a synthetic positively charged polymer that causes agglutination, by neutralising the negative charge on the surface of the red cells.

Table 13.2 Additional Investigations

DAGT	Negative
IAGT	Negative
Heinz prep.	Negative
Ham/Sucrose lysis test	Negative
Urinary haemosiderin	Negative
G6PD (IU/g Hb)	14.6
TCR-receptor	Normal bands only
IgG (g/l)	8.4
IgA (g/l)	1.72
IgM (g/l)	7.30
Serum iron (μmol/l)	6.9
Ferritin (μg/l)	6
Serum B12 (ng/l)	140
Serum folate (μg/l)	14

Initial Assessment

The patient was not anaemic, and we could not find serological evidence supporting a diagnosis of AIHA. However, she was iron deficient and she had a reduced vitamin B12 level. Iron and B12 deficiency could be nutritional, but the patient belonged to a socio-economic group in which this did not seem likely, and she certainly did not seem malnourished.

Further Investigations

Haemoglobin electrophoresis revealed a sickle cell trait, with an Hb S level of 31%; this finding and the slightly low the red cell indices suggested coexisting α-thalassaemia; indeed, analysis of the α-globin gene cluster revealed that the patient was heterozygous for α^+-thalassaemia (i.e. α–/αα). An assay for G6PD yielded an elevated level (see Table 13.2), in keeping with a young population of red cells. Additional investigations (Table 13.2) were negative or normal, except for a high serum IgM level; but we knew it might be within range in Uganda.

A spleen scan using Technetium (99Tm)-labelled red cells revealed a marginal increase in splenic volume (503 ml). Because of the patient's prior DVT, we checked her levels of protein S, protein C and anti-thrombin III, and these were all normal.

In view of the low serum vitamin B12, a Schilling test was performed (see Table 13.3): part I (cyanocobalamin alone) was very low, and in part II (with intrinsic factor: IF) there was a 10-fold increase. Since tropical sprue

Table 13.3 Schilling Test

Schilling test:	Part I (%)[a]	0.3
	Part II (%)	3
	Part III (%)	0.3
Anti-parietal cell antibody		Positive ++
Anti-intrinsic factor antibody		Negative
Gastrin[b] (pmol/l)		400

[a] Normal excretion of radioactive vitamin B12 is ≥10%.
[b] Reference range: 0–40 pmol/l.

is endemic in regions of Africa [2], we proceeded to the so-called part III Schilling test; a two week course of tetracycline failed to correct the abnormal result seen in the part I test. The serum gastrin level was also markedly increased and, most important, the patient's serum contained anti-parietal cell antibodies.[2]

Comments

The challenge in this case was to identify the cause of a very severe anaemia "after the fact," because when we saw the patient there was no anaemia. With low serum B12, an abnormal Schilling test, anti-parietal cell antibodies and hypergastrinaemia, the diagnosis of pernicious anaemia (PA) is well supported.

We tried to work out retrospectively what may have happened. Upon further enquiries from colleagues in Uganda, we learned that the patient's initial treatment in 1991 had included vitamin B12, to which she responded; only to relapse one year later after B12 had been discontinued. In 1992, she had also received two injections of cobalamin (1 mg), some 3–5 days before being transferred to Nairobi. Thus, we interpreted the massive outpouring of reticulocytes and immature erythroid cells in the peripheral blood observed in Nairobi as a valid response by the bone marrow to cobalamin therapy; however, the MCV still betrayed the megaloblastic nature of her anaemia. This sequence of events also provided an explanation for the puzzling dramatic difference between her blood count in September 1992 in Nairobi and only two months later in London; by that time, the patient had clearly had a full response to B12. Although we do not have the bone

[2] It is true that even with IF we only got a B12 excretion of 3%. However, a 10-fold increase in B12 excretion signifies that IF was the rate-limiting factor for B12 absorption, and sub-normal increments of B12 excretion in PA have previously been reported [3, 4].

marrow aspirate slide from Uganda, we can imagine it may have looked like this (see Figure 13.3).

A further smoke screen on PA in this patient was the coexistence of an α-thalassaemia gene, and of associated iron deficiency. That α-thalassaemia limits the increase in MCV characteristic of PA has been well documented previously [3] and indeed, may have resulted in misdiagnoses in the past (see also Case 4). In this respect, the one MCV value of 114 fl recorded in Nairobi becomes even more significant; in the absence of α-thalassaemia, that value might have been even higher (perhaps 125 fl!).

In relation to the patient being from Uganda, it is pertinent to note that in the past PA has been regarded as very rare in Africa [5, 6]. However, work from Nigeria suggests that this may have been a myth [7]; and work from southern Africa has found that PA is actually the commonest cause of megaloblastic anaemia [8], and this coincides with personal recent experience of one of us in Tanzania. It is also interesting that the age of onset of PA may be earlier in Africa [4, 9, 10].

In retrospect, it seems likely that the patient never had AIHA; however, in fairness to the referral diagnosis, data from ancient history of haematology have shown that red cell survival is in fact shortened in PA [11]; and studies of erythrokinetics in PA have led to developing the very concept of *ineffective erythropoiesis* [12].

Whether the patient has antibodies against IF or against parietal cells, PA is essentially an auto-immune disorder, and we are still largely ignorant as to why it arises in an individual patient. A recent genome-wide association study has identified five genes that increase the risk of PA; the one with the highest odd ratio is, not surprisingly, the *AIRE* gene [13], that regulates the negative selection of autoreactive T-cells in the thymus.

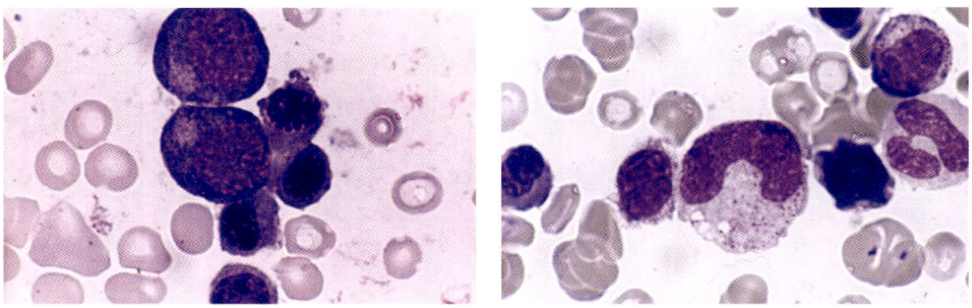

(a) (b)

Figure 13.3 Bone marrow aspirate from patient with pernicious anaemia: showing (a) megaloblasts; (b) giant metamyelocyte.

Follow-up

The patient was started on iron tablets, and two months later, her serum iron had increased considerably (44.4 μmol/l) and her ferritin level had normalized (23 μg/l); her haemoglobin level and red cell indices remained relatively unchanged. The patient's clinical progress has been good; the steroid side effects gradually reversed, and after about one year, she no longer looks cushingoid. Colleagues in Uganda made sure to provide 1 mg vitamin B12 parentally once a month, indefinitely; and we recommended to continue taking ferrous sulphate tablets (one every other day) until she reaches the menopause.

Conclusion

Pernicious anaemia.

Acknowledgements

Referred by Dr. R. Musoke, Nairobi hospital, Kenya.

References

1. Lalezari, P. (1968). A new method for detection of red blood cell antibodies. *Transfusion* 8, 372–380.
2. Guerra, R., Wheby, M.S., and Bayless, T.M. (1965). Long term antibiotic therapy in tropical sprue. *Ann. Intern. Med.* 63, 619–634.
3. Green, R., Kuhl, W., Jacobson, R. et al. (1982). Masking of macrocytosis by alpha-thalassemia in blacks with pernicious anemia. *N. Engl. J. Med.* 307, 1322–1325.
4. Abdalla, S.H., Corrah, P.T., and Mabey, D.C.W. (1986). Severe megaloblastic anaemia due to vitamin B12 deficiency in The Gambia. *Trans. R Soc. Trop. Med. Hyg.* 80, 557–562.
5. Friedlander, R.D. (1934). The racial factor in pernicious anemia; a study of five hundred cases. *Am. J. Med. Sci.* 187, 634–642.
6. Hoffbrand, A.V. (1981). Megaloblastic anaemias. In: Hoffbrand, A.V. and Lewis, S.M. editor. *Postgraduate Haematology*. London: William Heinemann Medical Books Ltd. p. 84.
7. Akinyanju, O.O. and Okany, C.C. (1992). Pernicious anemia in Africans. *Clin. Lab. Haematol.* 14, 33–40.
8. Savage, D., Gangaidzo, I., Lindenbaum, J. et al. (1994). Vitamin B12 deficiency is the primary cause of megaloblastic anaemia in Zimbabwe. *Br. J. Haematol.* 86, 844–850.

9. Carmel, R. and Johnson, C.S. (1978). Racial patterns in pernicious anemia. Early age at onset and increased frequency of intrinsic-factor antibody in Black Women. *N. Engl. J. Med*. 298, 647–650.
10. Solanki, D.L., Jacobson, R.J., Green, R. et al. (1981). Pernicious anemia in blacks. A study of 64 patients from Washington D.C., and Johannesburg, South Africa. *Am. J. Clin. Pathol*. 75, 96–99.
11. Hamilton, H.E., Degowin, E.L., Sheets, R.F. et al. (1954). Studies with inagglutinable erythrocyte counts. VI. Accelerated destruction of normal adult erythrocytes in pernicious anemia; contribution of hemolysis to the oligocythemia. *J. Clin. Invest*. 33(2), 191–205.
12. Harris R.W. (1963). *The Red Cell - Production, Metabolism, Destruction: Normal and Abnormal*. Cambridge, MA: Harvard University Press.
13. Laisk, T., Lepamets, M., Koel, M. et al. (2021). Genome-wide association study identifies five risk loci for pernicious anemia. *Nat. Commun*. 12(1), 3761.

See also related Case 4.

Case 14

Sicily in My Blood

Patient Details

Age: 46 *Sex:* F
Ethnic background: English
Occupation: Personal Secretary

Reason for Refaerral

Investigation of elevated haemoglobin F (blood sample only).

History and Clinical Findings in Brief

The patient has been healthy all her life and she has been a regular blood donor. At the age of 24, her first pregnancy ended with an early miscarriage. One year later, she gave birth to a healthy daughter and four years later to a healthy son. At the age of 43, she was investigated for anaemia and persistent menorrhagia; she had fibroids, and she underwent hysterectomy. Her anaemia resolved, but she was noticed to have a microcytic, hypochromic blood picture. The patient reported that "mild anaemia" had been seen in members of her family, and she was anxious to find the cause. Her physical examination was reported as being currently normal.

Laboratory Findings

Haemoglobin and reticulocyte count were normal, but the patient had microcytic, hypochromic red cells (see Table 14.1). On the blood film (see Figure 14.1), the red cells looked small, but otherwise quite unremarkable; there was only minimal anisocytosis and an occasional target cell.

The patient's iron status was normal (see Table 14.2). Haemoglobin electrophoresis revealed, in addition to the normal Hb A and Hb A_2 components, a distinct band in the Hb F position (see Figure 14.2). This was quantitated to about 10% (see Table 14.1).

Table 14.1 Haematology Data

Hb (g/dl)	13.0
RBC ($\times 10^{12}$/l)	5.72
MCV (fl)	73.1
MCH (pg)	22.7
MCHC (g/dl)	31.1
RDW (S.D.)	55.4
Retic (%)	0.7
Retic ($\times 10^9$/l)	40
Hb A_2 (%)	2.1
Hb F (%)	10.5

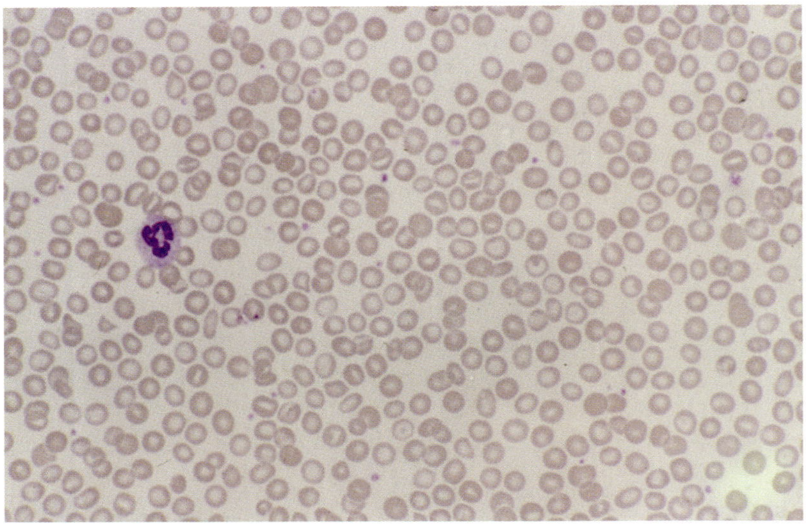

Figure 14.1 Peripheral blood film.

Table 14.2 Iron Status

Serum iron (µmol/l)	24.6
Transferrin (g/l)	2.22
Tfn. Saturation Index (%)	42

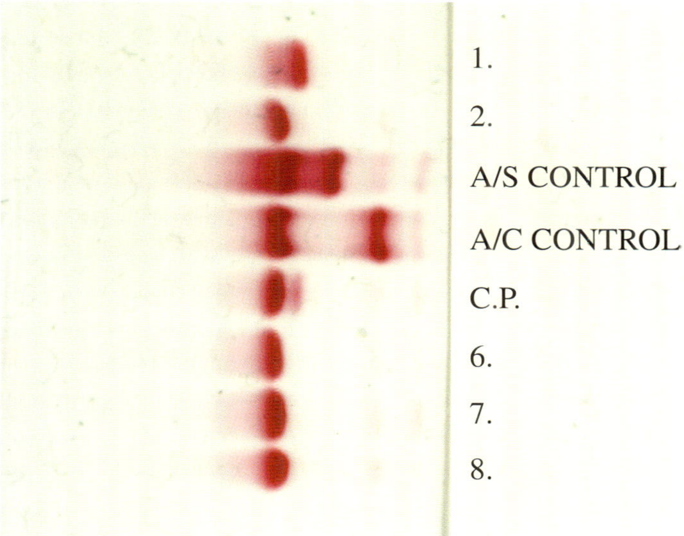

Figure 14.2 Haemoglobin electrophoresis on cellulose acetate membrane; the migration of the haemoglobin fractions is from right to left. An A/S control and A/C control are in lanes 3 and 4, respectively. A cord blood control is in lane 1. The patient (C.P.) is in lane 5.

A blood film stained by the acid elution cytochemical method of Kleihauer, Braun and Betke [1] revealed a heterocellular distribution of foetal haemoglobin (see Figure 14.3).

In order to find out whether we were dealing with a genetic abnormality, we tested the patient's relatives. A family study showed that her two sisters (one of whom was a twin), and some of the descendants through three generations, also had a raised level of Hb F (see Figure 14.4).

Initial Assessment

This patient had red cell indices compatible with mild iron deficiency, which she might have had in the past due to her menorrhagia; however, at the moment, her iron status is entirely normal. There was no suggestion of systemic illness or of any acquired disorder in this patient that may have

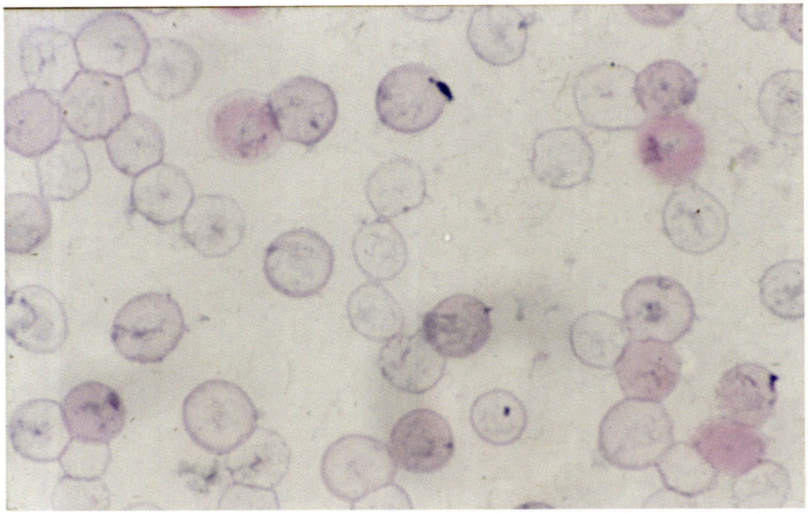

Figure 14.3 Blood film showing heterocellular distribution of haemoglobin F.

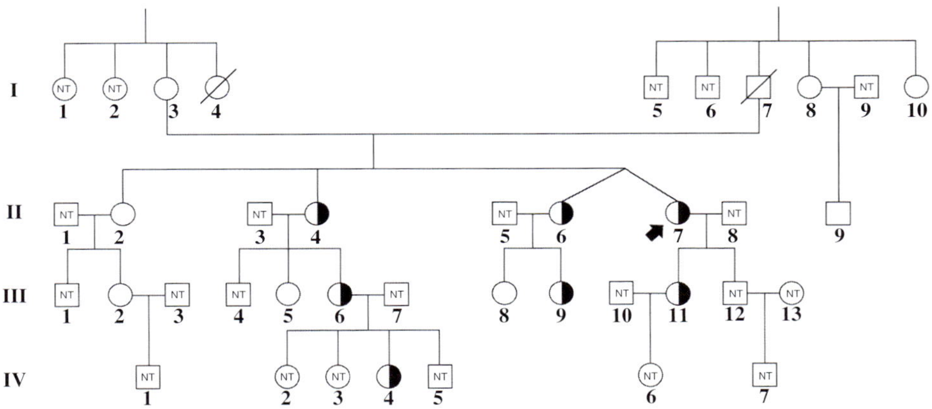

Figure 14.4 Family pedigree. Our patient is indicated by an arrow. Family members with a raised Hb F level are shown as half-filled circles, indicating they are heterozygous for the mutation causing this phenotype. The fact that they are all female is not genetically significant: it is merely due to the fact that we seem to have had little success in getting blood samples from males (NT stands for not tested).

caused a high Hb F level. The normal Hb A_2 excludes any ordinary type of β-thalassaemia trait. The patient is not known to have ancestry from any population where haemoglobinopathies are prevalent; however, the red cell indices, together with increased Hb F, would be compatible with either HPFH or δβ-thalassaemia.

Further Investigations

A sample of the patient's haemolysate was electrophoresed on a triton-urea gel (see Figure 14.5) to estimate the level of expression of the two γ-globin genes, $^{A}\gamma$ and $^{G}\gamma$. The results are illustrated below, clearly showing comparatively greater expression of the $^{A}\gamma$-globin chains compared with $^{G}\gamma$-globin chains. The observed increase may be due to a deletion, partial deletion of the $^{G}\gamma$-globin gene, or a promoter mutation leading to the upregulation of the $^{A}\gamma$-globin chains. Although this is only a semi-quantitative technique, the banding pattern would be quite in keeping with a non-deletional form of HPFH; however, this alone, would not explain the microcytic, hypochromic indices, which would be more in keeping with a deletional δβ-thalassaemia (in the case of the latter, the $^{G}\gamma$:$^{A}\gamma$ ratio is usually 60:40).

Southern blot analysis showed the patient to have a normal α-globin genotype. Only normal fragments were revealed by a γ-globin probe when hybridized to genomic DNA digested with *Xba I* and *BamH I*. Southern blot analysis of the β-globin gene cluster revealed only normal fragments following the hybridization of *Bgl II* and *Hind III* digested genomic DNA with a β-globin probe (not shown). However, the intensity of the bands in the tracks with the patient's and her sister's DNA were reduced in comparison to those in the control lane (despite having equal amount of DNA in all three lanes), implying a deletion of one of the β-globin alleles. This was confirmed by PCR analysis that revealed, in addition to the expected normal product, an abnormal fragment of 1.8 Kb. The latter was consistent with a 13.3 Kb deletion, which has previously been reported as the "Sicilian" δβ-thalassaemia deletion (see Figure 14.6). The deletion extends from intron II of the δ-globin gene to a position downstream the β-globin gene, thus removing the β-globin gene completely. Moreover, no δ-globin chains are synthesized from the partially deleted allele; hence the normal Hb A_2 value, which is typically found in δβ-thalassaemia.

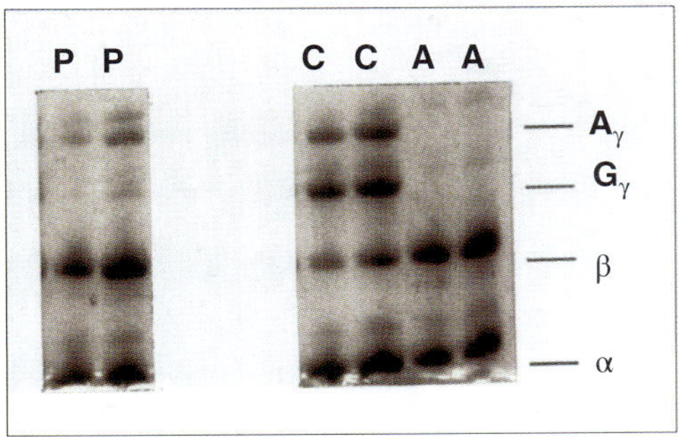

Figure 14.5 Triton-urea Globin chain electrophoresis. Position of the globin chains is indicated on the right. Lysates prepared from the patient's (P), normal umbilical cord (C) and normal adult (A) peripheral blood is loaded at two concentrations. The high proportion of the γ-globin chains in the cord blood is clearly observed. The increase in the γ-globin chains, particularly $^{A}\gamma$, is clearly seen in the P lanes.

Comments

The demarcation between δβ-thalassaemia and HPFH is somewhat arbitrary [3]. Classically, one would use the designation HPFH when red cell indices are normal, indicating that the increased synthesis of γ-chains compensates fully for a decreased synthesis of β-chains. This is seen in the deletional type of HPFH first reported from Ghana [4]. With this genetic abnormality, both heterozygotes and homozygotes are haematologically normal, and the distribution of Hb F is pancellular. In δβ-thalassaemia, instead, the derepression of the γ-chain genes is only partial; therefore Hb F synthesis fails to compensate for the deficit in β-chain synthesis and the distribution of Hb F is heterocellular. Heterozygotes have a haematological picture quite similar to β-thalassaemia trait, whereas most homozygotes have a clinical picture of thalassaemia intermedia [3].

Why some deletions within the β-globin gene cluster produce the δβ-thalassaemia phenotype, whereas others cause the HPFH phenotype has been puzzling for a long time. A recent study has highlighted that in this respect, a critical element is the presence or absence of the β-globin gene promoter [5]; this is removed by the deletion in this patient. This matter is discussed more in detail under Case 17.

The molecular data clearly show the inheritance in this English family of a mutant gene regarded as "Sicilian." Of course, we cannot say whether that gene did indeed reach these shores all the way from Sicily, or whether it happened to arise independently.

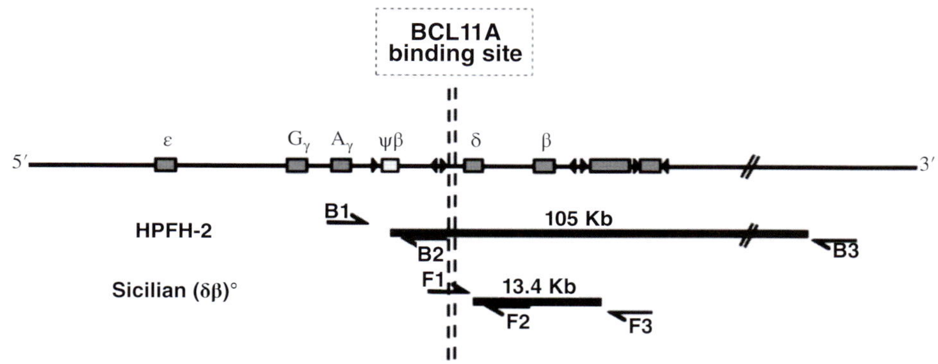

Figure 14.6 Diagram of the β-globin gene cluster, showing the position of two gene deletions, one causing HPFH, the other causing δβ-thalassaemia. [2]/with permission of SAGE Publications.

Follow-up

The patient and her family were fully reassured by what was communicated to them.

Conclusion

Heterozygous for Sicilian δβ-thalassaemia.

Acknowledgements

Referred by Dr. M. Saary, Haematology Department, JSPS House, Harley Street, London, UK.
Dr. S. L., Thein, MRC Molecular Haematology Unit, John Radcliffe Hospital, Oxford, UK.

References

1. Kleihauer, E., Braun, H., and Betke, K. (1957). Demonstration of fetal hemoglobin in erythrocytes of a blood smear. *Klin Wochenschr*. 35(12), 637–638.
2. Fornari, T.A., Lanaro, C., Albuquerque, D.M. et al. (2017). Featured article: modulation of fetal hemoglobin in hereditary persistence of fetal hemoglobin deletion type-2, compared to Sicilian deltabeta-thalassemia, by BCL11A and SOX6-targeting microRNAs. *Exp. Biol. Med*. (Maywood) 242, 267–274.
3. Wood, W.G. (2001). Hereditary persistence of fetal hemoglobin and db thalassemia. In: Steinberg, M.H., Forget, B.G., Higgs, D.R. et al. editor. *Disorders of Hemoglobin*. Cambridge: Cambridge University Press. pp. 356–388
4. Bethlenfalvay, N.C., Motulsky, A.G., Ringelhann, B. et al. (1975). Hereditary persistence of fetal hemoglobin, beta thalassemia, and the hemoglobin delta-beta locus: further family data and genetic interpretations. *Am. J. Hum. Genet*. 27, 140–154.
5. Topfer, S.K., Feng, R., Huang, P. et al. (2022). Disrupting the adult globin promoter alleviates promoter competition and reactivates fetal globin gene expression. *Blood* 139, 2107–2118.

See also related Case 12.

Case 15

A Storm of Half-ghosts

Patient Details

Age: 2 *Sex:* M
Ethnic background: Italian/Ghanaian

Reason for Referral

Investigation of severe anaemia.

History and Clinical Findings in Brief

This two year old boy with no significant past medical history was admitted to hospital because of a high fever. On examination, he was pyrexial (39.2 °C), extremely pale and jaundiced. His spleen was just palpable.

Laboratory Findings

The blood count revealed a very severe normocytic, hypochromic anaemia, with elevated white cell count and reticulocyte count (see Table 15.1). The blood film (see Figure 15.1) was rather spectacular, with a large number of very dense cells and contracted cells; many of these appeared to have a separate area which was totally lacking in colour;

Table 15.1 Haematology Data

	Patient
Hb (g/dl)	2.9
RBC ($\times 10^{12}$/l)	1.22
MCV (fl)	86.9
MCH (pg)	23.8
MCHC (g/dl)	27.4
RDW (S.D.)	39.3
Retic (%)	10.0
Retic ($\times 10^9$/l)	122
WBC ($\times 10^9$/l)	27.4
"Corrected" WBC	19.4
Neuts ($\times 10^9$/l)	11.5

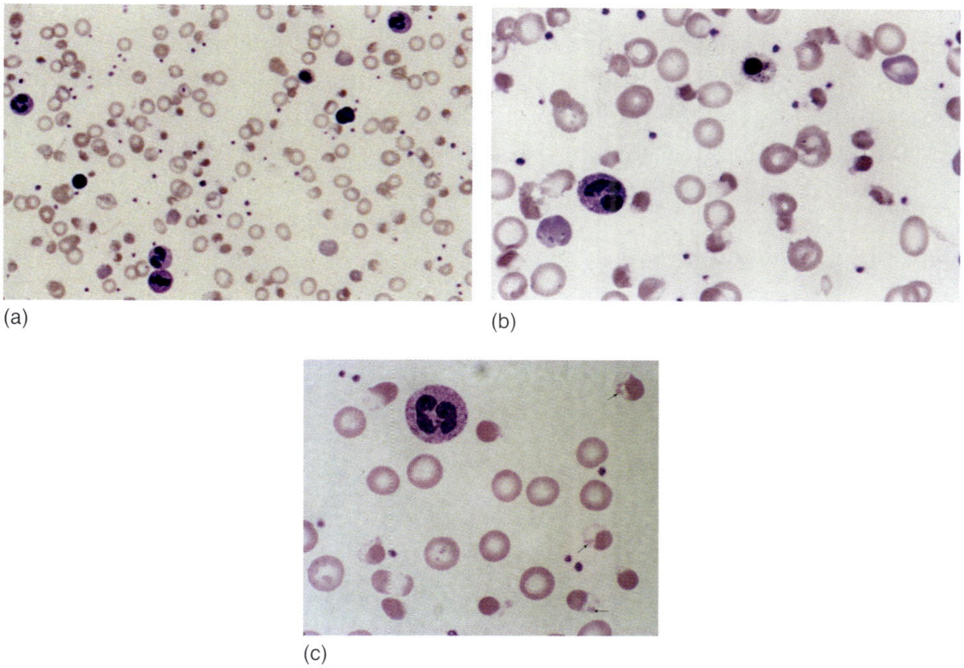

Figure 15.1 Peripheral blood film: (a) medium power view; (b) high power view; (c) high power view; Heinz bodies in hemighost cells arrowed.

these "hemighost" accounted for about 10% of the red cells. Bite cells and fragmented cells were also seen. Polychromasia was very evident. A "white cell" differential count revealed that in fact, 29% were nucleated red blood cells (NRBC).

In addition, the patient's bilirubin level was increased (65 μmol/l). Haemoglobin electrophoresis was normal and the DAGT was negative.

Initial Assessment

Based on the above findings, there seemed little doubt that this boy's sudden anaemia was haemolytic. The negative Coombs test was against autoimmune haemolytic anaemia (AIHA). As for the cause, the abnormal red cell morphology was strongly suggestive of oxidative damage, with a high number of hemighosts; this would suggest G6PD deficiency in the first place.

Further Investigations

A G6PD enzyme assay yielded an activity of 3.7 IU/g Hb (reference range 7.0–10.4 IU/g Hb); thus, the patient was definitely G6PD deficient in spite of his reticulocytosis. On electrophoresis (see Figure 15.2), the G6PD had a fast mobility (110% of the control), typical of the G6PD variant known as G6PD A−. Assay of G6PD on the mother yielded a value of 5.6 IU/g Hb and on electrophoresis, one normal band and one band with fast mobility were detected; this was in keeping with a heterozygous deficiency.

Clinical Course

The patient was given a broad spectrum antibiotic and was transfused with 250 ml of concentrated red blood cells. After three weeks, surprisingly, there was again a moderate drop in Hb and another bout of reticulocytosis; he

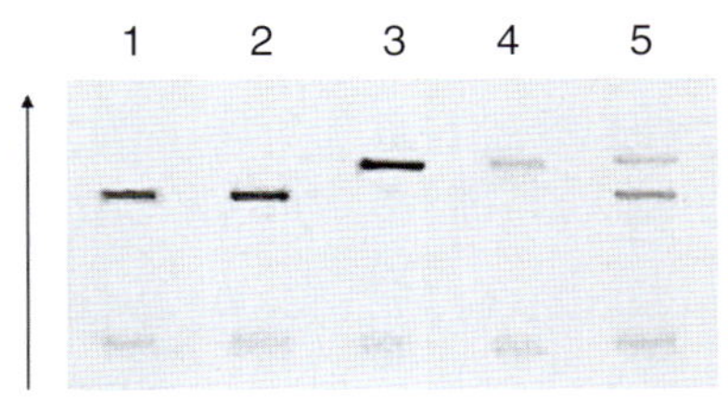

Figure 15.2 G6PD electrophoresis on Cellogel® (black and white image). The gel was stained for G6PD activity, giving a deposition of formazan. Patient's sample (lane 4); mother's (lane 5); normal (G6PD-B) (lanes 1 and 2); normal G6PD A control (lane 3). The arrow shows the direction of electrophoresis. The slowly migrating band at the bottom of the gel is haemoglobin.

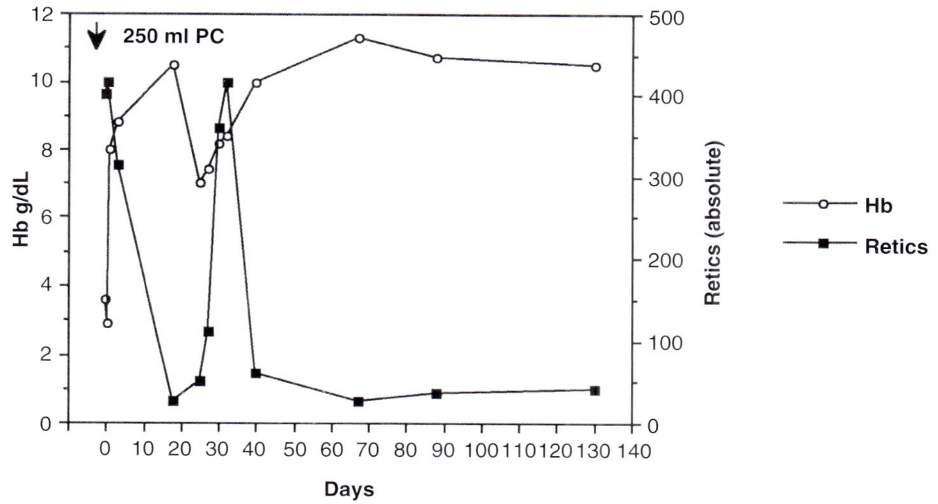

Figure 15.3 Progress chart showing haemoglobin concentration (Hb) and reticulocyte count following blood transfusion.

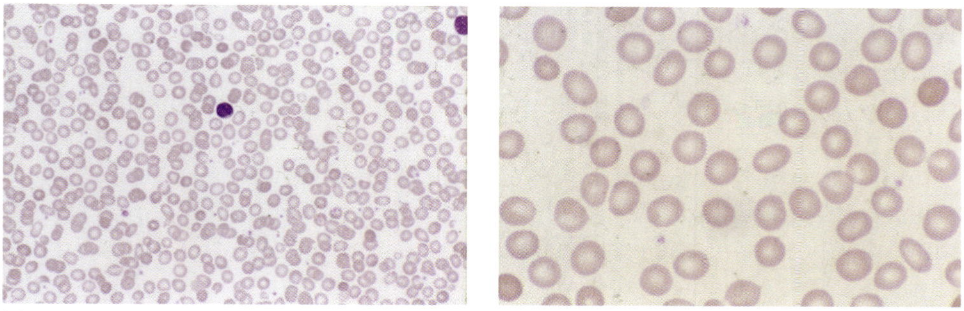

(a) (b)

Figure 15.4 Steady-state peripheral blood film (day 68): (a) medium power view; (b) high power view.

then reverted to a steady state haemoglobin of 10–11 g/dl (see Figure 15.3). On a follow-up blood film, a few poikilocytes and hypochromic microcytes could be seen. We could only find a very occasional dense cell, and did not see a single hemighost cell (see Figure 15.4).

Comments

The diagnosis in this boy was not difficult. In many parts of the world, the most likely trigger for such a sudden and severe acute haemolytic anaemia (AHA) in a G6PD deficient boy would be a meal of fava beans, i.e. an attack of favism [1]. However, this was denied in this case; nor could we elicit any history of administration of any potentially dangerous medicine. The third potential trigger of haemolysis in G6PD deficient persons (probably more common than it might appear from the literature) is infection [2]; although we could not pinpoint the nature of infection in this boy, he had a high fever and a high neutrophil leucocytosis. We regret not having carried out more extensive microbiological investigations, but there was urgency.

G6PD deficiency is vastly heterogeneous, as many different mutant alleles can underlie this phenotype [2]. From the boy's Italian surname, we might have expected G6PD Mediterranean; but we were wrong. Surnames in most countries are inherited in a Y-linked pattern; G6PD, on the other hand is X-linked, and therefore this boy's G6PD came from his mother, who is Ghanaian. G6PD A− is, of course, the common variant in Africa, although it is also found in Southern Italy, Greece and elsewhere. In the past, the view has been held by some that the clinical course of haemolysis with G6PD A− is "mild." This case history on its own disproves such contention; this boy's haemoglobin had dropped to 2.9 g/dl, and his life was certainly at risk had he not been promptly transfused. The recently revised WHO classification has merged the former class II and class III into class B, that includes G6PD A− [3].

The finding of such a large number of hemighosts on the peripheral blood film is not common, and we have not seen it other than in AHA associated with G6PD deficiency. Fisher et al. [4] have analyzed in detail these cells, and they found that the haemoglobin was confined to one part of the cell only, leaving the other part as transparent as a Hb-free ghost. In this empty part, the membranes appeared tightly bonded, and artificial swelling of the erythrocytes could not peel apart the bonded membranes. These authors have shown compellingly that in a haemolytic attack in a G6PD deficient person red cell destruction *in vivo* occurs through a summation of extravascular haemolysis due to erythrophagocytosis, and intravascular haemolysis consequent on reduced surface area followed by osmotic lysis.

Conclusion

Acute haemolytic anaemia in an infant with G6PD deficiency.

Acknowledgements

Dr. Irene Roberts, Haematology Department, Hammersmith Hospital, London, UK.

References

1. Luzzatto, L. and Arese, P. (2018). Favism and glucose-6-phosphate dehydrogenase deficiency. *N. Engl. J. Med.* 378, 60–71.
2. Luzzatto, L., Ally, M., and Notaro, R. (2020). Glucose-6-phosphate dehydrogenase deficiency. *Blood* 136, 1225–1240.
3. Luzzatto, L., Bancone, G., Dugue, P.A. et al. (2024). New WHO classification of genetic variants causing G6PD deficiency. *Bull. World Health Organ.* 102, 615–617.
4. Fischer, T.M., Meloni, T., Pescarmona, G.P. et al. (1985). Membrane cross bonding in red cells in favic crisis: a missing link in the mechanism of extravascular haemolysis. *Br. J. Haematol.* 59, 159–169.

Case 16

Honora Medicum

Patient Details

Age: 28 *Sex:* M
Ethnic background: Nigerian
Occupation: Physician

Reason for Referral

Patient with known sickle cell anaemia moving to UK.

History and Clinical Findings in Brief

The patient had had his first sickle cell pain crisis at the age of three. He grew up, attended school and trained as a doctor in Nigeria. On the whole, he regards himself as having clinically mild sickle cell anaemia (SCA). Until now, he has needed hospital admission approximately once every 12–18 months; his steady-state haemoglobin level is between 8.5 and 9.5 g/dl.

Three days after arriving to London from Nigeria, he was admitted as an emergency to another hospital suffering from pain in his right hip and left shoulder. After two days, he developed a fever, 38.3 °C, and pain over the left lower lateral chest wall. His chest remained clear clinically and radiologically, but a throat swab grew a β-haemolytic strep; he was treated with penicillin and made a quick recovery. Two years later, the patient was referred to the Hammersmith Hospital. He reported that over the past several months, since moving to London, he has suffered from "minor" but disturbing crises when he wakes up in the middle of the night with bone pains and also intermittent painful penile erections. On examination, his general condition was good. The only physical findings were a degree of pallor, minimal jaundice and markedly enlarged tonsils.

Laboratory Findings

The patient had a mild microcytic, hypochromic anaemia (see Table 16.1). On the blood film (see Figure 16.1), we found a large number of target cells, which made the hypochromia especially prominent; on the other hand, many of the red cells showed normal haemoglobinization. Polychromatic cells were also present, and anisocytosis was prominent, yielding a high RDW. There was a very occasional cell in which the haemoglobin had retracted away from the edge of the cell leaving one half of the cell empty ("hemi-ghost"). We saw several cells that were elongated, curved, dense, lacking central pallor: we had little doubt as to what they were although, even after looking hard, we did not find one that met the ultimate criterion for an irreversibly sickled cell, namely the pointed ends. A single Howell-jolly body was seen in a small proportion of red cells.

Table 16.1 Haematology Data

	Presenting	Episode 1	Episode 2
Hb (g/dl)	10.0	7.9	4.9
RBC ($\times 10^{12}$/l)	4.07	2.97	1.87
MCV (fl)	74.1	86.2	86.6
MCH (pg)	24.6	26.6	26.2
MCHC (g/dl)	33.2	30.9	30.2
RDW (S.D.)	64.1	68.1	68.1
Retic (%)	6.4	–	–
Retic ($\times 10^{9}$/l)	260	–	–
Hb A_2 (%)	2.5	–	–
Hb F (%)	1.7	–	–
G6PD	7.2	–	–
α thal	α-/αα	—	—

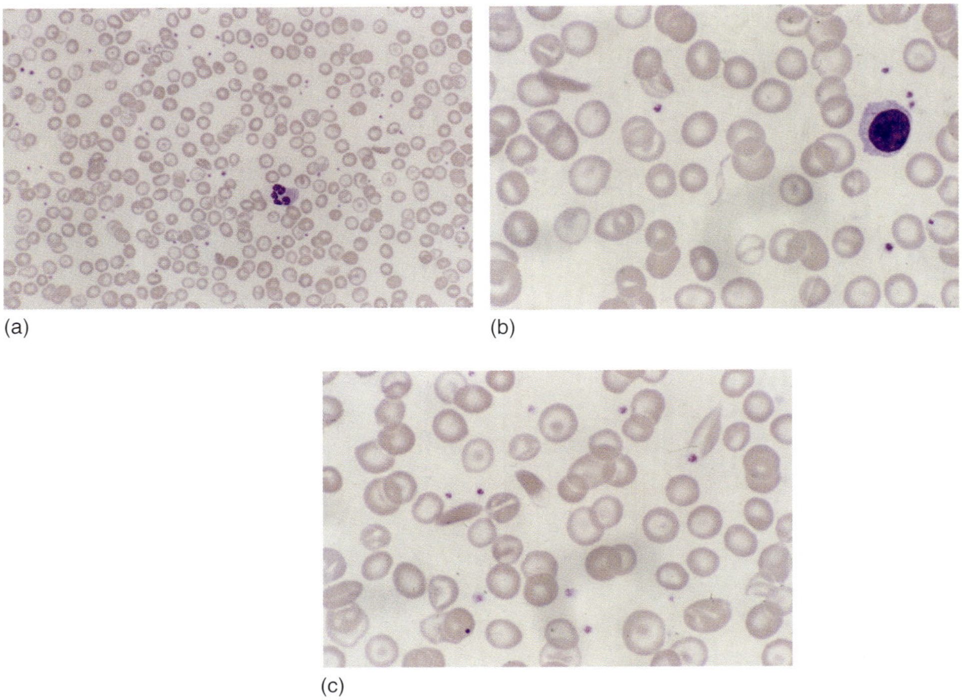

Figure 16.1 Peripheral blood film: (a) medium power view; (b) and (c) high power view.

Initial Assessment

The findings in this patient were entirely consistent with the diagnosis of homozygous SCA previously made in Nigeria; the patient was also known to have G6PD deficiency, due to a unique variant [1]. Two points of note were: (i) Why was his anaemia microcytic?; (ii) Was there a link between his enlarged tonsils, that might have caused oxygen desaturation during sleep [2], and his nocturnal stuttering priapism?

Further Investigations

The microcytosis could be quickly explained; the patient was heterozygous for alpha thalassaemia. As for his enlarged tonsils, there had been at least one episode of proven streptococcal throat infection. After an ENT consultation, a tonsillectomy was planned; in preparation for which, the patient was given a three units exchange blood transfusion, followed by exchange of two further units one week later. Eight days after the second exchange, there was a sharp fall in the patient's haemoglobin, associated with very dark urine, which tested positive for haemoglobin.

The differential diagnosis of this episode had to include the following: (i) intravascular haemolysis associated with G6PD deficiency; (ii) exacerbation of haemolysis of SCA; (iii) haemolytic transfusion reaction.

Because of the time relationship between the exchange blood transfusion and the haemoglobinuria, we were highly suspicious of the third possibility. In fact, the other two possibilities were ruled out by haemoglobin electrophoresis of a urine sample, which was found to contain Hb A but no Hb S. Clearly, the red cells that had undergone intravascular haemolysis were from the transfused blood.

In view of this serious episode, the need for tonsillectomy was reassessed. On three consecutive all night studies, there was no evidence of oxygen desaturation, and the tonsillectomy was cancelled.

The patient gradually reverted to his steady state, but over the next two years, he continued to suffer with episodes of priapism which were getting progressively worse, and which he had virtually every night, causing him much distress. He developed his own treatment; if he undertook fairly strenuous physical exercise (i.e. running 1–2 miles), he would eventually achieve detumescence. However, on some occasions, a more prolonged episode of priapism required hospitalization, and required aspirations of blood from the *corpora cavernosa*; on one occasion, this was followed by an exchange blood transfusion. In spite of a "clear" cross-match before-hand, the patient had a massive, life-threatening, transfusion reaction. His haemoglobin fell to 4.9 g/dl and many nucleated red blood cells were seen in his peripheral blood (see Figure 16.2); this was highly suspicious of bone marrow necrosis.

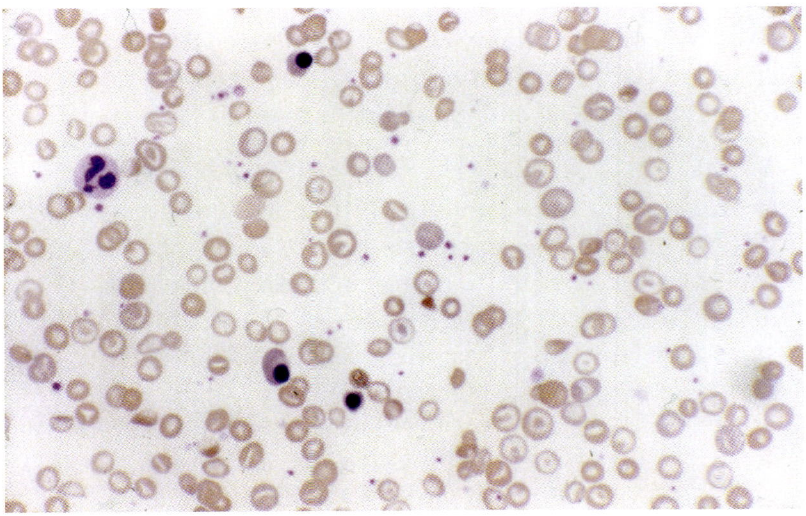

Figure 16.2 Blood film at the time of severe exacerbation of anaemia: showing nucleated red cells, polychromasia and contracted red cells.

Table 16.2 Blood Group Phenotype of Patient's Red Cells

ABO	C	Cw	c	D	E	e	M	N	S	s
B	–	–	+	+	+	–	+	–	–	+
P_1	Lu^a	K	Le^a	Le^b	Fy^a	Fy^b	Jk^a	Jk^b		
+	–	–	–	+	–	–	+	+		

Table 16.3 Reaction of Cold Agglutinin with Adult and Cord Cells at Various Temperatures

Cell type	4 °C	20 °C	30 °C	37 °C
Adult cells	256	128	2	0
Adult cells[a]	512	128	32	4
Cord cells	16	1	0	0

[a] Enzyme-treated red cells.

In view of two episodes of severe intravascular haemolysis, extensive *serological investigations* were carried out. The results can be summarized as follows.

1. An extended phenotype of the patient's red cells was obtained (Table 16.2).
2. The patient had anti-HI, anti-Kell and anti-S allo-antibodies. A weak anti-E auto-antibody was also detected. The Donath-Landsteiner test was negative. Instead, the serum contained a cold agglutinin with anti-I specificity (Table 16.3).
3. The DAGT was intermittently weakly positive (complement only); and a weak, warm complement-binding antibody, showing no specificity, was detectable by IAGT (after acidification of the serum), with anti-C3d only.

These findings did not enable us to pinpoint the precise mechanism of the patient's haemolytic transfusion reactions/hyper-haemolytic syndrome. Therefore, we resorted to a time-honoured *in vivo* test. A small aliquot of group B, cde/cde donor cells that were negative for the S and K antigens was labelled with ^{51}Cr and injected into the patient. Sequential blood samples (see Figure 16.3) showed a markedly reduced *in vivo* survival (T_{50} = 1.5 days), with complete disappearance of donor red cells by six days after infusion. This confirmed rapid *in vivo* haemolysis, but it could not be attributed to his known allo-antibodies.

In the hope of finding a suitable donor for future emergencies, the patient's sister volunteered. A similar ^{51}Cr study carried out with a small

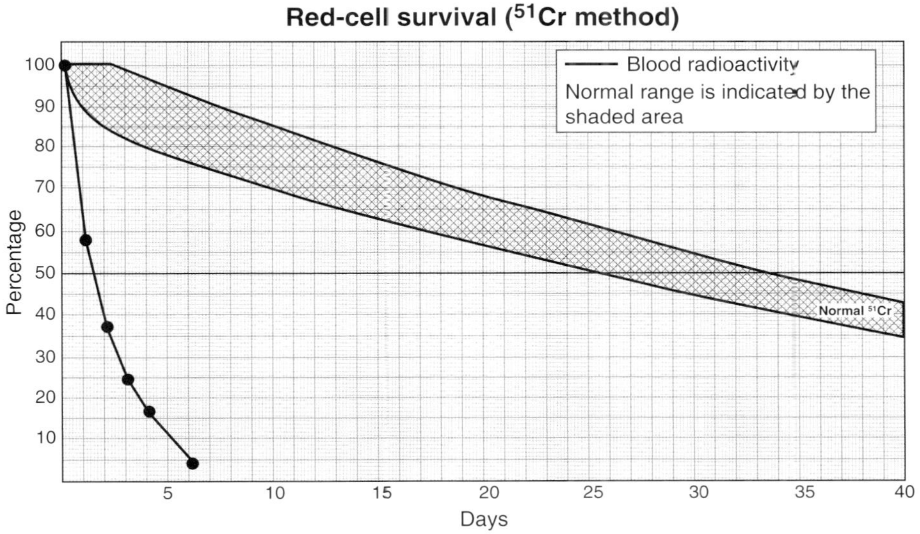

Figure 16.3 Survival curve of donor red cells.

sample of her blood (which had proven compatible by standard techniques) showed a normal survival up to day 15; after that, there was rapid destruction that we could not explain. We decide to refrain from any further blood transfusions, and four weeks later, the patient was well enough to be discharged.

Apart from episodes of severe bone pains at the time, the patient felt persistent tingling and right-sided pain in his chin, lower lip and gum, corresponding with the distribution of the mandibular nerve. It seems likely that the neuropathy resulted from a local vaso-occlusive crisis as from a publication by the patient himself [3]. There were no other neurological abnormalities.

In summary, it became clear we had to confront two issues: (i) the patient was un-transfusable, and (ii), on top of his steady-state SCA, he had recurrent significant clinical manifestations. To deal with (i), as soon as the patient's haemoglobin was back to 8 g/dl, in order to provide for possible future emergencies, we started monthly phlebotomy followed by cryopreservation. On test samples, although the recovery of red cells after thawing and subsequent washings was only 48%, the T_{50} of autologous fresh or cryopreserved blood was 20 days (thus confirming once again the role of allo-antibodies, rather than auto-antibodies, in the previous haemolytic episodes). With respect to (ii), we were fortunate that by then it had become known that hydroxyurea (HU) increases Hb F, and anecdotal reports on clinical benefit in SCA had appeared [4]; the patient was started on HU (off label for SCD at the time), and within weeks his Hb F increased from 1.7 to 5.5%.

Comments

This patient illustrates several important issues associated with SCA; first and foremost, how erratic and unpredictable the clinical course of this condition can be. For the first 25 years of his life, this patient would have been certainly classified as mild, with few problems and a steady-state Hb of 10 g/dl; his α-thalassaemia trait might have been beneficial, whereas his low baseline Hb F was not. After this relatively benign course, that did not seriously interfere with the patient's development and lifestyle, whereby he trained successfully as a doctor in Nigeria and as a haematologist in the UK, the patient started suffering from a number of severe pain crises and from recurrent priapism; until he also experienced life-threatening complications.

Episodes of priapism in SCA are triggered by vaso-occlusive phenomena in the blood supply to the *corpora cavernosa*. Severe priapism has been often contrasted with mild "stuttering priapism," but unfortunately this patient had both. Like for other manifestations of SCA, it is remarkable that priapism may be a major recurrent problem for some, and may be unknown to others. This fact has motivated gene association studies, suggesting that a *TGFBR3* allelic gene in the transforming growth factor-beta pathway may be involved [5, 6]. Our patient was remarkably resourceful and brave in dealing with the problem on his own; he also benefited from pharmacological intervention with alpha-blockers (procyclidine), and on several occasions he actually required surgical intervention. Such interventions are often regarded as eventually leading to impotence; but this is not always correct, and it was very gratifying that subsequently our patient had two children.

There is a vast literature on the occurrence in SCA of *delayed haemolytic transfusion reactions* (DHTR [7–12]); and of a *hyper-haemolytic syndrome* (HHS) [13] that may occur after blood transfusion. The two terms are often used interchangeably: however, the former applies to events when one or more allo-antibodies[1] destroy transfused cells, whereas the latter is defined by a fall of the haemoglobin to a lower level after transfusion than before, implying that not only the transfused red cells, but also some proportion of the patient's own red cell must have been destroyed.[2] In DHTR, the allo-antibodies most frequently involved are anti-Rh and anti-Kell, but others have been encountered; and sometimes antibody identification has failed. It is not always clear why DHTR occurs only in a small proportion

---

[1] It has been suggested that one reason for the occurrence of this complication in Europe might be the considerable genetic difference between the mostly European blood donor population and the African ancestry of SCA patients. However, multiple allo-antibodies are a well-recognized problem in Italian patients with beta thalassemia regularly transfused from Italian donors [14].

[2] It is also important to avoid confusion with the "hyper-haemolytic phenotype": a term that has been used to designate a group of SCD patients who, in the steady state, have unusually high rate of haemolysis [15].

of transfused SCA patients; recently, an association was discovered with a loss of function mutation of the *MBL2* gene, that encodes a serum mannose-binding lectin [16]. In order to prevent DHTR long term cryo-preservation of autologous red cells for the purpose of auto-transfusion is a logical approach that, even in the face of chronic anaemia, in our experience with this patient has proven feasible: but we have to admit that it has practical limitations, for instance, when the patient moves.

In HHS, an important and characteristic feature (that may or may not occur in DHTR), is haemoglobinuria, together with a very high serum LDH: this signifies intravascular haemolysis, and it betrays an abrupt and rather massive activation of complement. With certain allo-antibodies the antigen–antibody reaction may have activated complement via the "classic" pathway; when no antibody is found, complement activation in a patient with SCA may have taken place through the alternative pathway [17], especially since a chronic inflammatory state is part and parcel of SCA [18]. We still don't know what exactly triggers HHS and why, under these circumstances, CD55 and CD59, complement regulators present on the surface of red cells, prove unable to protect them from lysis; but the history of our patient tells us loudly that HHS is a life-threatening emergency, and that complement activation plays a crucial role in its pathogenesis. Since powerful C5 and C3 inhibitors are now available[19], a logical emergency therapeutic procedure is complement blockade: in individual cases, the anti-C5 monoclonal antibody eculizumab has been used successfully [20, 21].

That this patient with SCA was also G6PD deficient had been first discovered while conducting a deliberate study on the clinical implications of this particular genotypic combination [22]. It emerged from that study and from other subsequent studies [23] that, in most cases, G6PD deficiency as such does not much influence the clinical course of SCA. The relatively frequent coexistence of the two conditions can be explained in general by the high frequency of both the *HBB S* gene and the *G6PD* A− gene in West Africa. However, this is not the explanation in this particular case, because our patient turned out to have a unique G6PD variant G6PD Ilesha, rather than G6PD A− [24].

Follow-up

Our patient was one of the first in the UK, in 1992, to start taking HU (1 g/day), on an off-label basis; it was a few years later that clinical benefit was proven by a controlled multi-centre trial [25], of which recently the thirty year anniversary has been celebrated [26]. The priapism, although still recurring, became much less bothersome; he had a single episode of transient mild thrombocytopenia, and only one hospital admission in the following seven years. The dose of HU was increased to 1.5 g/day, with regular monitoring of his blood counts. Our patient attested himself to the fact that HU was the first really good thing that happened in the medical management of SCA, since it had become known as a molecular disease.

The patient progressed in a successful professional career: among other things, he published several papers, most of them on SCA, including the most authoritative currently available review on priapism in this condition [27]. The patient became a respected consultant Haematologist in Northern England. Subsequently, the patient was offered and accepted an academic Faculty position in Northern Canada. He remained generally well until, out of a blue sky, in 2013, he suddenly observed massive haemoglobinuria associated with acute worsening of anaemia. We learnt that very sadly he died on the fourth day of hospital admission, at the age of 50. In Canada the patient's research work was on multiple myeloma: a paper published several years later [28] was dedicated by his co-authors to the memory of their colleague, who had designed the study.

This brief report cannot make justice to the unique history of a colleague who was able to discuss SCA and to teach about SCA in depth, both as a patient and as a senior haematologist. A lasting testimony to his passionate concern for his fellow patients is, among other things, a wonderful book written by this patient, together with O. Akinyanju, addressed to SCA patients themselves: *How to Live with Sickle Cell Disorder* (Ibadan, Nigeria, ISBN 978 8088 36 8).

Conclusion

Homozygous SCA with α-thal trait and a rare type of G6PD deficiency; multiple red cell antibodies and hyper-haemolytic syndrome.[3]

Acknowledgements

Dr. George Marsh, Department of Haematology, North Middlesex Hospital, London, UK.
Dr. Ruth Warwick, The North London Blood Transfusion Service, London, UK.
Mr. Gordon Williams, Department of Urology, Hammersmith Hospital, London, UK.

[3] Quite apart from the objective problems inherent in this case, reviewing and writing up this clinical history was very hard emotionally. In fact, we have recurrently debated whether or not to include this patient in this book, and we have also discussed the matter with members of his family. As stated above, the patient was a highly valued colleague, who had not hesitated to publish several papers based on his own experience of sickle cell disease; in the end, we felt this meant that he wished for all of us to continue learning on both the advances and the setbacks that we are still experiencing.

References

1. Luzzatto, L., Usanga, E.A., Bienzle, U. et al. (1979). Imbalance in X-chromosome expression: evidence for a human X-linked gene affecting growth of haemopoietic cells. *Science* 205, 1418–1420.
2. Samuels, M.P., Stebbens, V.A., Davies, S.C. et al. (1992). Sleep related upper airway obstruction and hypoxaemia in sickle cell disease. *Arch. Dis. Child.* 67, 925–929.
3. Gregory, G. and Olujohungbe, A. (1994). Mandibular nerve neuropathy in sickle cell disease. Local factors. *Oral. Surg. Oral. Med. Oral. Pathol.* 77, 66–69.
4. Platt, O.S., Orkin, S.H., Dover, G., et al. (1984). Hydroxyurea enhances fetal hemoglobin production in sickle cell anemia. *J. Clin. Invest.* 74, 652–656.
5. Elliott, L., Ashley-Koch, A.E., De Castro, L. et al. (2007). Genetic polymorphisms associated with priapism in sickle cell disease. *Br. J. Haematol.* 137, 262–267.
6. Cintho Ozahata, M., Page, G.P., Guo, Y. et al. (2019). Clinical and genetic predictors of priapism in sickle cell disease: results from the recipient epidemiology and donor evaluation study III Brazil cohort study. *J. Sex Med.* 16, 1988–1999.
7. Bowen, D., Devenish, A., Dalton, J. et al. (1988). Delayed haemolytic transfusion reaction due to simultaneous appearance of anti-Fya and anti-Fy5. *Vox Sang.* 55, 35–36.
8. Hmida, S., Mojaat, N., Maamar, M. et al. (1994). Red cell alloantibodies in patients with haemoglobinopathies. *Nouv. Rev. Fr. Hematol.* 36, 363–366.
9. Halverston, G., Shanahan, E., Santiago, I. et al. (1994). The first reported case of anti-Dob causing an acute hemolytic transfusion reaction. *Vox. Sang.* 66, 206–209.
10. Cullis, J.O., Win, N., Dudley, J.M. et al. (1995). Post-transfusion hyperhaemolysis in a patient with sickle cell disease: use of steroids and intravenous immunoglobulin to prevent further red cell destruction. *Vox Sang.* 69, 355–357.
11. Garratty G. (1997). Severe reactions associated with transfusion of patients with sickle cell disease [editorial; comment] [see comments]. *Transfusion* 37, 357–361.
12. Vidler, J.B., Gardner, K., Amenyah, K. et al. (2015). Delayed haemolytic transfusion reaction in adults with sickle cell disease: a 5-year experience. *Br. J. Haematol.* 169, 746–753.
13. Petz, L.D., Calhoun, L., Shulman, I.A. et al. (1997). The sickle cell hemolytic transfusion reaction syndrome. *Transfusion* 37, 382–392.
14. Franchini, M., Forni, G.L., Marano, G. et al. (2019). Red blood cell alloimmunisation in transfusion-dependent thalassaemia: a systematic review. *Blood. Transfus.* 17, 4–15.
15. Dubert, M., Elion, J., Tolo, A. et al. (2017). Degree of anemia, indirect markers of hemolysis, and vascular complications of sickle cell disease in Africa. *Blood* 130, 2215–2223.
16. Mwesigwa, S., Moulds, J.M., Chen, A. et al. (2018). Whole-exome sequencing of sickle cell disease patients with hyperhemolysis syndrome suggests a role for rare variation in disease predisposition. *Transfusion* 58, 726–735.
17. Tampaki, A., Gavriilaki, E., Varelas, C. et al. (2021). Complement in sickle cell disease and targeted therapy: I know one thing, that I know nothing. *Blood Rev.* 48, 100805.
18. Conran, N. and Belcher, J.D. (2018). Inflammation in sickle cell disease. *Clin. Hemorheol. Microcirc.* 68, 263–299.

19. Gavriilaki, E., de Latour, R.P., Risitano, A.M. (2022). Advancing therapeutic complement inhibition in hematologic diseases: PNH and beyond. *Blood* 139(25), 3571–3582.
20. Boonyasampant, M., Weitz, I.C., Kay, B. et al. (2015). Life-threatening delayed hyperhemolytic transfusion reaction in a patient with sickle cell disease: effective treatment with eculizumab followed by rituximab. *Transfusion* 55, 2398–2403.
21. Lapite A, Bhar S, Fasipe T. (2024). Eculizumab for management of hyperhemolysis syndrome in pediatric patients with sickle cell disease: A single-center case series. Pediatr *Blood Cancer* 71(8):e31061.
22. Bienzle, U., Sodeinde, O., Effiong, C.E. et al. (1975). Glucose 6-phosphate dehydrogenase deficiency and sickle cell anemia: frequency and features of the association in an African community. *Blood* 46, 591–597.
23. Bernaudin, F., Verlhac, S., Chevret, S. et al. (2008). G6PD deficiency, absence of alpha-thalassemia, and hemolytic rate at baseline are significant independent risk factors for abnormally high cerebral velocities in patients with sickle cell anemia. *Blood* 112, 4314–4317.
24. Vulliamy, T.J., D'Urso, M., Battistuzzi, G. et al. (1988). Diverse point mutations in the human glucose-6-phosphate dehydrogenase gene cause enzyme deficiency and mild or severe hemolytic anemia. *Proc. Natl. Acad. Sci. USA*. 85, 5171–5175.
25. Charache, S., Terrin, M.L., Moore, R.D. et al. (1995). Effect of hydroxyurea on the frequency of painful crises in sickle cell anemia. Investigators of the Multicenter Study of Hydroxyurea in Sickle Cell Anemia. *N. Engl. J. Med*. 332, 1317–1322.
26. Costa E, Ware R, Tshilolo L, Luzzatto L. (2025). Thirty years of hydroxyurea for sickle cell anemia - scientific progress, global health gaps. *N Engl J Med*. 393(16):1556–1559.
27. Olujohungbe, A. and Burnett, A.L. (2013). How I manage priapism due to sickle cell disease. *Br. J. Haematol*. 160, 754–765.
28. Rangel-Pozzo, A., Yu, P.L.I., La, L.S. et al. (2021). Telomere architecture correlates with aggressiveness in multiple myeloma. *Cancers (Basel)*. 13(8), 1969.

Case 17

Failing to Switch

Patient Details

Age: 35 *Sex:* F
Ethnic background: India (Gujarati)

Reason for Referral

Investigation of anaemia (blood sample only).

History and Clinical Findings in Brief

There was no relevant clinical history apart from some fatigue. The patient knew about "anaemia in the family," but no specific data could be obtained. Patient had had one previous normal pregnancy.

Laboratory Findings

The patient had a mild to moderate microcytic anaemia (see Table 17.1). The blood film (see Figure 17.1) confirmed microcytosis, and showed marked anisocytosis and poikilocytosis, including "tear-drop" poikilocytes and others with a tail-like appendage ("ichthiocytes"). There were many target cells,

Table 17.1 Haematology Data

Hb (g/dl)	9.8
RBC ($\times 10^{12}$/l)	4.58
MCV (fl)	72.0
MCH (pg)	21.4
MCHC (g/dl)	29.8
Hb F (%)	100

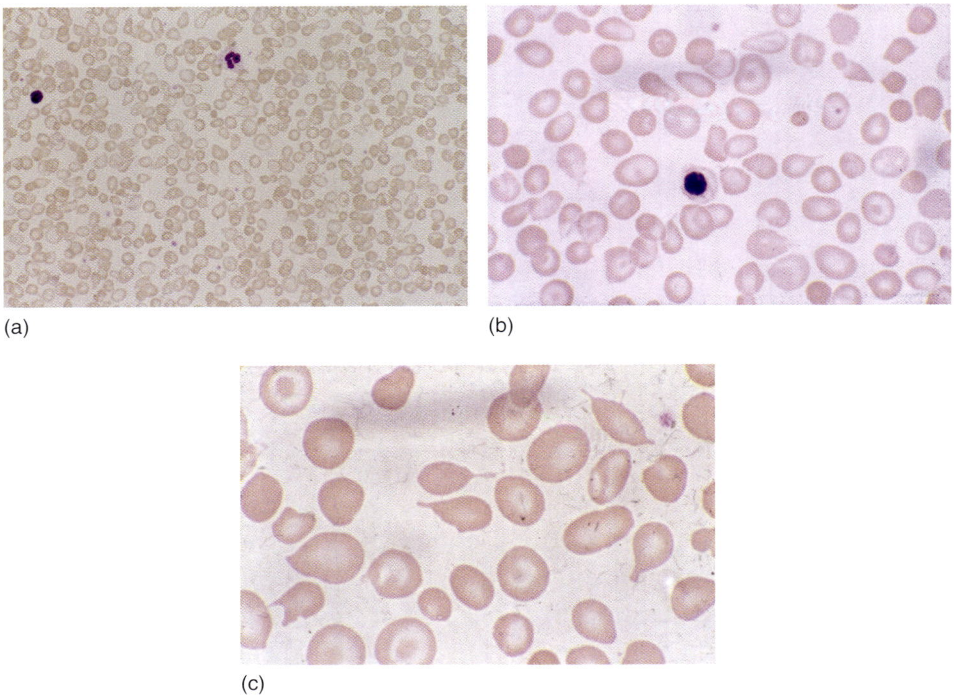

Figure 17.1 Peripheral blood film: (a) low power view; (b) medium power view; (c) high power view.

microspherocytes and irregularly shaped very dense (pyknotic) cells. Some of the red cells were extremely hypochromic and had the appearance of ghost cells. There were occasional polychromatic cells and nucleated red cells.

Because of the abnormal red cell indices and morphology, haemoglobin electrophoresis on cellulose acetate membrane was performed (see Figure 17.2). This showed only Hb F; Hb A and Hb A_2 were undetectable.

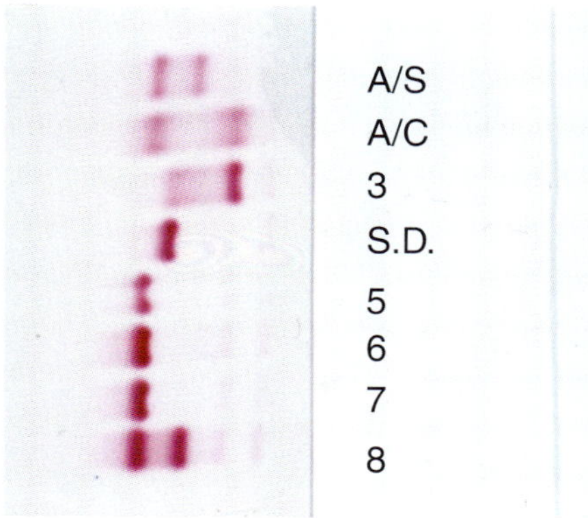

Figure 17.2 Haemoglobin electrophoresis on cellulose acetate membrane; the migration of the haemoglobin fractions is from right to left. An A/S and A/C control are in lanes 1 and 2, respectively. The patient (S.D.) is in lane 4.

Initial Assessment

The red cell indices, morphology and electrophoresis suggested the patient was homozygous for either HPFH or δβ thalassaemia. Since not only MCV and MCH were low, but MCHC was also low (29.8 g/dl), there might be super-imposed iron deficiency.

Further Investigations

A Kleihauer test showed, not surprisingly, a pancellular distribution of Hb F (see Case 12, Figure 12.2).

Patient's genomic DNA Southern blot hybridization studies using γ and β probes implied a major disruption to the normal arrangement of the β-globin gene cluster. The β-globin probe Southern blot analysis revealed only abnormal fragments, suggesting the patient was homozygous for a major rearrangement (Figure 17.3a and b). The hybridization analysis with the γ-globin probe yielded normal fragments with two of the three restriction enzymes (Figure 17.4). These normal fragments are consistent with both $^{G}\gamma$-globin genes being intact, while the $^{A}\gamma$ globin genes on the two chromosomes were disrupted. The fragments observed following Southern blot analysis with β- and γ-globin probes were consistent with molecular studies previously reported for a patient, also of Indian origin, who was diagnosed with homozygous $(^{A}\gamma\delta\beta)^0$ thalassaemia [1, 2]. Therefore, we concluded our patient had the same molecular lesion. Southern blot analysis of the α-globin gene cluster revealed only normal fragments with both α- and ζ-globin probes (not shown).

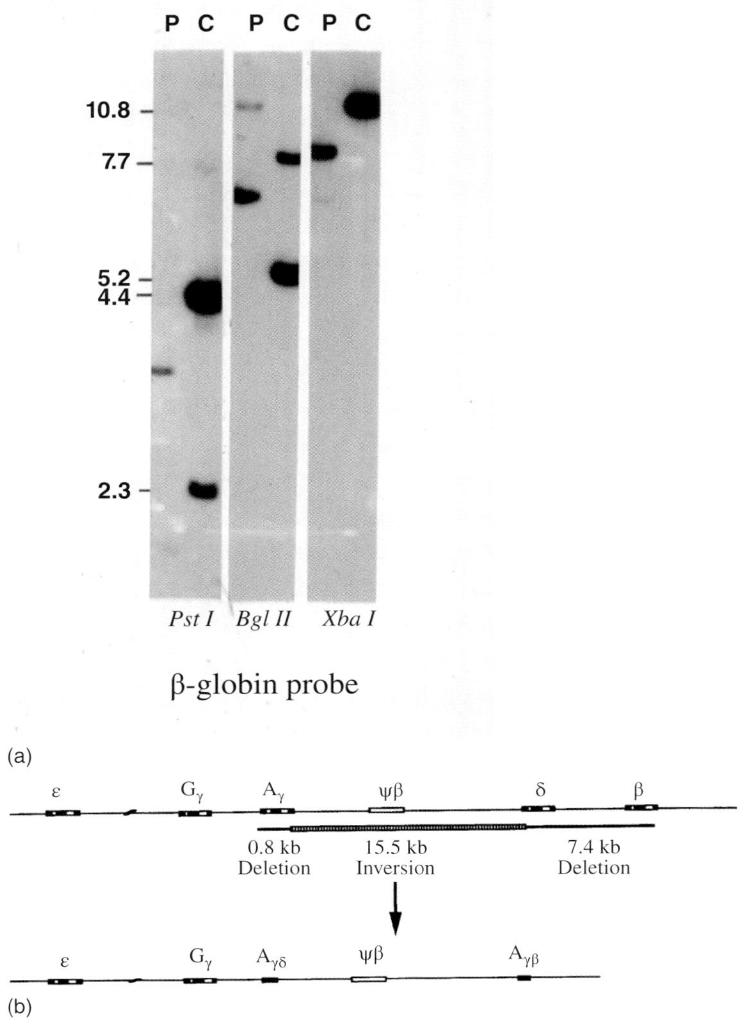

Figure 17.3 (a) Southern blot analysis of the β-globin gene. The results of the Southern blot analysis are shown following the hybridization of genomic β-globin probe to DNA digested by three different restriction enzyme as indicated. The expected normal fragment sizes are indicated on the left. The patient's DNA yielded only abnormal faint fragments consistent with the inversion/deletion commonly observed among Indians. P: patient; C: normal control. (b) Schematic representation of the normal β-globin gene and the molecular lesions deleted. The relative positions of the 0.8 and the 7.4 Kb deletions are shown and also the inverted region of the β-globin gene cluster giving rise to $(^{A}\gamma\delta\beta)^{0}$ thalassaemia for which the patient is homozygous. [3]/John Wiley & Sons.

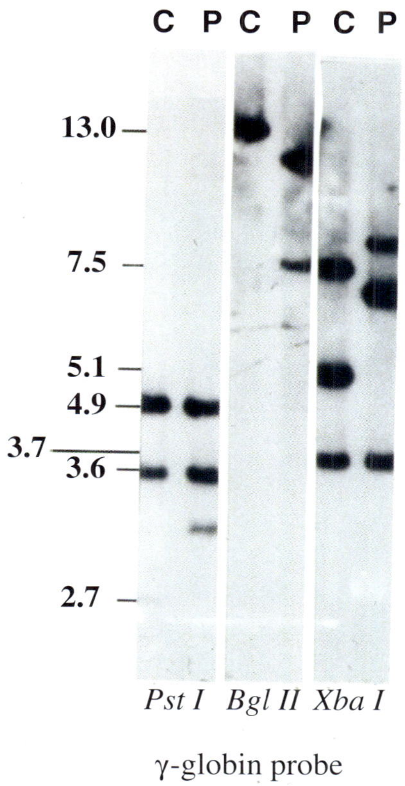

Figure 17.4 The autoradiograph shows the results of the Southern blot analysis on hybridization to a γ-globin probe after digestion with *Pst I*, *Bgl II* and *Xba I* restriction enzymes. The fragment sizes revealed are consistent with the patient being homozygous for the Asian-Indian inversion/deletion rearrangement of the β-globin gene cluster, giving rise to $^{G}\gamma^{A}(\gamma\delta\beta)^{0}$ thalassaemia. The presence of the normal fragments 4.9, 3.7 and 3.6 Kb with *Pst* and *Xba I* restriction enzymes respectively, confirm that the $^{G}\gamma$ gene is intact. P: patient; C: normal control.

Comments

This patient has 100% Hb F in her blood, because she is homozygous for a complex deletion–inversion mutation that disrupts the δ-globin and β-globin genes. Her hematologic data are very similar to those in the first patient reported who almost certainly had the same genotype (family B in Ref. [1]). As outlined in our comments to Case 12, the absence of the β-globin promoter is key to the derepression of the γ-globin genes; however, since the $^{A}\gamma$ genes are also disrupted, the production of Hb F relies on the $^{G}\gamma$ genes only; therefore, the clinical phenotype is more similar to δβ-thalassaemia than to HPFH, and indeed the patient has a mild to moderate anaemia.

We could find in the literature, only two instances of patients with nearly 100% Hb F who had had successful pregnancies. One was a previously asymptomatic patient who was heterozygous for HPFH and β-thalassaemia [4]. She had three pregnancies: and during each, she developed severe anaemia in her second trimester, requiring several blood transfusions to enable her to reach term. Thus she had in fact, mainly Hb A during the second half of her pregnancies. The other patient was reported to have thalassaemia major [5], and on electrophoresis was found to have Hb F only. She delivered a normal baby weighing 3120 g at term. In retrospect, she probably had thalassaemia intermedia, and may have been similar to our patient, who did not receive any blood transfusion before, during or after her pregnancy. She had had a normal pregnancy two years previously and had delivered a normal male infant weighing 2895 g. The outcome of this second pregnancy was also satisfactory.

We must infer that the difference in O_2 affinity of Hb A and Hb F is not an absolute requirement for adequate oxygen supply to the foetus; the oxygen pressure gradient across the placenta appears to be sufficient at least in some cases (see also Case 12).

The foetal to adult "haemoglobin switching" has been the title and the theme of biennial research meetings held regularly since 1978: the main aim of these basic science conferences was to understand the mechanism of the switch, a prototype example of a discrete molecular event in human developmental biology. In the last few meetings *BCL11A* emerged as crucial in producing the switch (see Figure 12.6), and therefore as a potential target for possibly reversing the switch. This is the rationale of a currently approved protocol for gene therapy of both sickle cell anaemia [6] and thalassemia major [7]. Although these trials are recent, it is reasonable to expect that the patients thus treated are cured; and it is in the best tradition of haematology that what we learn in basic science is turned into clinical practice.

It seems both intriguing and gratifying that, through clever genetic engineering of stem cells, the γ-globin genes, present but normally non-functional in adults, can be used in patients as a back-up for β-globin genes that have pathogenic mutations. Indeed, it has been known for a long time that an adult can do very well with only Hb F [8, 9]; and in a woman this very unusual situation is compatible even with a successful pregnancy.

Follow-up

If pregnancy for a woman having only Hb F can be uneventful, quite a different issue are possible implications with respect to acquired anaemia. An increase in BPG in red cells is an important adaptive mechanism that improves tolerance of anaemia by shifting to the right the O_2 dissociation curve; but this is hardly applicable to Hb F. Fortunately, this patient has tolerated well her mild anaemia; we have recommended she should have her blood counts checked regularly.

Conclusion

Homozygous $(^{A}\gamma\delta\beta)^{0}$ thalassaemia (thalassaemia intermedia).

Acknowledgements

Referred by Dr. Keshava Prasad, Department of Haematology, King Khalid Hospital, Najran, Saudi Arabia.
Some data on this patient have been previously published [3].

References

1. Amin, A.B., Pandya, N.L., Diwin, P.P. et al. (1979). A comparison of the homozygous states for G gamma and G gamma A gamma delta beta thalassaemia. *Br. J. Haematol.* 43(4), 537–548.
2. Jones, R.W., Old, J.M., Trent, R.J. et al. (1981). Major rearrangements in the human beta-globin gene cluster. *Nature* 291, 39–45.
3. Kaeda, J.S., Prasad, K., Howard, R.J. et al. (1994). Management of pregnancy when maternal blood has a very high level of fetal haemoglobin. *Br. J. Haematol.* 88(2), 432–434.
4. Necheles, T. (1973). Obstetric complications associated with hemoglobinopathies. *Clin. Hematol.* 2, 497–511.
5. Perkins, R.P. (1971). Inherited disorders of hemoglobin synthesis and pregnancy. *Am. J. Obstetr. Gynecol.* 111, 120–159.
6. Frangoul, H., Locatelli, F., Sharma, A. et al. (2024). Exagamglogene Autotemcel for Severe Sickle Cell Disease. *N Engl J Med.* 390(18), 1649–62.
7. Locatelli, F., Lang, P., Wall, D. et al. (2024). Exagamglogene Autotemcel for Transfusion-Dependent beta-Thalassemia. *N. Engl. J. Med.* 390(18), 1663–76.
8. Conley CL, Weatherall DJ, Richardson SN. et al. (1963). Hereditary persistence of fetal hemoglobin: a study of 79 affected persons in 15 Negro families in Baltimore. *Blood* 21, 261–81.
9. Ringelhann B, Acquaye CT, Oldham JH., et al. (1977). Homozygotes for the hereditary persistence of fetal hemoglobin: the ratio of G gamma to A gamma chains and biosynthetic studies. *Biochem. Genet.* 15(11–12), 1083–96.

See also related Case 12.

Case 18

Rosettes Without a Trophy

Patient Details

Age: 40 *Sex:* F
Ethnic background: Scottish
Occupation: School teacher living in Dubai

Reason for Referral

Investigation of anaemia.

History and Clinical Findings in Brief

The patient had a long history of menorrhagia and anaemia. Five months earlier, in Dubai, she had been treated with iron, vitamin B12 and progesterone. The patient subsequently developed tiredness and breathlessness and was admitted to hospital as an emergency after she had collapsed. Her Hb was found to be 4.7 g/dl. She was transfused three units of blood and started on prednisolone (75 mg per day). The Coombs test was reported as negative on two occasions. The patient was referred to the Hammersmith hospital. On examination, the patient was generally well, but she was pale and mildly icteric. Her heart rate was 100, with a systolic murmur, but not in heart failure; there was no hepatosplenomegaly. An important unexpected finding was that, although the patient seemed not to be aware of it, she was 16 weeks pregnant. When she learnt this, she requested termination.

Laboratory Findings

The patient had a severe macrocytic anaemia with moderate reticulocytosis (see Table 18.1). The white cell and platelet counts were normal. On the blood film (see Figure 18.1), the majority of the red cells looked normal in shape and were generally macrocytic. However, we found a few spherocytes; as well as some polychromatic cells and a rare nucleated red cell (Figure 18.1a). An occasional metamyelocyte and band-form neutrophil were also seen. Blood films were prepared at different temperatures. At 37 °C, the appearance was similar to that described above; however, at 4 °C, there was, in addition to rouleaux formation, a striking phenomenon of red cell rosetting around neutrophils (Figure 18.1b), which could be seen also at room temperature; it seemed to be neutrophil-specific, since it did not occur around monocytes (Figure 18.1c). We also observed erythrophagocytosis by neutrophils in the peripheral blood (Figure 18.1d and e).

Additional baseline studies (see Table 18.2) revealed a moderately increased bilirubin and a reduced level of haptoglobins. Serum B12 and folate levels were within normal limits. In view of the macrocytic anaemia with normal B12 and folate, a diagnostic bone marrow aspirate was indicated (see Figure 18.2). This was extremely cellular and showed erythroid hyperplasia (myeloid–erythroid ratio 1 : 2). There was slight dyserythropoiesis, and occasional foamy macrophages. No primary marrow disorder was evident.

Table 18.1 Haematology Data

	Presenting	Follow-up
Hb (g/dl)	6.6	11.0
RBC ($\times10^{12}$/l)	1.82	3.71
MCV (fl)	110.4	97.7
MCH (pg)	36.3	32.1
MCHC (g/dl)	32.8	32.8
RDW (S.D.)	62.9	57.2
Retic (%)	8.2	1.2
Retic ($\times10^9$/l)	149	45
WBC ($\times10^9$/l)	8.4	6.9
PLT ($\times10^9$/l)	290	586

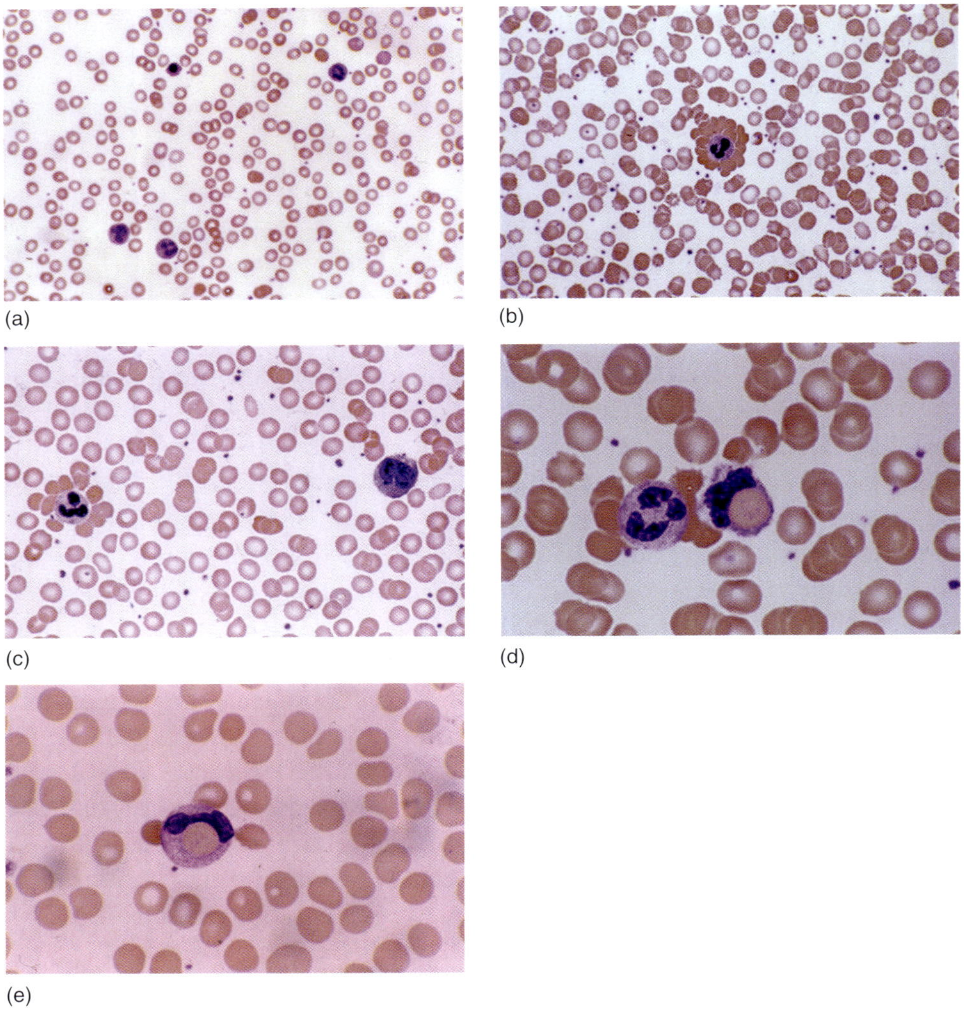

Figure 18.1 Peripheral blood films. (a) Routine blood film, showing spherocytes, polychromatic cells and nucleated red cell; (b) film prepared at 4 °C, showing red cell rosetting around a neutrophil; (c) film prepared at the same time at room temperature, showing no demonstrable red cell rosetting around monocytes; (d) and (e), films also prepared at room temperature, showing erythrophagocytosis by neutrophils.

Initial Assessment

The patient has a severe macrocytic anaemia associated with erythroid hyperplasia in her bone marrow. The overall picture is consistent with haemolytic anaemia; the haemoglobinuria indicates that haemolysis was at least in part intravascular. Red cell rosetting around neutrophils and erythrophagocytosis in the peripheral blood are strong pointers to autoimmune haemolytic anaemia (AIHA).

Table 18.2 Additional Baseline Studies

Bilirubin (µmol/L)	64
B12 (ng/L)	246
Serum folate (µg/L)	9.2
Haptoglobins (mg/dL)	<35
Ham test	Negative
Autoantibodies	Negative
DAGT[a]	Negative
Urinary-Hb	Positive ++ (No microhaematuria)

[a] When tested at room temperature.

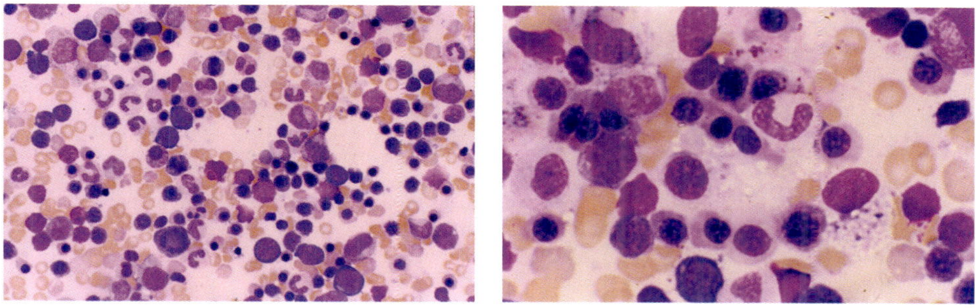

(a) (b)

Figure 18.2 Bone marrow aspirate: (a) medium power view; (b) high power view.

Table 18.3 Serological Investigations

Serum screen	Weak antibody detectable by IAT (at 20 °C)
	IgG – IgM, C-binding
	Pan-reactive biphasic lysin
	No anti-P specificity
DAGT	Positive for IgG at 4 °C
	Negative at 25 °C
	Negative for IgM and complement

Further Investigations

When the DAGT was carried out at 4 °C, it was positive, for IgG (negative for IgM and complement). The Ham test was negative, excluding PNH. Further serological studies (Table 18.3) revealed that the patient had a biphasic Donath–Landsteiner-like lytic antibody that, however, did not have anti-P specificity.

The patient was treated with intravenous immunoglobulin, prednisolone and azathioprine: however, her anaemia failed to correct. A ^{51}Cr radioisotope study showed that her erythrocytes had a reduced survival of 36 days, with a half-life (T_{50}) of 15 days. Body-surface counting performed during the following 10 days revealed the site of red cell destruction to be mainly the spleen; the spleen : liver ratio was greater than 3 : 1 (see Figure 18.3).

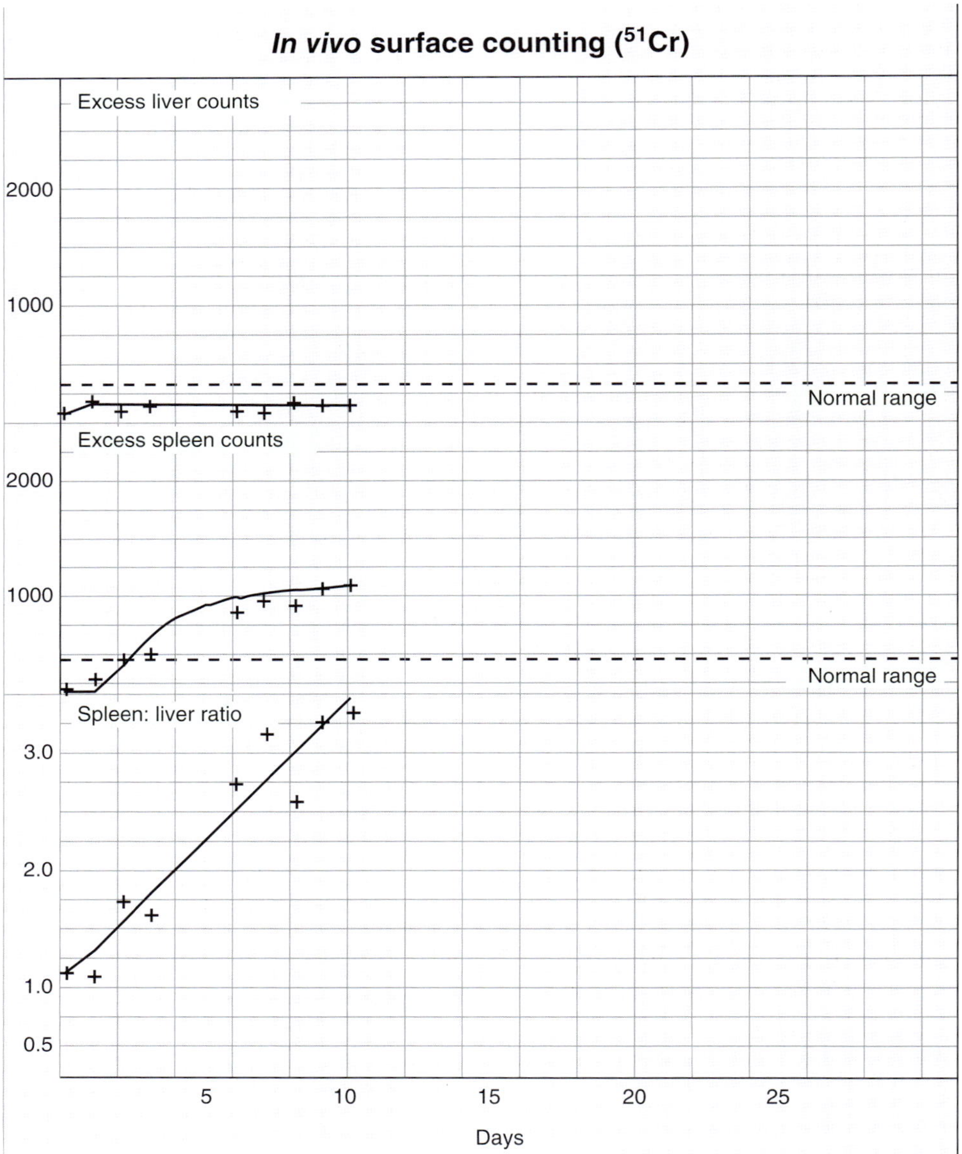

Figure 18.3 Locating site of preferential red cell destruction by radio-isotope studies. After labelling the patient's own red cells with ^{51}Cr, surface counting was carried out over the liver (top) and the spleen (middle); the spleen/liver count ratios were then plotted against time (bottom).

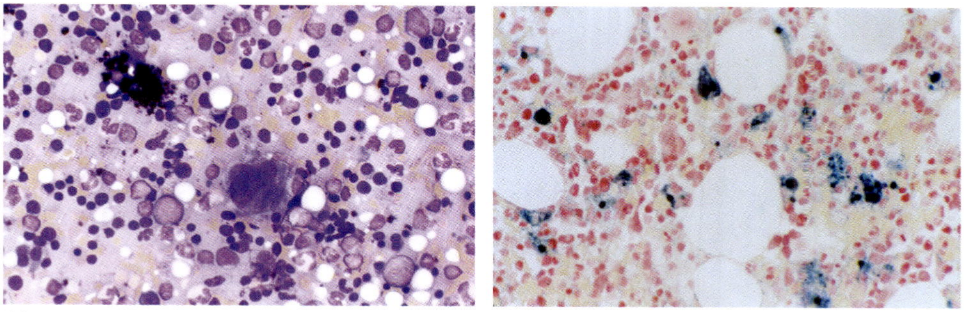

(a) (b)

Figure 18.4 Appearance of splenic dab: (a) showing extramedullary erythropoiesis; (b) pigment-laden macrophages stained by Perl's Prussian-blue reaction.

In compliance with the patient's request, termination of pregnancy was performed; and in view of the above data, including the ^{51}Cr-labelled red cell surface count results and failure of steroid treatment, a splenectomy was performed at the same time. The splenic dab (see Figure 18.4) showed erythroid and myeloid cells, as well as megakaryocytes, consistent with extramedullary haemopoiesis. In addition, we found large numbers of pigment-laden macrophages, which stained strongly with iron: evidence that they had actively phagocytosed red cells.

Comments

In an adult with severe haemolytic anaemia of apparently abrupt onset AIHA is near the top of the list of differential diagnoses; yet, this diagnosis had been rejected because the DAGT was repeatedly negative. Once again, the blood film is at least as important as any other test: we don't know of any condition, other than AIHA, in which you find red cell rosetting around neutrophils; erythrophagocytosis by neutrophils in the peripheral blood is seen in AIHA as well as with malaria (Figure 18.5): but no malaria parasites were present in this case.[1] This prompted our further serological investigations, which proved that the negative DAGT result was not due to a low number on the red cell surface of molecules of antibody [1]; but rather to its unusual serological properties.

In our patient, the past history of anaemia may mean that her AIHA was already in the making; but it is also possible that initially, she really did have iron deficiency anaemia consequent on menorrhagia. The clinical and

[1] To see erythrophagocytosis (by monocytes or neutrophils) in the peripheral blood is a rare phenomenon; but it can be seen in malaria (see Figure 18.5), and in rare cases of chemical poisoning or of severe septicaemia. Rosetting around neutrophils is seen, as far as we know, only with AIHA.

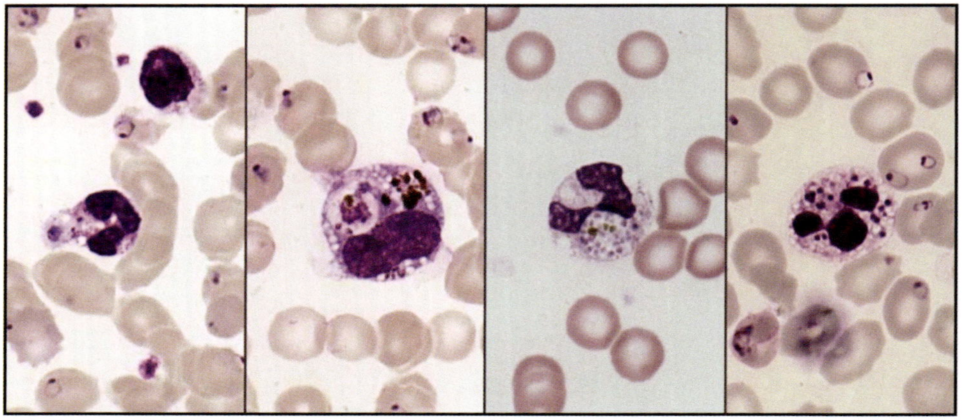

Figure 18.5 Phagocytosis of red cells parasitized by malarial parasites.

haematologic picture is highly reminiscent of the rare disease paroxysmal cold haemoglobinuria (PCH), of which the Donath–Landsteiner antibody is regarded as the landmark; its specificity is classically anti-P, but in one series, this specificity was lacking in 10% of cases [2]. PCH is much more common in children but it occurs also in adults; it is often but not always triggered by a viral infection; it is usually but not always self-limiting [3]. In PCH, haemolysis is both intravascular and extravascular [3]; neutrophil rosetting and erythrophagocytosis by neutrophils – most unusual in other forms of AIHA [4] – have been reported in several cases [5–8]; and the antibody is by definition biphasic; all features present in this patient. However, whether we should attribute to our patient the PCH label is a matter of semantics; we prefer to say that she had AIHA with some special features. A diagnosis of PCH is not regarded as an indication for splenectomy; but given the ^{51}Cr data and no response to steroids, we thought it was indicated in this patient.

The positive DAGT at 4 °C only, points to a "cold-reactive" antibody. In most cases, this is IgM, but occasionally it may be IgG, as in our patient. Usually, it is "warm-reactive" antibodies that cause sequestration of sensitized erythrocytes by the spleen; whereas cold-reacting antibodies usually cause complement-mediated intravascular destruction (as in cold agglutinin disease). The antibody in this case was able to fix complement; thus, we have a reasonable explanation as to why there was evidence of both intravascular and extravascular haemolysis. The relatively modest absolute increase in reticulocytes in the face of severe anaemia may indicate that even reticulocytes were suffering haemolysis.

Phagocytosis by macrophages in the spleen, liver and bone marrow is of course, the major mechanism for removal of erythrocytes that are coated and have been damaged by auto-antibodies. We had a histopathological image of this in the patient's spleen when it was removed. In this respect, what we see in the peripheral blood may be just like the tip of the iceberg. Red cell rosetting means that red cells were coated (at 4 °C or at 20 °C) with antibody that mediated binding to the Fcγ receptor on neutrophils. Complement was activated through the classic pathway, and C3b binding to the complement receptor CD35 on red cells enabled the formation of several layers of red cells. Lysis did not occur because this requires activation of the terminal complement pathway at 37 °C; indeed, lower temperature generally favours antigen-antibody combination, but not the enzymatic steps that lead to haemolysis. The reason why rosetting occurred with neutrophils and not with monocytes is probably that the nature and density of Fcγ receptors differ in these two cell types. The rather spectacular phenomenon of rosetting thus depends on a combination of the properties of the antibody involved, of the receptors involved, the extent of complement activation and temperature.

There are previous reports in the literature of AIHA occurring in pregnant women who were in perfect health before conception [9, 10], but this of course does not necessarily mean that pregnancy was the trigger (in our case, the trigger may have been her upper respiratory tract infection). If the pregnancy comes to term and whenever the antibody is IgG one should be alert to possible signs of haemolytic disease of the newborn, in order to institute treatment promptly as indicated in this condition.

Follow-up

After splenectomy and three months of treatment with steroids, the patient made a clinical recovery. Although her serology remained unchanged, her blood counts were near normal (with an expected increase in platelets; see Table 18.1). The morphology of the red cells has become almost normal apart from an occasional crenated red cell. The patient was given Penicillin V and antimalarial prophylaxis.

Conclusion

AIHA with intravascular and extravascular haemolysis manifesting during early pregnancy.

Acknowledgements

Referred by Dr. P. Gravett, Harley Street, London, UK.

Dr. M. Marashi, Specialist Physician, Department of Health & Medical Services, Rashid Hospital, Dubai.

Irene Owen, Blood Transfusion Laboratory, Hammersmith Hospital, London, UK.

References

1. Petz, L.D. and Garratty, G. (1980). *Acquired Immune Hemolytic Anemias*. New York, NY: Churchill Livingstone.
2. Sokol, R.J., Booker, D.J., and Stamps, R. (1999). Erythropoiesis: paroxysmal cold haemoglobinuria: a clinico-pathological study of patients with a positive Donath-Landsteiner test. *Hematology* 4, 137–164.
3. Shanbhag, S. and Spivak, J. (2015). Paroxysmal cold hemoglobinuria. *Hematol. Oncol. Clin. North. Am*. 29, 473–478.
4. Lee, J.H. (2017). A rare case of erythrophagocytosis by neutrophils on the peripheral blood smear. *Blood. Res*. 52, 74–75.
5. Pettit, J.E., Scott, J., and Hussein, S. (1976). EDTA dependent red cell neutrophil rosetting in autoimmune haemolytic anaemia. *J. Clin. Pathol*. 29, 345–346.
6. Dacie, J.V. (1992). *The Haemolytic Anaemias*. 3 ed. III. The Auto-immune Haemolytic Anaemias. England: Churchill Livingstone.
7. Gocke, C.B. and Shanbhag, S. (2018). Neutrophil-red blood cell rosetting in a patient with autoimmune hemolytic anemia. *Transfusion* 58, 2102–2103.
8. Yadav, G., Rahman, K., and Gupta, R. (2016). Neutrophil erythrocyte rosettes: an unusual manifestation of autoimmune hemolytic anemia. *Indian J. Hematol. Blood Transfus*. 32, 309–310.
9. Champlin Jr., H., Cohen, R., Bloomberg, G. et al. (1973). Pregnancy and idiopathic autoimmune haemolytic anaemia: a prospective study during 6 months gestation and 3 months post-partum. *Br. J. Haematol*. 24, 219–229.
10. Sokol, R.J., Hewitt, S., and Stamps, B.K. (1982). Erythrocyte autoantibodies, autoimmune haemolysis and pregnancy. *Vox Sang*. 433, 169–176.

Case 19

Too Little Beta and Too Much Alpha

Patient Details

Age: 50 *Sex:* F
Ethnic background: Portugal

Reason for Referral

Investigation of chronic anaemia (blood sample only).

History and Clinical Findings in Brief

The patient was the mother of two children and had felt generally quite well up until seven years previously. However, she had anaemia and was treated with vitamins and iron both p.o. and i.m. She improved considerably and remained symptom-free until her menopause, when she became quite disturbed by hot-flushes and intermittent vaginal bleeding. Now, she presented at her local hospital with profound asthenia, palpitations and a dull ache in the left hypochondrium. Physical examination revealed an obese woman, pale, with a slight jaundiced tinge. The pulse was regular 72/min., BP 130/80 mmHg, and no ankle oedema. The liver was palpable at 3 cm and the spleen was palpable at 6 cm below the costal margin.

Laboratory Findings

The patient had a moderate microcytic anaemia (see Figure 19.1). On the blood film (see Figure 19.2), we could see tear-drop and "hand-mirror" cells, target cells, and bizarre poikilocytes; some that were not quite fragments (because they still had an area of central pallor) and others with a tail-like appendage. Occasional cells with punctate basophilia, which ranged from fine to very coarse, were quite noticeable.

Initial Assessment

The elevated Hb A_2 and the low MCV were in keeping with β-thalassaemia trait, inherited from the patient's father (I-1 in Figure 19.1). However, her overall clinical picture, her anaemia, and her red cell morphology suggested that this may not be the entire diagnosis.

Further Investigations

By PCR amplification of the beta globin (see Figure 19.3a and b), the mutation accounting for β-thalassaemia was identified as IVS 1 nt 1 (G→A), a β^0 point mutation for which the patient is heterozygous.

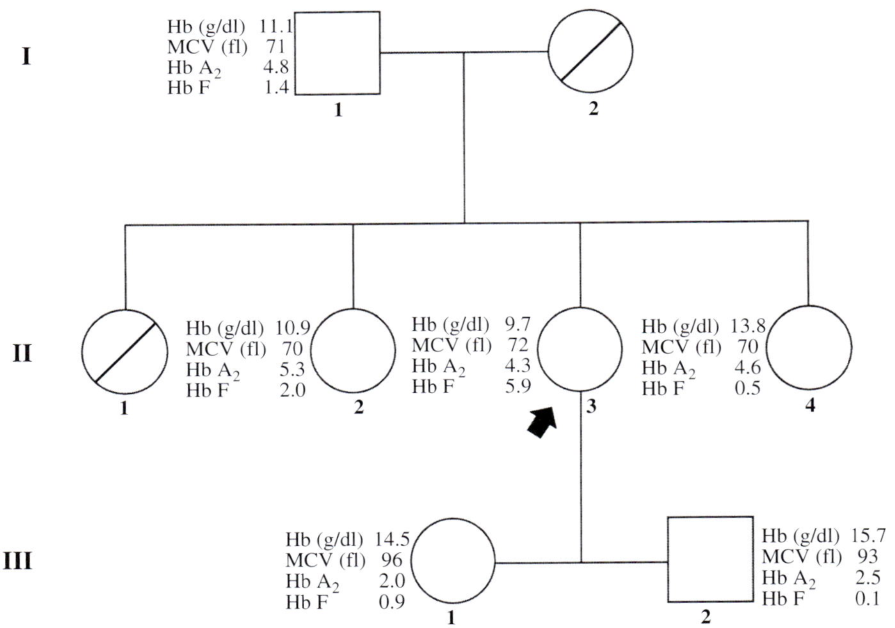

Figure 19.1 Family pedigree: our patient is arrowed.

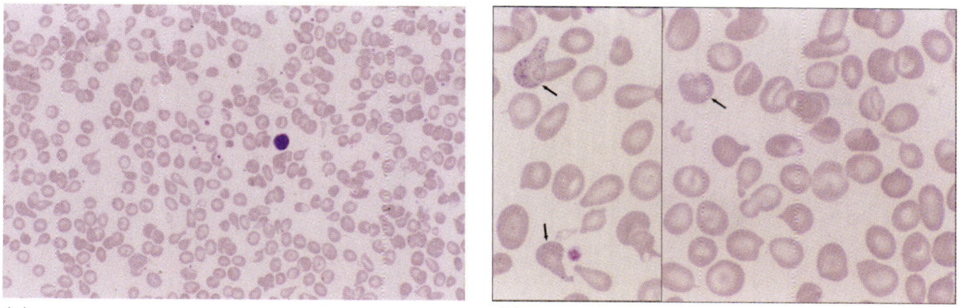

(a) (b)

Figure 19.2 Peripheral blood film: (a) medium power view; (b) high power view (composite) with punctate basophilia arrowed.

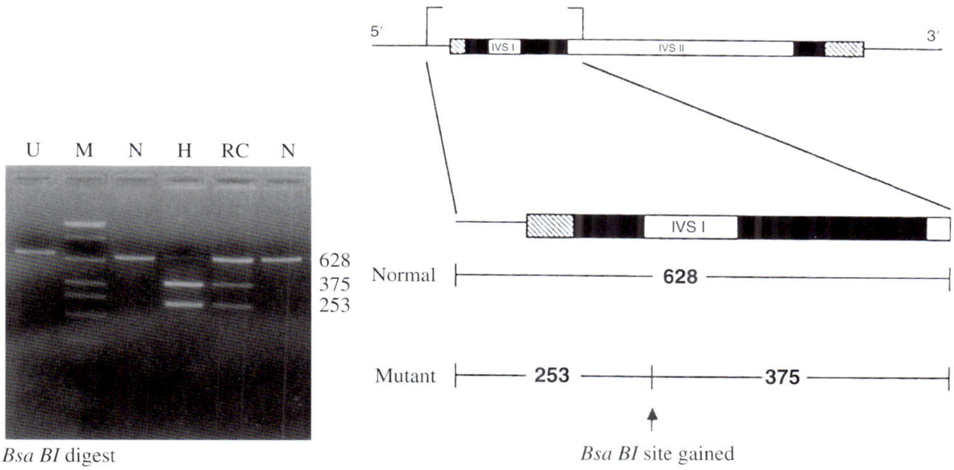

(a) (b)

Figure 19.3 Detection of the IVS 1 nt 1 (G→A) mutation. A portion of the β-globin gene was PCR-amplified with appropriate primers, yielding a 628 bp product. (a) Ethidium bromide stained agarose gel, displaying the fragments generated after digestion with the restriction enzyme, *Bsa BI*. U: undigested PCR product; M: molecular size markers; N: normal controls; H: homozygote for IVS 1 nt 1 (G→A) mutation; RC: patient. (b) Diagram of the β-globin gene and of the PCR product. The IVS 1 nt 1 (G→A) mutation creates a *Bsa BI* restriction site: whereby, when the mutation is present, the 628 product is digested by the enzyme into two fragments, 253 and 375 bp in size. RC, showing both the undigested PCR product and the two products of the digestion, is clearly heterozygous for the IVS 1 nt 1 (G→A) thalassaemia mutation.

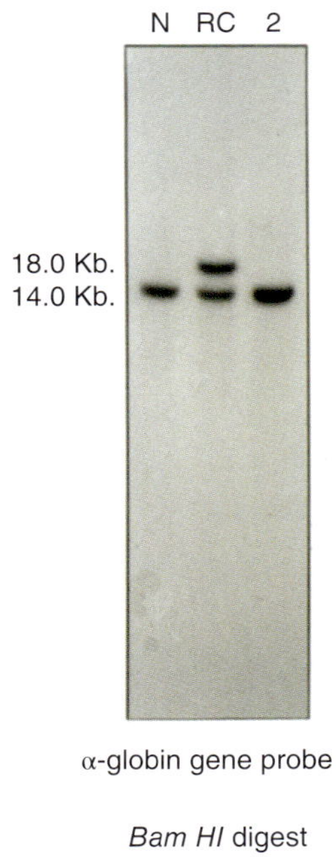

Figure 19.4 Triplicated α-globin gene. Southern blot analysis of a *Bam HI* digest of genomic DNA following hybridization to an α1-globin probe. The normal control DNA (αα/αα) yielded the expected 14.0 kb fragment. The patient's DNA revealed in addition to the normal 14 kb fragment, a band corresponding to 18.0 kb. The 18.0 kb *Bam HI* fragment is characteristic of a triplicated α-globin gene, i.e. ααα; thus, the patient's *HBA* genotype is ααα/αα.

Globin chain biosynthetic analysis gave a β : α ratio of 0.3, considerably lower than is generally seen in β-thalassaemia heterozygotes. Therefore, we proceeded to examine the α-globin genes as well. By Southern blot analysis (Figure 19.4), we found that this patient was also heterozygous for triplication of the α-globin gene (genotype ααα/αα).

Comments

The spectrum of clinical-haematologic severity of thalassaemia intermedia, or non-transfusion dependent thalassaemia (NTDT) is very wide; not surprisingly, since the underlying genotypes are many [1]. In β-thalassaemia, erythropoiesis is affected by two abnormalities: (i) an absolute deficit in β chains is the reason why in β-thalassaemia the red cells are small; they adapt to the reduced amount of haemoglobin; (ii) the consequent excess of α chains, that are intrinsically unstable (so much so that they require an alpha globin-specific chaperone, the alpha haemoglobin stabilizing protein [AHSP]) [2], is responsible for the β/α chain imbalance: this may result from either a decreased output of β-chains, or an increased output of α-chains, or both, as in this case. The serious chain imbalance is, in turn, the major factor responsible for ineffective erythropoiesis [3].

From the data in Figure 19.1, we infer that the patient's father (I-1) and her two sisters (II-2 and II-4) have the β-thal mutation, but an αα/αα genotype; that is why they did not develop thalassaemia intermedia; and the triplicated ααα may have come to II-3 from her mother (I-2). The two children III-1 and III-2 have apparently not inherited the β-thal mutation; whether their α globin genotype is ααα/αα or αα/αα is not clinically relevant in the absence of a β-thal gene [4].

The genotypic combination observed in our patient had already been recognized as one of the many that can cause thalassaemia intermedia [4, 5]. We have been able to compare the findings in four additional patients with thalassaemia intermedia who were heterozygous for β-thalassaemia and had the ααα/αα genotype (see Table 19.1).

All of them had red cell morphology very similar to that shown here (Figure 19.2), and they had mild to moderate anaemia. However, there was variability, which cannot be explained merely by whether the β-thalassaemia mutation was β^+ or β^0 [6]. One might surmise that genetic polymorphism of the AHSP chaperone might play a role, but this has not been substantiated hitherto [7].

The triple α-globin gene presumably arises through misaligned crossover on chromosome 16, being the reciprocal product of deletional alpha thalassaemia (α−/αα). The ααα allele is polymorphic in several populations, e.g. in Cypriots [8], in Iranians [9], and in Polynesians [10]. The αα/ααα genotype, and even the ααα/ααα genotype are, on their own (i.e. in the absence of a β-thalassaemia gene) essentially asymptomatic [11]. However, there is no known selective advantage associated with the triplicated alpha gene; unlike for α-thal genes, that are subject to malaria selection, and therefore have far higher frequencies in many populations, and in some they come close to fixation [12].

Table 19.1 β-thalassaemia Trait Plus Triplicated α-globin Gene

	JR	AF	CF	FM
Hb (g/dl)	9.6	8.3	10.3	11.2
RBC ($\times 10^{12}$/l)	4.55	4.74	5.28	5.57
MCV (fl)	67.5	54.8	64.3	63.3
MCH (pg)	21.1	17.5	19.5	20.1
MCHC (g/dl)	31.2	31.9	30.4	31.7
Hb A_2 (%)	4.6	5.5	4.8	5.8
Beta mutation	IVS1nt5	NT	IVS1nt5	IVS1nt1
Alpha genotype	ααα/αα	ααα/αα	ααα/αα	ααα/αα

NT, not tested.

In medical genetics, monogenic *versus* polygenic disorders is a classic dichotomy. In this patient, although thalassaemia is a typical monogenic disorder, the clinical picture is clearly determined by at least two genes (*HBA* and *HBB*); in such cases, thalassaemia intermedia must be regarded as a *digenic* disorder.

Follow-up

The patient was commenced on folic acid treatment (10 mg daily); she remains symptom free.

Conclusion

Thalassaemia intermedia, mild, resulting from interaction of triplicated alpha gene and heterozygous state for the β-thalassaemia mutation IVS 1 nt 1 (G→A).

Acknowledgements

Referred by Dr Gabriel Tamagnini, Centro Hospitalar de Coimbra, Coimbra, Portugal.
Dr George Hughes, Haematology Department, West Middlesex Hospital, London, UK.
Dr S. Kenny, Haematology Department, St. Helier Hospital, Surrey, UK.
Dr David Lewis, Department of Haematology, Oldchurch Hospital, Romford, UK.
Dr E. Moffat, Department of Haematology, Royal Gwent Hospital, Newport, Wales, UK.

References

1. Musallam, K.M., Taher, A.T., and Rachmilewitz, E.A. (2012). Beta-thalassemia intermedia: a clinical perspective. *Cold Spring Harb Perspect. Med.* 2, a013482.
2. Kihm, A.J., Kong, Y., Hong, W. et al. (2002). An abundant erythroid protein that stabilizes free alpha-haemoglobin. *Nature* 417(6890), 758–763.
3. Weatherall, D.J. and Clegg, J.B. (1981). *The Thalassaemia Syndromes*. 3 ed. Oxford: Blackwell Scientific Publications.
4. Kanavakis, E., Metaxotou-Mavromati, A., Kattamis, C. et al. (1983). The triplicated alpha gene locus and beta thalassaemia. *Br. J. Haematol.* 54, 201–207.
5. Sampietro, M., Cazzola, M., Cappellini, M.D. et al. (1983). The triplicated alpha-gene locus and heterozygous beta thalassaemia: a case of thalassaemia intermedia. *Br. J. Haematol.* 55, 709–710.

6. Kulozik, A.E., Thein, S.L., Wainscoat, J.S. et al. (1987). Thalassaemia intermedia: interaction of the triple alpha-globin gene arrangement and heterozygous beta-thalassaemia. *Br. J. Haematol.* 66, 109–112.
7. Viprakasit, V., Tanphaichitr, V.S., Chinchang, W. et al. (2004). Evaluation of alpha hemoglobin stabilizing protein (AHSP) as a genetic modifier in patients with beta thalassemia. *Blood* 103(9), 3296–3299.
8. Goossens, M., Dozy, A.M., Embury, S.H. et al. (1980). Triplicated alpha-globin loci in humans. *Proc. Natl. Acad. Sci.* USA. 77(1), 518–521.
9. Moosavi, S.F., Amirian, A., Zarbakhsh, B. et al. (2011). The carrier frequency of alpha-globin gene triplication in an Iranian population with normal or borderline hematological parameters. *Hemoglobin* 35(4), 323–330.
10. Trent, R.J., Mickleson, K.N., Wilkinson, T. et al. (1985). Alpha globin gene rearrangements in Polynesians are not associated with malaria. *Am. J. Hematol.* 18(4), 431–433.
11. Galanello, R., Ruggeri, R., Paglietti, E. et al. (1983). A family with segregating triplicated alpha globin loci and beta thalassemia. *Blood* 62(5), 1035–1040.
12. Modiano, G., Morpurgo, G., Terrenato, L. et al. (1991). Protection against malaria morbidity: near-fixation of the alpha-thalassemia gene in a Nepalese population. *Am. J. Hum. Genet.* 48(2), 390–397. PMID: 1990845; PMCID: PMC1683029.

Case 20

Missing Something You Never Knew You Ought to Have

Patient Details

Age: 1 month *Sex:* M
Ethnic background: British

Reason for Referral

Investigation of anaemia and jaundice (blood sample only).

History and Clinical Findings in Brief

This baby was delivered at 37 weeks gestation by emergency Caesarian section, because of failure to engage following spontaneous rupture of membranes. At 12 days of age, the patient presented with jaundice and marked anaemia, but he was otherwise well. There was no splenomegaly. There was no family history of anaemia or jaundice. The baby's older brother (two and a half years of age) had no clinical or haematological problems during infancy.

Laboratory Findings

The patient had a severe macrocytic anaemia with marked reticulocytosis (see Table 20.1). On the blood film (see Figure 20.1), the degree of polychromasia and anisocytosis was quite striking. Many of the red cells appeared exceedingly dense, and had an irregular outline; occasional cells looked

Table 20.1 Haematology Data

Age	1 month	7 months
Hb (g/dl)	6.5	13.2
RBC ($\times 10^{12}$/l)	1.98	4.97
MCV (fl)	102.5	76.9
MCH (pg)	32.8	26.6
MCHC (g/dl)	32.0	34.6
RDW (S.D.)	65.5	38.3
Retic (%)	18.0	1.5
Retic ($\times 10^{9}$/l)	356	75

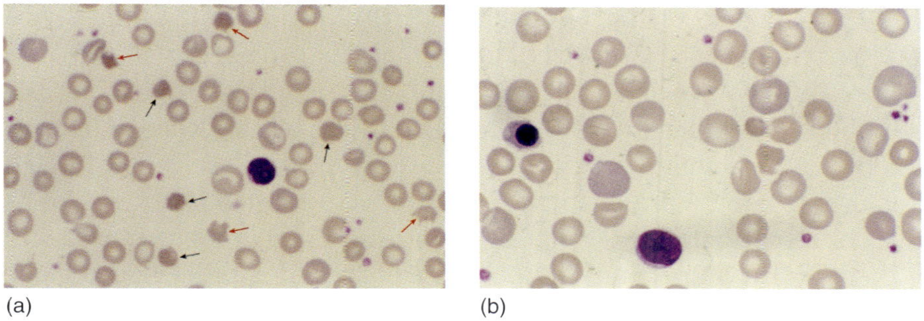

Figure 20.1 Peripheral blood film: (a) medium power view; note dense cells with irregular outline (black arrows) and "bite cells" (red arrows); (b) high power view.

precisely like spherocytes. Some of the cells had ragged edges and appeared as if they had had pieces removed from their membrane ("bite-cells"). In a few of the cells, the haemoglobin appeared to be retracted to either pole, leaving a clear band across the centre of the cell ("puddle-cell"). An occasional nucleated red blood cell was also seen.

Because the mother and child were both found to be group O Rhesus negative, the referring hospital ruled out an ABO or Rhesus blood group incompatibility. The DAGT on the patient's red cells was negative. His bilirubin level was 109 μmol/l. Blood counts and film morphology on the child's parents were all normal.

Initial Assessment

On the basis of the baby's age and of his red cell morphology, the picture fitted very well with cases previously referred to in the literature as "infantile pyknocytosis."

Further Investigations

Infantile pyknocytosis (IP) is a haematological syndrome defined as above, for which no defined underlying defect has been established as yet. Since there was no evidence of isoimmune or autoimmune haemolysis, we thought we should investigate the patient as though he had an early presentation of a congenital haemolytic anaemia. Therefore, our next line of tests included the following. (i) Haemoglobin electrophoresis on cellulose acetate membrane and on agar gel, which showed Hb A and an appropriate amount of Hb F for the patient's age; there were no abnormal haemoglobin bands detected (not shown). (ii) An autohaemolysis test[1] that showed a moderate increase (10.7%) and full correction with glucose (0.8%). (iii) G6PD and pyruvate kinase enzyme assays gave high and normal values, respectively (see Table 20.2). (iv) Tests for an unstable haemoglobin (heat stability and isopropanol precipitation) were negative. (v) A Heinz body preparation was positive, with few cells (<1%) containing a single, small Heinz body. Thus, most of the tests were normal, but the presence of Heinz bodies supported the notion of "oxidative damage," that may have justified the abnormal autohaemolysis.

Therefore, having excluded low G6PD activity and unstable haemoglobins, we proceeded to test for one of the rarer abnormalities of oxidative metabolism. Assay of glutathione (GSH) yielded a result above the normal range (110 mg/dl) which rules out most possible defects of glutathione metabolism, specifically glutamyl cysteine synthetase, glutathione synthetase and glutathione reductase. The only related enzyme defect it would not eliminate is glutathione peroxidase (GPX) deficiency; therefore, we next assayed this enzyme. The patient had only about 30% of the activity compared to the mean level obtained from simultaneously testing 10 members of staff; the patient's mother and father had normal levels of this enzyme (see Table 20.2).

Thus, the patient did have a GPX deficiency; but since both parents had normal values, it did not seem to be an inherited deficiency. Since GPX is a selenoprotein (see Figure 20.2), we next obtained an assay of selenium; the level was only 0.23 μmol/l, i.e. 37% of normal.

Table 20.2 Enzyme Activities (IU/g Hb)

	Patient	Mother	Father	Control
G-6-PD	18.7	—	—	9.4
PK	11.2	—	—	8.0
GPX	4.8	11.9	14.7	13.9

[1] An age-matched control yielded normal values.

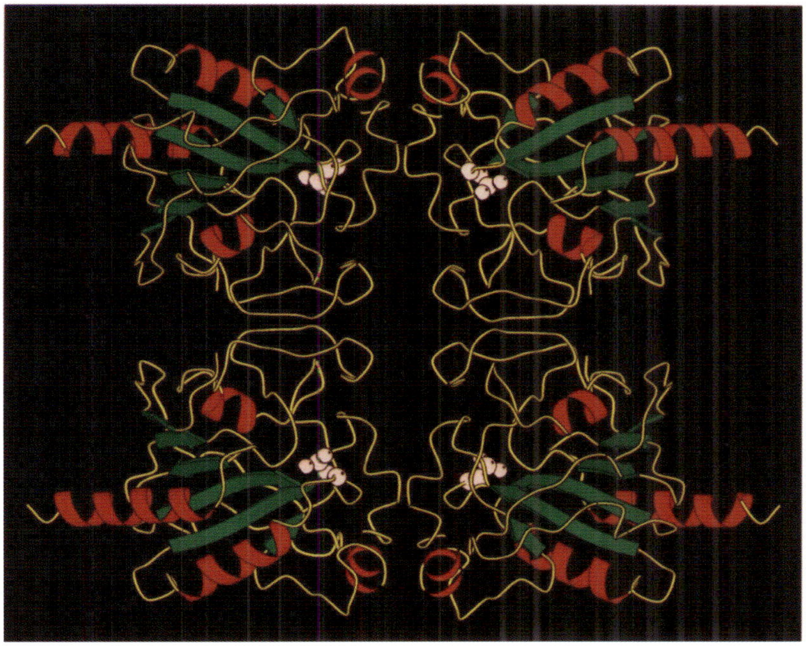

Figure 20.2 Ribbon diagram of the tetrameric form of human GPX. Helices are shown in red, β-strands in green and other elements in yellow. The active site residue, selenocysteine, is represented in pink ball-and-stick. Selenocysteine is incorporated into proteins through a unique co-translational mechanism that involves reprogramming the translation machinery to recognize the UGA codon, usually a stop codon, as a code for selenocysteine (courtesy Bin Ren, see Ref. [16]).

Comments

IP is a recognized entity, but the cause is still unknown [1–3]. The findings in this infant suggested to us that a low level of selenium might have limited his level of GPX enzyme activity, thus causing his haemolytic anaemia. Both parents had normal GPX activity, thus ruling out an inherited deficiency of this enzyme; and genetic testing has failed to identify a responsible defect in other cases [4, 5]. Interestingly, Lee et al. [6] found maternal plasma selenium concentrations significantly greater than foetal levels; placental selenium levels were four times that of foetal levels; and for unknown reasons male newborns had lower selenium levels than female newborns. In the erythrocytes of healthy newborns GPX levels are generally lower than in older children and adults [7]; and it has been suggested that low levels of GPX in newborns may be related to insufficient availability of selenium during pregnancy [8].

Glutathione peroxidase (GPX) and the thioredoxin pathway provide two mechanisms to detoxify hydrogen peroxide and organic hydroperoxides (see Figure 20.3). Buildup of these dangerous reactants causes hemichrome formation which often leads to the production of Heinz bodies. This might explain

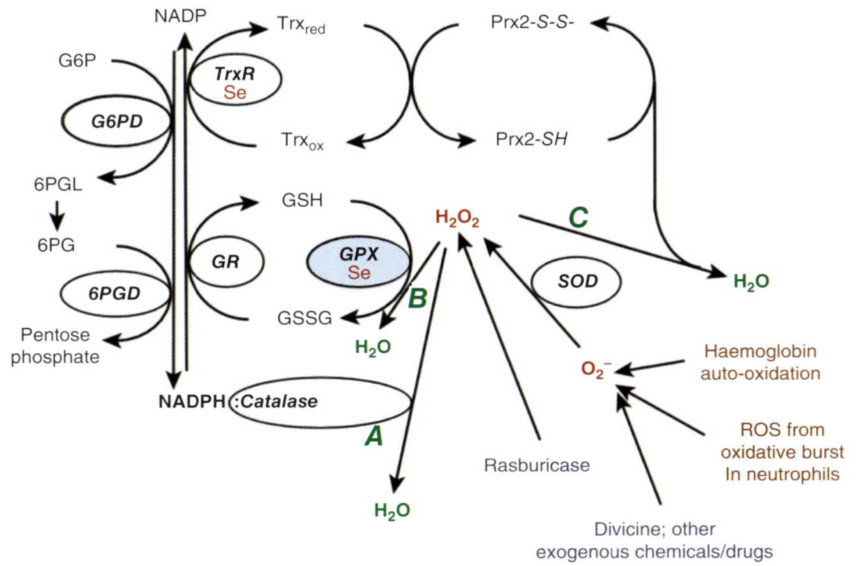

Figure 20.3 The red cell has several lines of defence against oxidative stress as illustrated by the different mechanisms whereby hydrogen peroxide (H_2O_2) can be converted to harmless H_2O. Mechanism A is catalase; mechanism B is glutathione peroxidase (GPX); mechanism C is peroxiredoxin, that depends in turn on thioredoxin and thioredoxin reductase (TrxR). It is noteworthy that both GPX and TrxR are selenoproteins. [10]/with permission of Elsevier.

the positive autohaemolysis test and the haemolytic anaemia in our patient. Remarkably, both GPX and thioredoxin reductase are selenoproteins; thus, selenium deficiency would affect both. Selenium deficiency in Great Britain is extremely rare, because the element is abundant within the soil; this is unlike New Zealand, for example, where the soil has a low content of this element [9].

Follow-up

IP is self-limiting and its spontaneous resolution is almost regarded as part of its definition. In our patient, a repeat blood count at the age of seven months revealed normal haemoglobin and reticulocytes (see Table 20.1). There were no contracted cells or polychromasia; indeed, we can say that the overall red cell morphology was normal (see Figure 20.4). By that time, the selenium level had risen to a level above the top of the reference range and the assay of GPX was now normal (see Table 20.3).

Thus, the patient fits the benign course seen in cases of IP.

Conclusion

IP in a child with GPX deficiency secondary to a neonatal deficiency of selenium.

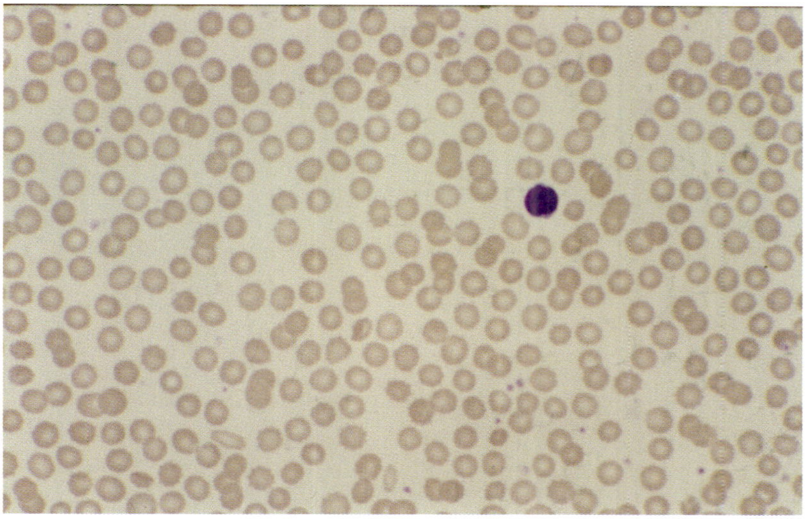

Figure 20.4 Peripheral blood film six months later.

Table 20.3 Glutathione Peroxidase Activity (IU/g Hb) and Selenium Level (μmol/l)

Time	GPX	Selenium
Presentation	4.8	0.23
After 6 months	10.7	0.99
(N/R)	(8.8–21.2)	(0.51–0.71)

Addendum

Since investigating this patient, we had referrals of two more neonates with severe anaemia and jaundice. Both babies had hyperbilirubinaemia and red cell morphology fitting the description of "infantile pyknocytosis." Blood samples were taken on about the third week for investigation (see Table 20.4), after which the babies were each given a blood transfusion. In both of these patients also, GPX and selenium levels were low; but subsequently, they became normal, and the anaemia and hyperbilirubinaemia resolved.

Thus, we seem to have at least a plausible pathogenetic hypothesis. Low selenium in the baby, possibly due to low level in the mother and/or sub-optimal transfer across the placenta; consequently, low level of GPX, a selenoprotein, and possibly of the other selenoprotein thioredoxin reductase; as a result, oxidative haemolysis.

A pathogenetic hypothesis must account not only for the haematologic picture of IP, but also for several additional non-trivial facts. (i) Spontaneous recovery is the rule; (ii) there are two case reports [11, 12], where only one of two non-identical twins was affected: thus, low Se in the mother is not sufficient to explain pyknocytosis; (iii) rarity of the condition. These facts

Table 20.4 Data on Two Additional Patients with "Infantile Pyknocytosis"

	Case 2[b] (male)		Case 3 (female)	
	Initial	After 6 months	Initial	After 3 months
Hb (g/dl)	6.8	12.6	6.4	9.1
GPX (IU/gHb)	2.9	12.7	5.1	15.4
Selenium[a] (μmol/l)	0.16	0.65	0.25	0.61
Retics ($\times 10^9$/l)	330	47	360	55
Bilirubin (μmol/l)	267	5	264	6

[a] Reference ranges for selenium: 0.36–0.46 μmol/l (at 1 - 3 months)
0.51–0.71 μmol/l (at six months)

[b] This infant also had a low level of vitamin E (3 μmol/l; reference range: 11.5–35.0 μmol/l), which became normal (23.1 μmol/l) at three months.

could be explained by considering that Se transfer across the placenta is mediated by the selenoprotein, SEPP1 in the mouse [13], and presumably also in humans. Before birth, supply of Se to the foetus will depend on SEPP1, and a hypo-functional variant of the gene encoding this protein might limit supply[2]: if the variant is rare it would explain the rarity of IP, and it might have been present in only one and not in the other twin in the cases above: discordance at birth between dizygotic twins is a pointer to a genetic difference between them. After birth, an infant with IP will receive Se in breast milk or in formula milk and will be cured.

Whereas the link between low selenium, low GPX and IP is well supported by our cases, the idea that a *SEPP1* mutation may be the underlying cause is purely hypothetical. We regret we have not tested for such mutations, and *SEPP1* would not be part of haemolytic anaemia gene panels that others have used; we hope in the near future somebody will do this in new cases, and thus will be able to confirm or refute our hypothesis that inadequate transfer of Se across the placenta is involved in the pathogenesis of IP.

Acknowledgements

Referred by Dr. Anne Miller, St., Peter's Hospital, Chertsey, Surrey, UK.
Dr. Richard Newton, St., Peter's Hospital, Chertsey, Surrey, UK.
Dr Giovanni Palazzi, Department of Pediatrics, University of Modena and Reggio Emilia, Modena, Italy.
Ren, B., (for Figure 20.2; unpublished data, 1998) Ribbon diagram of the tetrameric form of human plasma GPX. Karolinska Institute, Novum Center for Structural Biochemistry, Huddinge, Sweden [16].

[2] A missense mutation of *SEPP1* that produces an alanine to threonine amino acid replacement at position 234 has been found to modify response to dietary selenium [14]; and the same mutation is associated with the clinical course of retinopathy of prematurity [15].

Trace Element Laboratory, Department of Clinical Biochemistry and Clinical Nutrition, Guilford, Surrey, UK.
Dr Richard van Wijk, Central Diagnostic Laboratory, University Medical Center, Utrecht, Netherlands.

References

1. Català, L., Salazar, J.J., Pujol, M. et al. (2025). Infantile pyknocytosis as a cause of neonatal hemolytic anemia. *Indian J. Pediatr.* 92, 201.
2. Drouilly, M., Jourdan, L., Gérard, D. et al. (2024). Infantile pyknocytosis, a neonatal hemolytic anemia with Heinz bodies: a cohort study. *Pediatr. Blood Cancer* 71, e31078.
3. Rees, C., Lund, K., and Bain, B.J. (2019). Infantile pyknocytosis. *Am. J. Hematol.* 94(4), 489–490.
4. Spoorenberg, M.E., Wachters-Hagedoorn, R.E., van Wijk, R. (2021). Infantile pyknocytosis in a premature dichorionic diamniotic twin. *J. Pediatr. Hematol. Oncol.* 43(7), e1037–e1039.
5. Bahr, T.M., Knudsen, M.C., Lozano-Chinga, M. et al. (2020). Infantile pyknocytosis: end-tidal CO, %Micro-R measurements, next-generation sequencing, and transfusion avoidance with darbepoetin. *Biomed. Hub.* 5(3), 227–234.
6. Lee, A.M., Huel, G., Godin, J. et al. (1995). Inter-individual variation of selenium in maternal plasma, cord plasma and placenta. *Sci. Total Environ.* 159, 119–127.
7. Emerson, P.M., Mason, D.Y., and Cuthbert, J.E. (1972). Erythrocyte glutathione peroxidase content and serum tocopherol levels in newborn infants. *Br. J. Haematol.* 22, 667–680.
8. Perona, G., Guidi, G.C., Piga, A. et al. (1979). Neonatal erythrocyte glutathione peroxidase deficiency as a consequence of selenium imbalance during pregnancy. *Br. J. Haematol.* 42, 567–574.
9. Thomson, C.D. (2004). Selenium and iodine intakes and status in New Zealand and Australia. *Br. J. Nutr.* 91, 661–672.
10. Luzzatto, L., Ally, M., and Notaro, R. (2020). Glucose-6-phosphate dehydrogenase deficiency. *Blood* 136(11), 1225–1240.
11. Berardi, A., Balestri, E., Bonacorsi, G. et al. (2017). Neonatal pyknocytosis in a preterm dizygotic twin. *World J. Clin. Pediatr.* 6, 176–179.
12. Stephan, C., Phulpin, A., Steschenko, D. et al. (2018). Oxidative stress-related infantile pyknocytosis with Heinz bodies. *Transfusion* 58, 840–841.
13. Burk, R.F., Olson, G.E., Hill, K.E. et al. (2013). Maternal-fetal transfer of selenium in the mouse. *FASEB J.* 27, 3249–3256.
14. Kopp, T.I., Outzen, M., Olsen, A. et al. (2018). Genetic polymorphism in selenoprotein P modifies the response to selenium-rich foods on blood levels of selenium and selenoprotein P in a randomized dietary intervention study in *Danes. Genes Nutr.* 13, 20.
15. Strauss, E., Januszkiewicz-Lewandowska, D., Sobaniec, A. et al. (2023). SELENOP rs3877899 variant affects the risk of developing advanced stages of retinopathy of prematurity (ROP). *Int. J. Mol. Sci.* 24.
16. Ren, B., Huang, W., Akesson, B. et al. (1997). The crystal structure of seleno-glutathione peroxidase from human plasma at 2.9 Å resolution. *J. Mol. Biol.* 268, 869–885.

Case 21

Two Variants Walk into a Blood Cell

Patient Details

Age: 35 *Sex:* M
Ethnic background: Nigerian

Reason for Referral

Unusual findings in a blood sample from a haematologist (blood sample only).

History and Clinical Findings in Brief

There was no significant past medical history. The patient complained of painful swelling in his right foot and of feeling tired. His clinical examination was normal.

Laboratory Findings

The patient had a borderline microcytosis but was not anaemic (see Table 21.1). The blood film (see Figure 21.1) showed mild anisocytosis, poikilocytosis, target cells and red cells that had lost their central pallor but were not quite spherocytes ("quasi-spherocytes"). There were also occasional burr cells and polychromatic cells.

Table 21.1 Haematology Data

Hb (g/dl)	14.4
RBC ($\times 10^{12}$/l)	5.86
MCV (fl)	74.7
MCH (pg)	24.8
MCHC (g/dl)	32.9

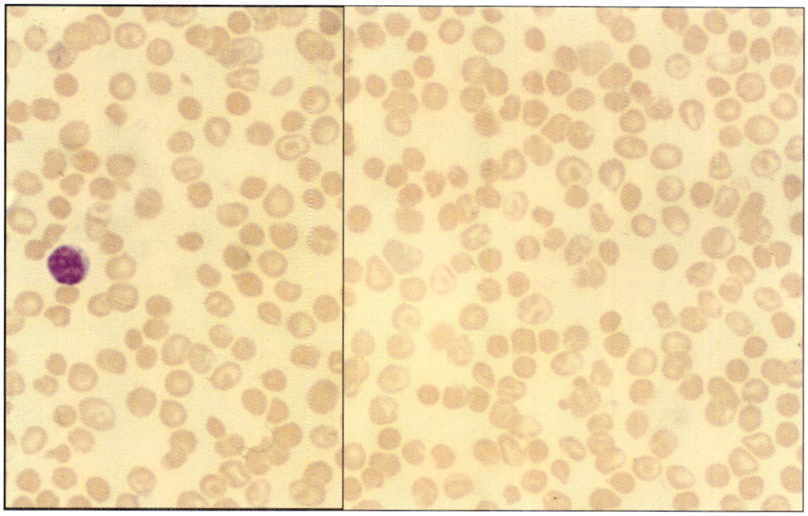

Figure 21.1 Peripheral blood film (composite).

Initial Assessment

There was no anaemia, but the blood was not normal. The mild microcytic, hypochromic picture might be compatible with chronic disease (e.g. rheumatoid) but could also be compatible with a mild form of thalassaemia. In view of the normal MCHC, iron deficiency seems unlikely.

Further Investigations

Haemoglobin electrophoresis revealed two major abnormal bands, in the absence of Hb A (see Figure 21.2). The more intense of the two bands was in the position of Hb C; the other, less intense haemoglobin band had an unusually slow mobility as it migrated behind Hb C, in the exact position of carbonic anhydrase. Hb F was not elevated. On alkaline globin chain electrophoresis (see Figure 21.3), three bands could be visualized: one was in the position of α^A; one in the position of the β^C control; the third appeared, from its position, to be an abnormal α-chain and by comparison with data in the literature [1], it was in the position of α^G. The band in the β^C position was the more intense of the three.

Comments

We had never come across this haemoglobin electrophoretic pattern, but the diagram below (Figure 21.4) shows a rather simple explanation.

The normal α chain pairs with β^C to give Hb C; the abnormal α chain (probably α^G) also pairs with β^C to form a hybrid haemoglobin (Hb X): since there are only two major haemoglobins, the person must be homozygous for Hb C gene HBB^{E6K}. Since the net charge of Hb C is −2 and the net charge of Hb G is −1, the net charge of Hb X $(\alpha_2{}^G\beta_2{}^C)$ will be −3, compared to Hb A. The patient appears to be heterozygous for α^G; this would account for the more intense band seen in the Hb C position on haemoglobin electrophoresis and for the more intense β^C band on globin chain electrophoresis. The finding of target cells and spherocytic cells is typical for Hb C disease. Although we have not definitively identified the alpha chain variant in this

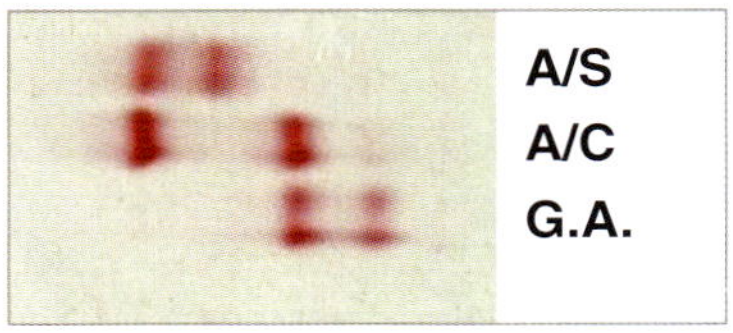

Figure 21.2 Haemoglobin electrophoresis on cellulose acetate membrane; the migration of the haemoglobin fractions is from right to left. An A/S and A/C control are in lanes 1 and 2, respectively. The patient (G.A.) is in lane 3.

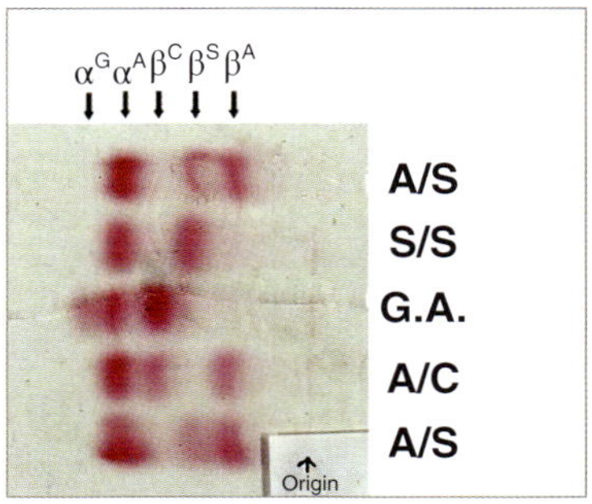

Figure 21.3 Alkaline globin chain electrophoresis on cellulose acetate membrane; the migration of the globin chains is from right to left; the application point (origin) is indicated. An A/S and A/C control are in lanes 1 and 4, respectively. The patient (G.A.) is in lane 3.

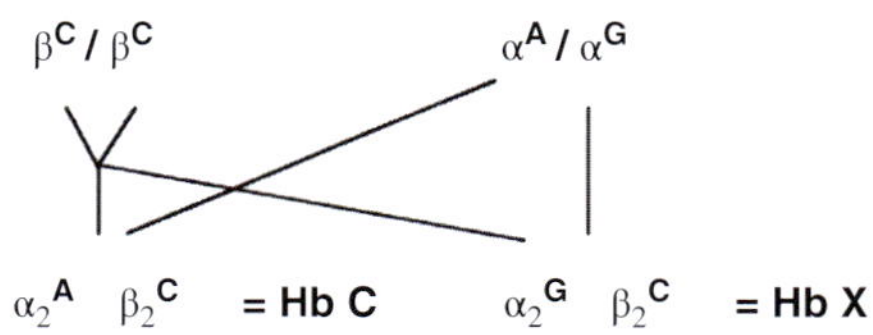

Figure 21.4 Schematic representation of genetic pairing of the globin genes that make up this unusual combination of haemoglobins.

patient, G Philadelphia is by far the commonest α chain variant in West Africa. In addition, α^G is linked to α-thalassaemia [2–5], accounting for the low Hb G/Hb A ratio usually seen in heterozygotes: with the genotype $-\alpha^A/-\alpha^G$, Hb G is on average 46%; whereas with the genotype $\alpha^A\alpha^A/-\alpha^G$ it is approximately 34%. In our patient, an α-thalassaemia gene linked to α^G would explain his low MCV and MCH.

The doubly heterozygous combination of haemoglobins C and G has been previously reported [6–8]. However, to the best of our knowledge, this patient is the first case of haemoglobin G in a person who is also *homozygous* for the haemoglobin C mutation.

Follow-up

We have not formally sought a follow up on this person since he had no clinical problems. In this age of HPLC, we presume Hb $\alpha_2{}^G\beta_2{}^C$ would elute as a major peak after Hb C, but we are not sure; and the HPLC elution pattern, without individual globin chain analysis, would not provide a full explanation.

Conclusion

Homozygous Haemoglobin C in combination with alpha G variant.

Acknowledgements

Referred by Dr. A M Akinsete, Haematology Department, Lagos University Teaching Hospital, Lagos, Nigeria.

References

1. Bunn, H.F. and Forget, B.G. (1986). *Hemoglobin: Molecular, Genetics and Clinical Aspects*. Philadelphia: W.B. Saunders Company.
2. Sancar, G.B., Tatsis, B., Cedeno, M.M. et al. (1980). Proportion of hemoglobin G Philadelphia ($\alpha_2{}^{268AsnLys}\beta_2$) in heterozygotes is determined by α-globin gene deletions. *Proc. Natl. Acad. Sci. USA*. 77, 6874–6878.
3. Surrey, S., Ohene-Frempong, K., Rappaport, E. et al. (1980). Linkage of to α-thalassaemia in African-Americans. *Proc. Natl. Acad. Sci. USA*. 77, 4885–4889.
4. Felice, A.E., Ozdonmez, R., Headlee, M.E. et al. (1982). Organisation of α-chain genes among Hb G-Philadelphia heterozygotes in association with Hb S, β-thalassaemia, and α-thalassaemia-2. *Biochem. Genet*. 20, 689–701.

5. Martinez, G., Ferreira, R., and Colombo, B., (1985). Linkage of the α^G Philadelphia locus to α-thalassaemia in the Cuban population. *Acta Haematologica* (Basel). 74, 186–188.
6. Raper, A.B., Gammack, D.B., Huens, E.R. et al. (1960). Four haemoglobins in one individual. A study of the genetic interaction of Hb G and Hb C. *Br. Med. J.* 2, 1257–1261.
7. Weatherall, D.J., Sigler, A.T., and Baglioni, C. (1962). Four haemoglobins in each of three brothers. Genetic & Biochemical significance. *Bull. Johns Hopk Hosp*. 11, 143–156.
8. McCurdy, P.R., Sherman, A.S., Kamuzora, H. et al. (1975). Globin synthesis in subjects doubly heterozygous for haemoglobin G-Philadelphia and haemoglobin S or C. *J. Lab. Clin. Med.* 85, 891–897.

See also related Case 42.

Case 22

Low GPI, High GPA

Patient Details

Age: 15 *Sex:* M
Ethnic background: Italian

Reason for Referral

Investigation of anaemia.

History and Clinical Findings in Brief

This boy was born, following an uneventful pregnancy, in Morcone, a small town on a hill in the Province of Benevento, Italy. There was no history of neonatal jaundice. At the age of one year, he was noted to be anaemic. There was no family history of note. When he was referred, at the age of 15, to the Haematology Department of the Federico II University in Naples, it emerged that he had been suffering from anaemia since birth, with haemoglobin values ranging from 7 to 11 g/dl, requiring occasional blood transfusions. Physical examination revealed pallor, mild jaundice and splenomegaly; he also had cholelithiasis. There were no neurological signs or muscle weakness.

Laboratory Findings

The patient had a moderate macrocytic anaemia (see Table 22.1). The blood film (see Figure 22.1) showed slight variation in red cell size with polychromasia and quite striking basophilic stippling in about 4% of red cells.

Additional baseline studies (see Table 22.2) were negative or normal, except for the autohaemolysis test, which showed increased lysis, not corrected (in fact further increased) by addition of glucose. Such a pattern is known as Type 2 autohaemolysis and is frequently associated with pyruvate kinase (PK) deficiency.

Table 22.1 Laboratory Data

	Age 15	Age 18
Hb (g/dl)	10.8	10.4
RBC ($\times 10^{12}$/l)	–	3.01
MCV (fl)	–	104.4
MCH (pg)	–	34.5
MCHC (g/dl)	–	33.1
Retic (%)	–	15.9
Retic ($\times 10^{9}$/l)	677	480
Bilirubin (μmol/l)[a]	144	86

[a] unconjugated.

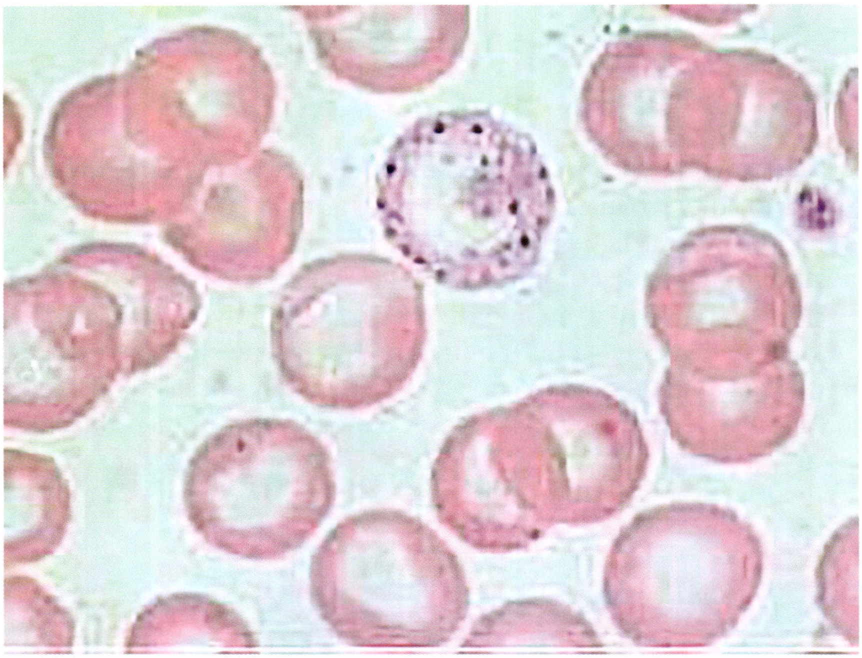

Figure 22.1 Peripheral blood film.

Table 22.2 Baseline Studies

DAGT	Negative
Ham test	Negative
Osmotic fragility	Normal
Haemoglobin separation	Normal
Autohaemolysis	Increased

Initial Assessment

Based on the history and blood findings, particularly the very high absolute reticulocytosis and abnormal autohaemolysis test, it seemed likely that the patient had a congenital haemolytic anaemia, probably due to a glycolytic enzyme abnormality.

Further Investigations

A Cr^{51} study showed reduced red cell lifespan with increased uptake in the spleen and liver. A panel of red cell enzyme assays (see Figure 22.2) revealed normal or increased activities in all, except for glucose-6-phosphate isomerase (GPI), which had an activity of only 15% of normal. The parents were not anaemic and their red cell GPI activity was about 50% of normal. Based on biochemical abnormalities, the enzyme variant was assigned the provisional name "GPI Morcone" [1].

DNA analysis revealed a 1028A → G mutation in exon 12 of the *GPI* gene, for which the patient is homozygous. This mutation causes a glutamine to arginine amino acid replacement in the enzyme protein (p.Q343R) [2].

Comments

At the time of diagnosis, this was the fourth case of glucose phosphate isomerase (GPI) deficiency found in Italy [1], in keeping with GPI deficiency being a rare autosomal recessive disorder that causes hereditary nonspherocytic haemolytic anaemia (HNSHA) of variable severity. It is the second most common erythro-enzymopathy of anaerobic glycolysis after pyruvate kinase deficiency [3]. GPI deficiency has been associated in some cases with neurological impairment [3], but fortunately not in this case. GPI is a homo-dimeric enzyme encoded by a housekeeping

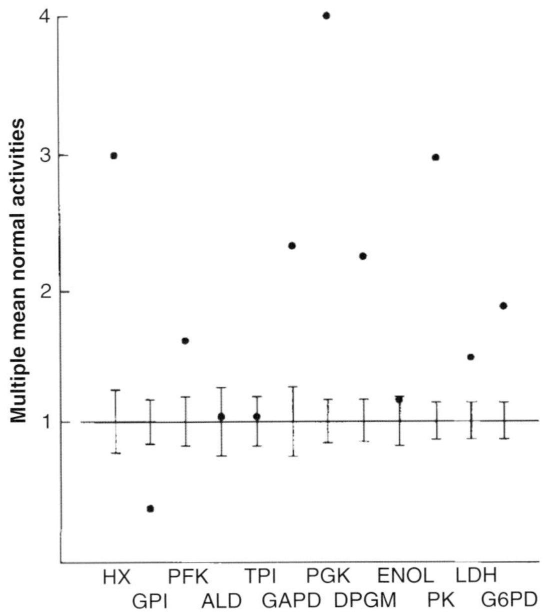

Figure 22.2 Activity of red cell enzymes tested in the patient's red cells. The horizontal line represents the mean control value; vertical bars are one standard deviation. Abbreviations are as follows: Hexokinase (HX), Glucose-6-phosphate isomerase (GPI), Phosphofructokinase (PFK), Aldolase (ALD), Triosephosphate isomerase (TPI), Glyceraldehyde phosphate dehydrogenase (GAPD), Phosphoglycerate kinase (PGK), Diphosphoglyceromutase (DPGM), Enolase (ENOL), Pyruvate kinase (PK), Lactate dehydrogenase (LDH) and Glucose-6-phosphate dehydrogenase (G6PD). Closed circles: activity in the propositus, expressed as multiples of normal. The increased activity of most enzymes is due to the reticulocytosis. [1]/John Wiley & Sons.

gene that maps to chromosome 19q13.1 [4]; it catalyses the reversible conversion of glucose-6-phosphate (G6P) to fructose-6-phosphate (F6P) in the second step of the Embden–Meyerhof glycolytic pathway. Since the first report of GPI deficiency by Baughan et al. [5] at least 57 *GPI* mutations have been reported [6]. The major clinical features include mild to severe normochromic anaemia, variable degrees of jaundice, slight-to-moderate splenomegaly and an increased incidence of gallstones.

Molecular characterization of GPI variants has revealed in most cases point mutations that lead to enzyme instability. The mutation in our patient is close to the substrate binding site [7]; it has been found to cause not only decreased activity but also decreased thermostability and decreased substrate affinity [8].

Although the parents were not aware of being consanguineous, both were born in Morcone, a town with a population of about 4,000; therefore, it is not unlikely that the patient's parents did have a common ancestor.

Follow-up

The patient continued to receive blood transfusions (packed red cells) whenever clinically indicated, and typically whenever his haemoglobin level fell below 7.0 g/dl (see Figure 22.3).

The patient began to suffer recurrent episodes of jaundice associated with severe colicky pain due to gallstones. At the age of 25, the patient suffered acute cholestasis; he underwent abdominal surgery that included cholecystectomy, choledochoduodenostomy and splenectomy. The spleen weighed 500 g; microscopic examination showed congestive features and foci of erythropoiesis. Liver biopsy revealed evidence of cholestasis. Despite this, he continued with his studies, and the following year he obtained a degree in Philosophy from the University of Naples.

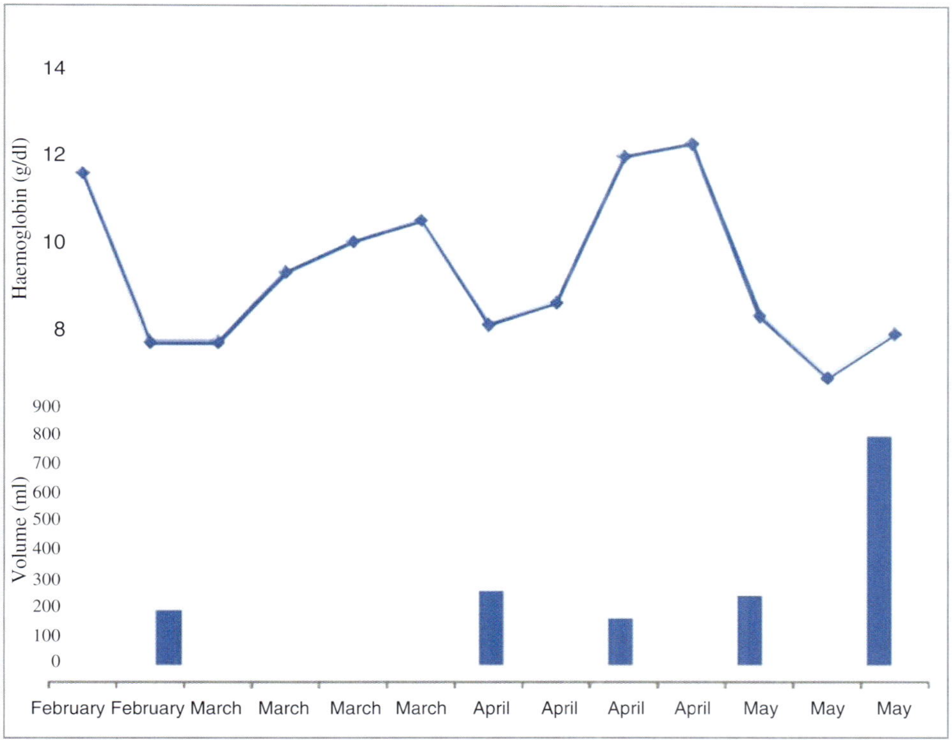

Figure 22.3 Excerpt of the patient's red cell transfusions (indicated by blue bars) at the age of 19 years.

Long-term Follow-up

At age 43, the patient was appointed Head Librarian in an academic institution in Rome. He has not required a blood transfusion since splenectomy and his general condition is good. An abdominal ultrasound scan was suggestive of an accessory spleen (splenunculus). At the age of 44, he had an episode of severe jaundice associated with abdominal pain and was admitted to hospital. His bilirubin level increased progressively up to a peak of 80 mg/dl (1368 μmol/l), and he required several blood transfusions; however, subsequently, his condition slowly improved and he made a gradual recovery. The patient was discharged with a diagnosis of severe cholestatic jaundice and subacute cholangitis in the presence of biliary-intestinal anastomosis and suspected biliary tract tumour. A liver biopsy revealed cholestasis and ballooned hepatocytes, probably from bilirubin toxicity; massive ceroidosis of Kupffer cells, possibly related to chronic haemolysis; moderate centrolobular perisinusoidal fibrosis, but no evidence of evolution to cirrhosis.

Quantitative magnetic resonance imaging (see Figure 22.4) studies revealed significant iron overload in the liver; deferoxamine was recommended as the iron-chelating agent least likely to be hepatotoxic.

At the age of 52, after four further episodes of severe jaundice, imaging studies revealed features of cholestasis, sclerosing cholangitis/cholangiolitis, iron overload, possibly slowly evolving to biliary cirrhosis. The patient underwent surgery to remove very numerous stones, including one single 20 mm diameter stone, reconstruction of the biliary intestinal anastomosis, and removal of the accessory spleen. Spleen histology revealed massive numbers of phagocytosing macrophages, and a new liver biopsy revealed lobular fibrosis and grade 4 iron overload. Since then, the patient has been stable clinically and haematologically, with a haemoglobin of about 11 g/dl, reticulocytes about four times the upper normal limit and mildly elevated bilirubin.

In the meantime, the patient, now aged 62, has published several books in the area of philosophy and political science. We have learnt from him several lessons regarding GPI deficiency, including the following. (i) Splenectomy can be highly beneficial, but it may not be definitive: an accessory spleen, that had been missed at the time of the first abdominal surgery, subsequently underwent significant growth; (ii) cholecystectomy was certainly indicated, but problems with bile outflow eventually required further surgery; (iii) haemolysis and numerous transfusions caused serious iron overload, and compliance with iron chelation was not easy. In view of the above, GPI deficiency must be regarded as a serious

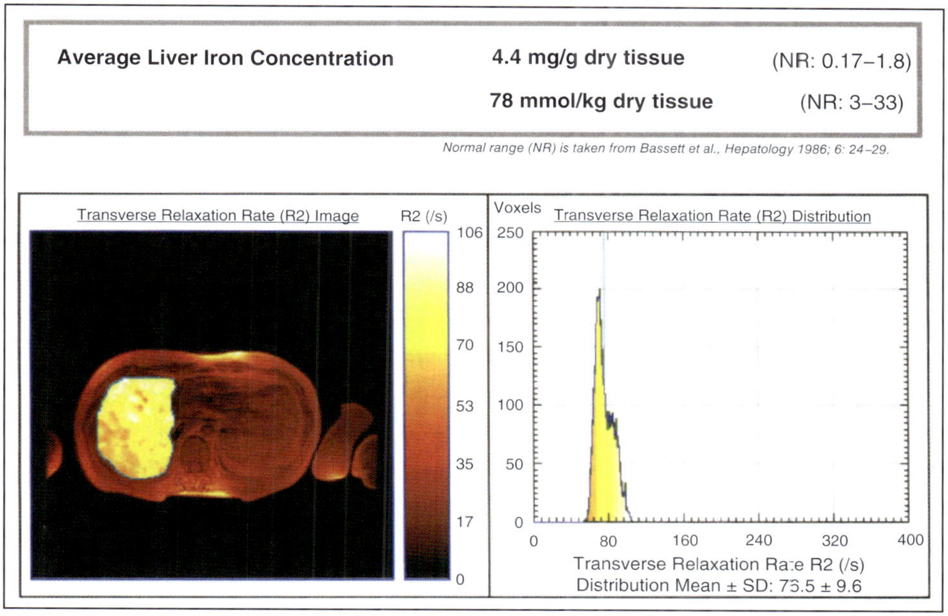

Figure 22.4 Excerpt from FerriScan liver iron concentration report. Diagnostic image from: Resonance Health Analysis Services. [1]/John Wiley & Sons.

condition, even when the patient is not transfusion-dependent or has become transfusion-independent after splenectomy. In spite of all the above, a patient with GPI deficiency may have a normal life span; and, most important, the patient can lead a productive life.

Some details of this case study have been published when the patient was a young man. [1].

Conclusion

Glucose-6-phosphate isomerase (GPI) deficiency.

Acknowledgements

This patient, before and after being seen at the Hammersmith in London, was investigated and managed by many colleagues from different countries; we extend thanks to all, and here we are acknowledging at least some. Bruno Rotoli and Fiorella Alfinito, in Naples, Italy; Alberto Zanella in Milano, Italy; Luciano Baronciani in La Jolla, CA, USA; Giuliano Ramadori in Gottingen, Germany; Renzo Galanello in Cagliari, Italy; Tanya Roskam in Leuven, Belgium; Daniele Antonio Pinna, in Bologna, Italy.

References

1. Alfinito, F., Ferraro, F., Rocco, S. et al. (1994). Glucose phosphate isomerase (GPI) “Morcone”: a new variant from Italy. *Eur. J. Haematol.* 52(5), 263–266.
2. Baronciani, L., Zanella, A., Bianchi, P. et al. (1996). Study of the molecular defects in glucose phosphate isomerase-deficient patients affected by chronic hemolytic anemia. *Blood* 88, 2306–2310.
3. Kugler, W. and Lakomek, M. (2000). Glucose-6-phosphate isomerase deficiency. *Best Pract. Res. Clin. Haematol.* 13(1), 89–101.
4. McMorris, F.A., Chen, T.R., Ricciuti, F. et al. (1973). Chromosome assignments in man of the genes for two hexosephosphate isomerases. *Science* 179(4078), 1129–1131.
5. Baughan, M.A., Valentine, W.N., Paglia, D.E. et al. (1968). Hereditary hemolytic anemia associated with glucosephosphate isomerase (GPI) deficiency–a new enzyme defect of human erythrocytes. *Blood* 32(2), 236–249. PMID: 5672849.
6. Dhankar, M., Mandal, P., Singh, R. et al. (2024). Unusual cause of hemolytic anaemia: glucose phosphate isomerase deficiency. *Pediatr. Hematol. Oncol. J.* 9(4), 283–286. ISSN 2468-1245.
7. Read, J., Pearce, J., Li, X. et al. (2001). The crystal structure of human phosphoglucose isomerase at 1.6 A resolution: implications for catalytic mechanism, cytokine activity and haemolytic anaemia. *J. Mol. Biol.* 309(2), 447–463.
8. Kanno, H., Fujii, H., and Miwa, S. (1998). Expression and enzymatic characterization of human glucose phosphate isomerase (GPI) variants accounting for GPI deficiency. *Blood Cells Mol. Dis.* 24(1), 54–61.

Case 23

Split A_2: A Cue to Q

Patient Details

Age: 29 *Sex:* F
Ethnic background: Pakistan

Reason for Referral

From antenatal clinic.

History and Clinical Findings in Brief

This was the patient's first pregnancy; there was no significant medical history either in her or in her immediate family members. At 12 weeks pregnant, she was clinically well, and her physical examination was normal. She was on no medication.

Laboratory Findings

The patient had a mild microcytic hypochromic anaemia (see Table 23.1). The blood film confirmed a microcytic picture (see Figure 23.1), with some extremely small red cells. There was anisocytosis and poikilocytosis; some of the cells were "tear-drops" and others pear-shaped, with also an occasional

Table 23.1 Baseline Data

Hb (g/dl)	10.0
RBC ($\times10^{12}$/l)	4.84
MCV (fl)	66.1
MCH (pg)	20.7
MCHC (g/dl)	31.3
RDW (S.D.)	38.4
Hb A_2 (%) (normal position)	3.6
Hb A_2 (%) (variant)	0.4
Hb F (%)	1.1
Serum iron (μmol/l)	21.5
Transferrin (g/l)	2.37
Tfn. Saturation index (%)	35
Ferritin (μg/l)	88

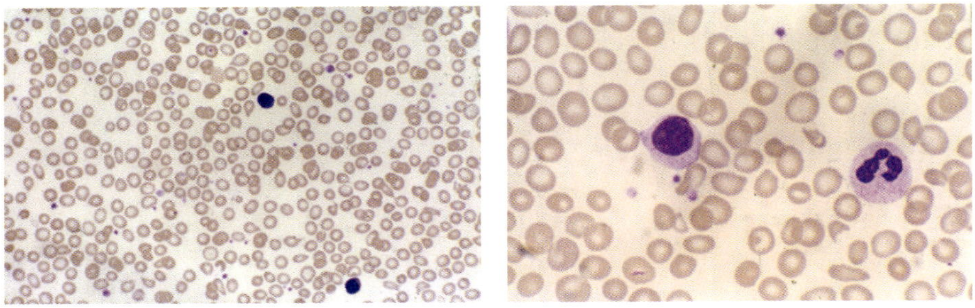

(a) (b)

Figure 23.1 Peripheral blood film: (a) medium power view; (b) high power view.

Figure 23.2 Haemoglobin electrophoresis on cellulose acetate membrane; the migration of the haemoglobin fractions is from right to left. An A/S control and A/S/C control are in lanes 1 and 2, respectively. The patient (S.A.) is in lane 7.

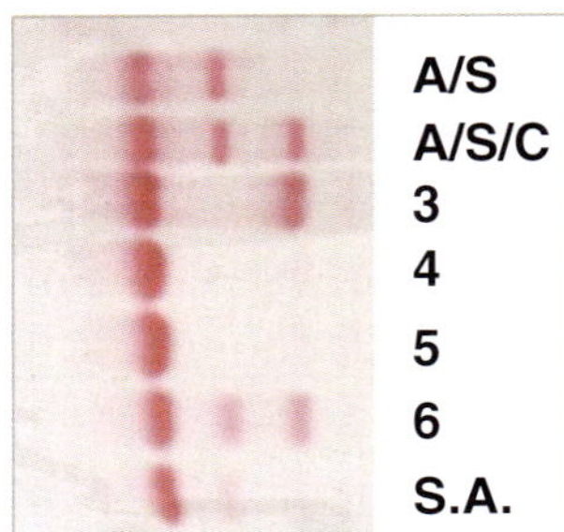

schistocyte and some very dense cells with an irregular but smooth outline. Occasional polychromatic cells and myelocytes could be seen.

Haemoglobin electrophoresis on cellulose acetate membrane (part of routine antenatal screening) revealed, in addition to the normal band of Hb A, a weaker band (9% of total) slightly ahead of the Hb S position (see Figure 23.2).

Quantitation of Hb A_2 was performed by electrophoresis followed by elution of the haemoglobin bands (this was the ICSH reference procedure, which entails applying a relatively large volume [20 μl] of patient's haemolysate across the cellulose strip). At the time of cutting out the individual haemoglobin fractions, we noticed that there were in fact two Hb A_2 bands (so-called "split-A_2"). The Hb A_2 in the normal position was the more intense of the pair and quantitated to 3.6%; the other migrated slightly more slowly than the normal and this quantitated to 0.4%. The combined Hb A_2 level, therefore, was 4.0%.

Initial Assessment

The red cell indices, red cell morphology and elevated Hb A_2 level were clearly in keeping with β-thalassaemia trait. In addition, the "split Hb A_2" raised the suspicion of an α-chain abnormality (arising from the combination of δ chains with either the normal or the abnormal α chains). Indeed, the abnormal band seen on electrophoresis was much below 50%, and therefore more likely an α-chain abnormality. These abnormalities did not necessarily justify the mild microcytic anaemia.

Further Investigations

On agar gel electrophoresis, the abnormal haemoglobin migrated between Hb S and Hb A, but much nearer to the latter (not shown). With globin chain (alkaline) electrophoresis (see Figure 23.3), three bands could be visualized: in addition to the normal bands in the positions of α^A and β^A we found a faint band ahead of the α^A, which was in the same position of the α^G control. This was in keeping with the suspected α-chain variant, and by comparison with data in the literature [1] we suspected the abnormal haemoglobin was probably Hb Q-India.

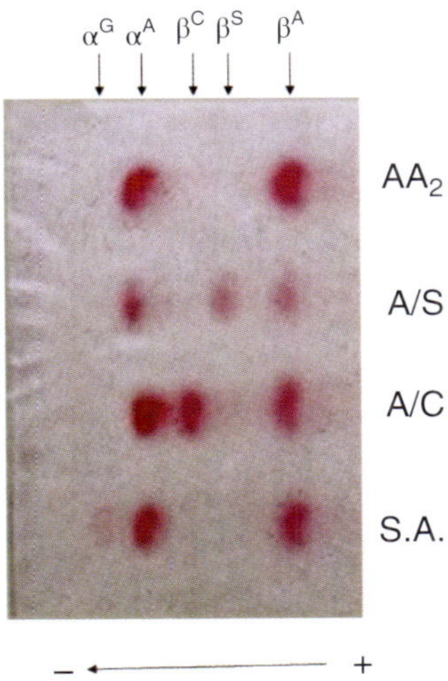

Figure 23.3 Globin chain (alkaline) electrophoresis on cellulose acetate membrane; the migration of the globin chains is from right to left. Normal (AA_2), A/S and A/C controls are in lanes 1, 2 and 3, respectively. The patient (S.A.) is in lane 4.

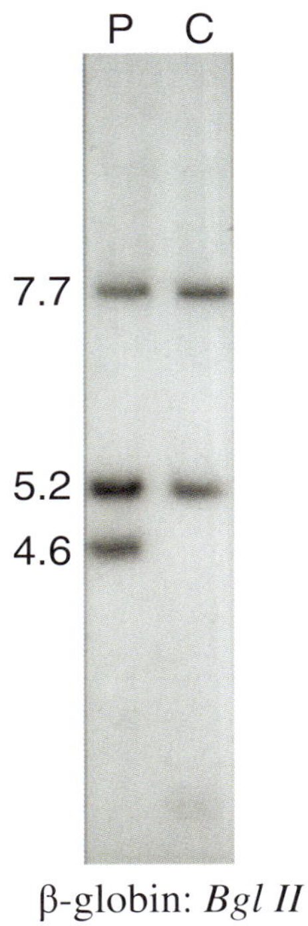

Figure 23.4 Autoradiograph of Southern blot. The genomic DNA from the patient (P) and a normal control (C) was digested with the restriction enzyme *Bgl II* and hybridized to a β-globin probe. The patient's DNA revealed, in addition to the normal 7.7 and 5.2 Kb fragments, a fragment of 4.6 Kb.

Southern blot analysis (see Figure 23.4) after hybridization to a β-globin probe, revealed, in addition to the normal fragments in size 7.7 Kb and 5.2 Kb, a fragment of 4.6 Kb. This is consistent with the patient being heterozygous for a previously known 619 bp deletion, which includes exon 3 of the β-globin gene. This deletion causes β-thalassaemia trait and it is seen in the Asian Indian population [2].

For the sake of completeness, the α-globin status was also assessed. Analysis of the alpha globin gene cluster revealed only normal fragments with *Bam H I* and *Bgl II* restriction enzymes, thus excluding coexistence of deletional α-thalassaemia. In view of the mild anaemia and borderline low MCHC, her iron status was also assessed (see Table 23.1); the data did not support iron deficiency.

Comments

From the point of view of genetic counselling, the β-thalassaemia was, of course, the more important finding in this pregnant woman. We offered for her partner to be tested, and the results were normal.

From the clinical point of view the abnormal haemoglobin was not a cause for concern. Although we have not identified the amino acid replacement, considering the ethnic origin of the patient we have assumed it is Q-India, as many cases have been reported from India [3, 4]: in fact, it is a good (perhaps the only) example of an α chain variant that is polymorphic in that population, although we have not been able to find an estimate of its population frequency. The amino acid replacement in this haemoglobin is Asp64His: thus, the charge change is the same as in haemoglobin G Philadelphia (Asn68Lys).

Patients heterozygous for Hb Q have normal haematology [5]. We ruled out iron deficiency in our patient, and we assume that her mild anaemia was related to haemodilution in pregnancy.

Qin et al. [6] have reported in heterozygotes for Hb Q a mean level of about 17%. This is in good agreement with the same value in a more recent paper by Sharma et al. [4] who also found 33% in homozygotes (this is of course because the α locus is duplicated, and homozygotes for Hb Q still have two normal α genes). These authors report a mean level of 10% in double heterozygotes for Q India and β-thalassaemia, almost exactly as in our patient. This genotypic combination had been previously described [6–8], and the haematological findings do not differ from those seen in β-thalassaemia heterozygotes without Hb Q. It has been suggested that the low level of Hb Q in this situation can be rationalized by considering that, when β-chains are in short supply, they associate preferentially with α^A rather than with α^G; the excess α^G will be degraded. Conversely, coexistence of α^+ thalassaemia, by reducing the available pool of α^A-chains, favours by default, the ${\alpha^Q}_2/{\beta^A}_2$ formation and increases haemoglobin Q to about 27%, which is the sort of level seen with the majority of heterozygous alpha chain variants.

Follow-up

The patient's pregnancy went to term uneventfully. Four years later, a blood count revealed a haemoglobin level of 11.9 g/dl; the red cell indices remained unchanged.

Conclusion

Double heterozygote for β^+ thalassaemia and Hb Q-India.

Acknowledgements

Professor M.G. Elder, Chairman, Division of Paediatrics, Obstetrics and Gynaecology, Hammersmith Hospital, London, UK.

References

1. Bunn, H. and Forget B.G. (1986). *Hemoglobin: Molecular, Genetics and Clinical Aspects*. Philadelphia: W.B. Saunders Company.
2. Varawalla, N.Y., Old, J.M., Sarkar, R. et al. (1991). The spectrum of beta-thalassaemia mutations on the Indian subcontinent: the basis for prenatal diagnosis. *Br. J. Haematol.* 78, 242–247.
3. Phanasgaonkar, S., Colah, R., Ghosh, K. et al. (2007). HbQ-India (HBA1:c.193G>C): hematological profiles and unique CE-HPLC findings of potential diagnostic utility in 65 cases. *Br. J. Biomed. Sci.* 64(4), 160–163.
4. Sharma, S., Sharma, P., Das, R. et al. (2017). Hb Q(India) and its interaction with beta-thalassaemia: a study of 64 cases from India. *Ann. Hematol.* 96(7), 1227–1229.
5. Huisman, T.H.J., Carver, M.F., and Efremov, G.D. (1996). *A Syllabus of Human Hemoglobin Variants*. Augusta, GA, USA: The Sickle Cell Anemia Foundation.
6. Qin, W.B., Baysal, E., Wong, K.F. et al. (1994). Quantities of alpha Q chain variants in heterozygotes with and without a concomitant beta thalassemia trait. *Am. J. Haematol.* 45, 81–83.
7. Schmidt, R.M., Bechtel, K.C., and Moo-Penn, W.F. (1976). Hemoglobin Q India, alpha 64 (E13) Asp → His, and beta thalassemia in a Canadian family. *Am. J. Clin. Path.* 66, 446–448.
8. Sukumaran, P.K., Merchant, S.M., Desai, M.P. et al. (1972). Hemoglobin Q India (alpha 64 (E13) aspartic acid histidine) associated with beta thalassemia observed in three Sindhi families. *J. Med. Genet.* 9, 436–442.

Case 24

A Celtic Trait?

Patient Details

Age: 54 *Sex:* F
Ethnic background: Welsh

Reason for Referral

Identification of abnormal haemoglobin (blood sample only).

History and Clinical Findings in Brief

The patient gave a family history of cystic fibrosis. This had previously prompted a detailed study of the family pedigree, going back over the last eight generations. The patient stated she came from a "pure-Welsh" background. The patient herself had a history of diabetes, but was reported to be well on examination, although slightly anaemic.

Laboratory Findings

A blood count revealed a moderate microcytic, hypochromic anaemia (see Table 24.1). The blood film (not shown) revealed a significant population of microcytes containing only a thin rim of haemoglobin; long, thin ("pencil") cells were present, and overall, the features were very suggestive of iron deficiency.

Because of suspected diabetes, a blood sample was sent for measurement of glycated haemoglobin. An abnormal peak was noticed on the high-performance liquid chromatography (HPLC) chromatogram. Haemoglobin electrophoresis on cellulose acetate membrane revealed, in addition to the normal haemoglobins A, A_2 and F, an abnormal haemoglobin with the mobility of Hb S, which quantitated to 29.0% (see Figure 24.1). The solubility test for sickle haemoglobin was negative.

Initial Assessment

The red cell indices and morphology of this patient are compatible with iron deficiency, which is not that uncommon in a 54-year-old woman in the Midlands. On the other hand, it is extremely unusual to find an abnormal haemoglobin in a person of Welsh ancestry. From the position on the electrophoretic strip, and having eliminated Hb S, the other most common variants are Hb D-Punjab or Hb G-Philadelphia. Hb Belfast and Hb Beograd (also known as Hb D-Camperdown) have the same electrophoretic mobility but are much rarer [1].

Table 24.1 Haematology Data

	Presenting	Follow-up
Hb (g/dl)	9.1	13.8
RBC ($\times 10^{12}$/l)	4.84	4.72
MCV (fl)	63.7	87.0
MCH (pg)	18.8	29.2
MCHC (g/dl)	29.6	33.5
Hb A_2 (%)	2.2	–
Hb F (%)	0.3	–

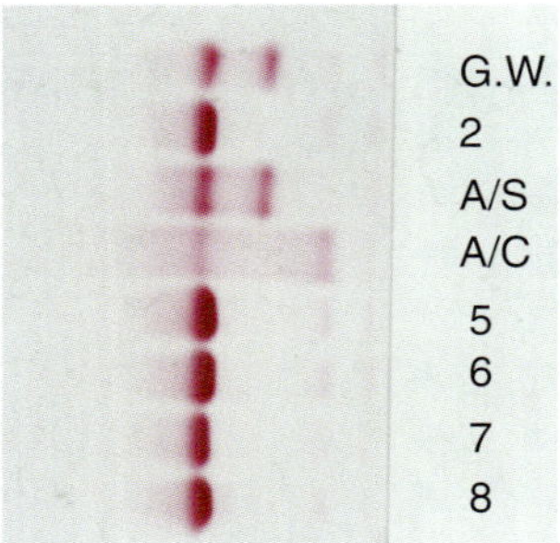

Figure 24.1 Haemoglobin electrophoresis on cellulose acetate membrane; the migration of the haemoglobin fractions is from right to left. An A/S control and A/C control are in lanes 3 and 4, respectively. The patient (G.W.) is in lane 1.

Table 24.2 Iron Status

Serum iron (μmol/l)	2.9
TIBC (μmol/l)	62.3
Tfn. saturation index (%)	5

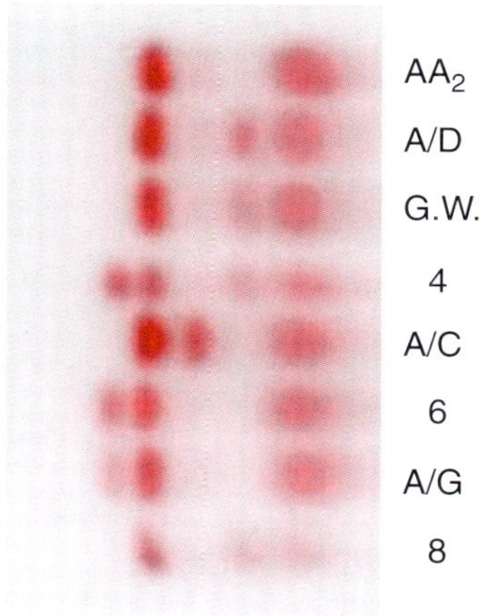

Figure 24.2 Globin chain (alkaline) electrophoresis on cellulose acetate membrane; the migration of the globin chains is from right to left. Normal (AA_2), A/D, A/C and A/G control samples are in lanes 1, 2, 5 and 7, respectively. The patient (G.W.) is in lane 3.

Further Investigations

Assessment of the patient's iron status confirmed iron deficiency (see Table 24.2).

Since citrate agar electrophoresis would not resolve Hb G or Hb D from Hb A, we went on to perform globin chain (alkaline) electrophoresis (see Figure 24.2), which showed three bands; one was in the position of α^A; one in the position of β^A, and the third was in the exact same position as the β^D of the control sample and therefore was identified as a β-chain variant; thus, Hb G Philadelphia was ruled out (we expected that, because with an α-chain variant we should have seen a "split Hb A_2").

By far the most common of the Hb D variants is Hb D-Punjab (also known as Hb D-Los Angeles). By sequence analysis we found indeed a G → C mutation in the first letter of codon 121 of the *HBB* gene (p.Glu121Gln), that identifies D Punjab (see also Figure 24.3). By restriction enzyme analysis we found no evidence of deletional alpha thalassaemia.

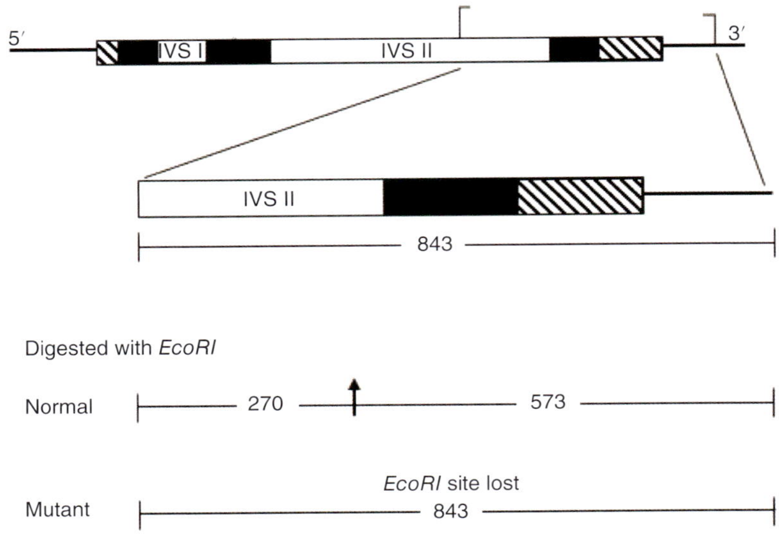

Figure 24.3 Schematic representation of the β-globin gene. The region indicated by brackets was PCR amplified. This diagram is shown because it is a good example of how, before routine sequencing, a point mutation could be easily identified by Southern blot analysis, as it abolishes a 6-base sequence recognized by the *EcoRI* restriction enzyme.

Comments

Haemoglobin D-Punjab gets its name from the north-western state of India where the frequency of heterozygotes is 1 to 3%. However, it is common also in the state of Odisha [2], and cases have been described in several other populations around the world (it is also known as Hb D-Los Angeles). Whether the gene reached Wales through the famous East India Trade route, or whether it was an independent mutation, we cannot say. Interestingly, a cluster of Hb D has been identified in south Wales (Personal communication: Dr. Alison May), from where this patient originates.

This abnormal haemoglobin was a chance finding during measurement of glycated haemoglobin in this patient with diabetes. Usually in heterozygotes the level of Hb D is between 35 and 40%. The lower level (29%) observed in this patient is not due to shortage of α chains (we have ruled out deletional α-thalassaemia); it could be related to iron deficiency whereby, just like Hb A_2 tends to decrease, the same may apply to an abnormal haemoglobin, presumably because the normal β^A chains have a competitive advantage over β^D chains for the available α chains (see Levere et al. [3]; Swarup et al. [4]; Wasi et al. [5]). Heterozygous Hb D is associated with no clinical or haematological abnormalities, although it has a somewhat decreased oxygen affinity [6]: this may be one reason why co-inheritance with Hb S gives rise to a clinical condition with a variable degree of severity, including serious vaso-occlusive crises, that qualifies as a form of sickle cell disease [7].

Follow-up

After a course of iron the patient's blood counts returned to normal (see Table 24.1).

Conclusion

Acquired iron deficiency in a Celtic heterozygous for haemoglobin D Punjab.

Acknowledgements

Referred by Dr. P.C. Srivastava, Haematology Department, South East Staffordshire Health Authority, West Midlanads, UK.

References

1. Huisman, T.H.J., Carver, M.F.H., and Efremav, G.D. (1996). *A Syllabus of Human Hemoglobin Variants*. Augusta, GA, USA: The Sickle Cell Anemia Foundation.
2. Patel, D.K., Mashon, R.S., Patel, S. et al. (2010). beta-globin gene haplotypes linked with the Hb D-Punjab [beta121(GH4)Glu-->Gln, GAA>CAA] mutation in eastern India. *Hemoglobin* 34, 530–537.
3. Levere, R., Lichtman, H.C., and Levine, J. (1964). Effect of iron-deficiency anaemia on the metabolism of the heterogenic haemoglobins in sickle cell trait. *Nature* 4931, 499–501.
4. Swarup, S., Ghosh, S.K., and Chatterjea, J.B., (1965). Effect of iron deficiency on the relative rates of synthesis of hemoglobin A and E studied in a hemoglobin E heterozygote. *Bull. Calcutta Sch. Trop. Med.* 13, 47–48.
5. Wasi, P., Disthasongchan, P., and Na-Nakorn, S., (1968) The effect of iron deficiency on the levels of hemoglobins A_2 and E. *J. Lab. Clin. Med.*, 71, 85–91.
6. Narayanan, S., Mathew, B., Srinivasu, B.Y. et al. (2020). Effect of point mutation on structure-function correlation of hemoglobin variants, HbE and HbD Punjab. *Amino. Acids.* 52, 893–904.
7. Torres, L.S., Okumura, J.V., Belini-Junior, E. et al. (2016). Phenotypic diversity of sickle cell disease in patients with a double heterozygosity for Hb S and Hb D-Punjab. *Hemoglobin* 40, 356–358.

Case 25

Cold May not be Cool

Patient Details

Age: 78 *Sex:* M
Ethnic background: Irish
Occupation: Retired underground conductor

Reason for Referral

Investigation of chronic anaemia (blood sample only).

History and Clinical Findings in Brief

The patient had been seen in our hospital originally in 1969, when he reported that his ears, nose and fingers tended to turn blue when he was out in cold weather. However, the patient has remained generally quite well, apart from dyspepsia for about 35 years, attributed to a duodenal ulcer. In 1988, when visiting his native Ireland, he took ill and may have had a myocardial infarction. In 1989, he had another hospital admission, during which he had a blood transfusion. Recently the patient was seen at his local hospital in London, where examination revealed cyanosis of the extremities: there was no lymphadenopathy or splenomegaly, but the liver was palpable just below the costal border.

Laboratory Findings

The initial blood count data generated by the analyzer did not make much sense. There was clearly an artefact, but the problem could be resolved by simply pre-warming the sample at 37 °C. This revealed the patient had a moderate macrocytic anaemia (see Table 25.1) with reticulocytosis and severe thrombocytopaenia. A marked effect of temperature on the blood cells could be also demonstrated on the blood film (see Figure 25.1), where, already under low power, auto-agglutination was most striking.[1] Sometimes with severe auto-agglutination, red cell clumps contrast strikingly with the surrounding free-standing red cells. Amongst the latter, spherocytes and polychromatic cells could be seen, together with an occasional nucleated red blood cell. There was also an absolute lymphocytosis.

Initial Assessment

The patient gave a history of Raynaud's-like symptoms, and he had evidence of haemolytic anaemia. With the blood findings described above, and since a test for cryoglobulins was negative, the overall picture was highly suggestive of cold agglutinin disease (CAD).

Table 25.1 Haematology Data

	RT[a]	37 °C[b]
Hb (g/dl)	7.9	8.0
RBC (×10^{12}/l)	1.32	2.42
MCV (fl)	112.6	101.7
MCH (pg)	59.8	33.1
MCHC (g/dl)	53.2	32.5
Retic (%)	–	6.0
Retic (×10^{9}/l)	–	145
WBC (×10^{9}/l)	24.2[c]	11.0
Lymphs (×10^{9}/l)	–	6.3
Neuts (×10^{9}/l)	–	4.5
PLT (×10^{9}/l)	30	31

[a] RT: analysis performed at room temperature.
[b] Analysis performed after pre-warming the sample to 37 °C.
[c] Spuriously elevated due to inclusion of large red cell agglutinates.

[1] To distinguish rouleaux from auto-agglutination may be impossible in the thicker part of the film, but looking near the tail, the difference is quite obvious. In rouleaux, the red cells are arranged – by definition – with their disc-like surfaces on top of each other, like a pile of coins; whereas auto-agglutinated red cells are juxtaposed or clumped altogether in a rather random fashion, regardless of their axes.

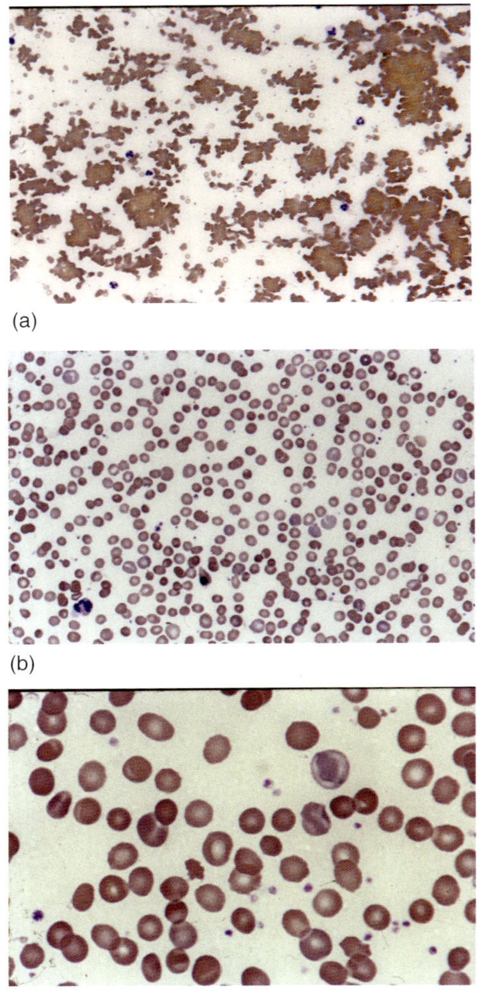

(a) (b) (c)

Figure 25.1 Peripheral blood film: (a) prepared at room temperature; (b) medium power view and (c) high power view, after pre-warming to 37 °C.

Further Investigations

We retrieved from the original records of the late Sheila Worlledge, serological data obtained in 1969 (see Table 25.2). Briefly, the direct antiglobulin test was positive due to complement (but not IgG) on the red cell surface. The patient's serum contained autoantibodies that reacted by the indirect antiglobulin test (IAT), by the two-stage papain technique and in saline against an extensive red cell panel; however, there was no significant activity against cord blood red cells, whence anti-I specificity was inferred. Upon titration, the antibody was found to have low thermal amplitude, and a high agglutinin titre with relatively low haemolytic activity. In theory the low platelets might be related to expression on platelets of the I antigen[1]: however, severe thrombocytopaenia is most unusual in CAD.

Table 25.2 Serological Investigations

	1969							1990	
	Agglutinin				Lysin			Agglutinin	
	4 °C	20 °C	30 °C	37 °C	20 °C	30 °C	37 °C	RT	
A[a]	2000	128	4	0	0	0	0	+	
B[b]	8000	32000	32	0	128	16	4	+	
C[c]	512	1	0	0	0	0	0	–	
		IgG	BS					IgG	C3
DAGT		–	+					–	+

[a] Group-compatible (adult) red cells.
[b] Enzyme-treated (adult) red cells.
[c] Cord-blood cells.
BS = broad spectrum anti-human globulin serum: this phrase was used in those days to indicate an antiserum that contained both anti-Ig and anti-C3.

More recent serological studies obtained from the NBTS (table 25.2, 1990) were entirely consistent with the findings of some 20 years earlier.

Thus, it appeared that the patient has had stable CAD, without much impact on his quality of life, for all this time. However, urine analysis now revealed the presence of Bence–Jones protein. In addition, the patient's total gamma globulin level was very high (67 g/l), and serum electrophoresis demonstrated a heavy paraprotein band (see Figure 25.2), which was identified by immunochemical analysis as IgMκ.

By the time of reassessment in 1990, a large proportion (about 50%) of the patient's lymphocytes were obviously abnormal, showing lympho-plasmacytoid features (see Figure 25.3). The bone marrow showed infiltration with similar cells (54%). Thus, the overall picture was suggestive of lymphoma. Indeed, flow cytometry studies of peripheral blood cells were consistent with a clonal B-cell disorder with lympho-plasmacytic differentiation (see Table 25.3). The lymphoma might now explain the severe thrombocytopenia.

Comments

The long history of acrocyanosis is typical of cold-mediated sludging of red cells affecting the cutaneous microvasculature, and this led to early diagnosis in this patient. In CAD cold agglutinins are able to agglutinate red cells at temperatures as high as 30 °C or even higher [2]; we obtained a proper blood count only after warming our patient's sample to 37 °C. The highest temperature at which such antibodies may cause detectable agglutination is known as the thermal amplitude. This value can vary from one patient to another, and in general, other things being equal, patients with

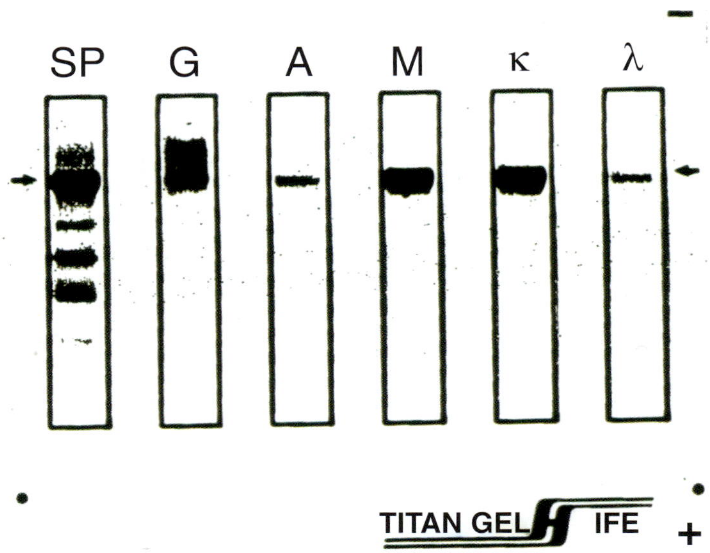

(a)

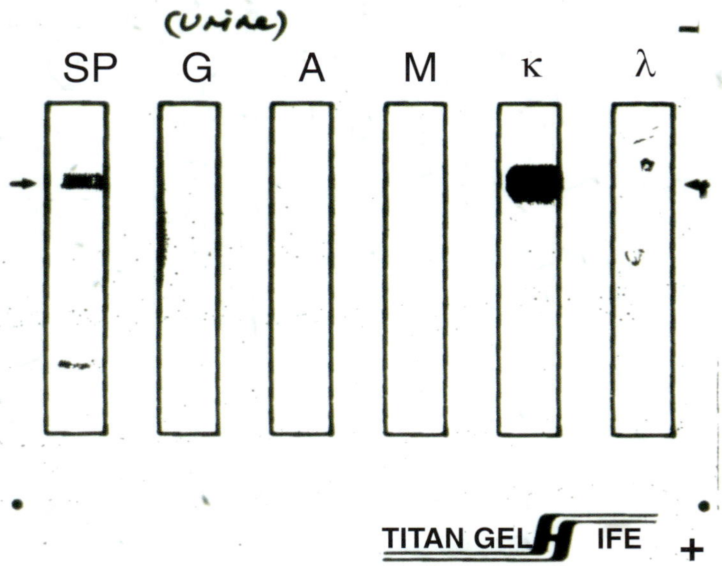

(b)

Figure 25.2 Electrophoresis of serum and urine: (a) serum protein electrophoresis displayed a heavy "spike" in the gamma region (see arrow), identified as IgM by immunoblot analysis; (b) a urine sample revealed the presence of a Bence–Jones protein, found by immunoblot analysis to consist of κ chains.

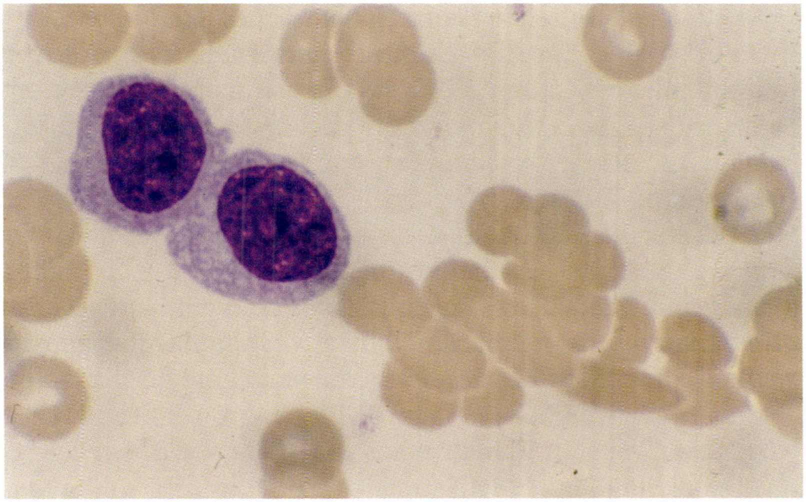

Figure 25.3 Lymphoplasmacytoid cells on peripheral film.

Table 25.3 Cell-marker Studies

B-cell markers	Score[a]	Immunoglobulins		T-cell markers	
CD10 (J5)	5/+	Memb. Igk	37/+++	CD5 (UCHT2)	74/+
FMC7	28/+	Memb. IgL	1/+++	CD2 (RFT11)	46/++
HLA.DR (GRB1)	42/++	IgM	32/+++		
CD19 (RFB9)	34/+				
CD23 (MHM6)	21/±				
L30	36/++				

[a] % positive cells/grading.

cold agglutinins with higher thermal amplitudes have more severe clinical manifestations [3]. Florid haemolytic anaemia, for example, has been reported in patients with cold agglutinins of only modest titre (e.g. 1 : 256) but of high thermal amplitudes [4]. The cold agglutinin in the serum from our patient had a low thermal amplitude, which may explain why he had a relatively mild chronic, stable condition. The pathogenicity of a cold agglutinin is dependent on its ability to bind to host red cells and to activate complement via the classical pathway. Agglutination is not a prerequisite for this, and in fact, the antibody tends to dissociate from red cells once rewarming in circulation takes place.

CAD straddles red cell and white cell haematology. CAD is caused by a B-cell clone that manifests itself because it produces an IgM anti-I red cell autoantibody that causes haemolysis; thus, it is prominent when it is still quite small, i.e. when otherwise most B-cell clones would not let us know about their existence. Since in CAD the anti-I IgM has a relatively high concentration (like any other IgM in Waldenström macroglobulinaemia, WM), and because WM is the manifestation of a plasma-lymphocytic lymphoma, a few decades ago one of us was tempted to surmise that "CAD is a special variant of WD, which is a special variant of lymphoma," [5] but I should have resisted temptation, because I was wrong. We now know that the *MYD88*^{L265P} mutation characteristic of WM is absent in CAD [6].

However, there is an analogy: an IgM MGUS with *MYD88*^{L265P} can become WM through the occurrence of an additional mutation, e.g. in *CXCR4* [7[. As for CAD, according to the most recent WHO classifications [8] it is "driven by an underlying clonal B-cell not fulfilling criteria for a B-cell lymphoma," currently referred to as CAD-associated lymphoproliferative disorder (LPD). The B cell clones of LPD causing CAD have somatic mutations (e.g. of *KMT2D* or *CARD11* [9, 10]), that presumably drive clonal growth. In a large multi-centric study of CAD patients (n = 232) [11], bone marrow histology revealed in the majority of cases only LPD; but a few had lymphoplasmacytic lymphoma (two of whom with the *MYD88*^{L265P} mutation). During follow-up eight patients (3.4%) developed diffuse large B cell lymphoma: it is reasonable to assume that this was caused by additional mutations, that have not yet been identified. Thus, similarly to WM evolving from IgM MGUS, B cell lymphoma can evolve from CAD.

This appears to have happened in our case, who must have had a CAD-associated lymphoid clone for at least 21 years. Since the probability of a spontaneous somatic mutation is proportional to the number of cell divisions D [12], the increasing size of the clone over that length of time must have made D quite high: enough for converting into reality the probability of at least one mutation transforming LPD into a B cell lymphoma.

As regards management, the common sense thermal protection precautions originally recommended to our patient (such as wearing extra clothing in cold weather and using gloves when reaching into a refrigerator) are still valid today; the indication for drug treatment depends on clinical severity. Sutimlimab, a humanized monoclonal antibody that inhibits C1s, a key component of the classical complement pathway that mediates anti-I induced haemolysis in CAD, was found to be effective [13]: in 2022 this good example of targeted therapy became the first approved drug specific for patients with CAD, and it is particularly indicated in those who have anaemia severe enough to require blood transfusion. Depending on individual response and side-effects, other alternatives are currently available, as from a very recent *ad hoc* algorithm [14].

Follow-up

After recovery from an episode of pneumonia that responded to antibiotics, our patient was found to have severe bronchiectasis; he declined chemotherapy for his lymphoma.

Conclusion

Cold agglutinin disease of 21 years duration with IgMκ monoclonal gammopathy: now B-cell lymphoma.

Acknowledgements

Referred by Dr. D. Thompson, Department of Haematology, Luton and Dunstable Hospital, Bedfordshire, UK.

Professor Sigbjørn Berentsen, Department of Research and Innovation, Haugesund Hospital, Helse Fonna Hospital Trust, Haugesund, Norway.

Professor D. Catovski, Department of Academic Haematology, Royal Marsden Hospital, London, UK.

Dr. P. M. de Silva, North London Blood Transfusion Center, London, UK.

References

1. Dunstan, R.A., Simpson, M.B., and Rosse, W.F. (1984). The presence of the Ii blood group system on human platelets. Am J Clin Pathol. 82(1), 74–77.
2. Dacie, J. (1992). *The Haemolytic Anaemias: The Autoimmune Haemolytic Anaemias*. Vol 3, 3 ed. New York, NY: Churchill Livingstone. pp. 210–362.
3. Schubothe, H. (1966). The cold hemagglutinin disease. *Semin. Hematol.* 3, 27–47.
4. Schreiber, A.D., Herskovitz, B.S., and Goldwein, M. (1977). Low-titre cold hemagglutinin disease. *N. Engl. J. Med.* 296, 1490–1494.
5. Oluboyede, O.A., Bademosi, O., David-West, A. et al. (1976). Monoclonal gammopathy (Waldenstrom's macroglobulinaemia) producing specific red cell antibody. *J. Clin. Pathol.* 29, 219–223.
6. Randen, U., Troen, G., Tierens, A. et al. (2014). Primary cold agglutinin-associated lymphoproliferative disease: a B-cell lymphoma of the bone marrow distinct from lymphoplasmacytic lymphoma. *Haematologica* 99(3), 497–504.
7. Xu, L., Hunter, Z.R., Tsakmaklis, N. et al. (2016). Clonal architecture of CXCR4 WHIM-like mutations in Waldenstrom Macroglobulinaemia. *Br J Haematol.* 172(5), 735–744.
8. Alaggio, R., Amador, C., Anagnostopoulos, I. et al. (2022). The 5th edition of the World Health Organization classification of haematolymphoid tumours: lymphoid neoplasms. *Leukemia* 36(7), 1720–1748.

9. Malecka, A., Troen, G., Tierens, A. et al. (2018). Frequent somatic mutations of KMT2D (MLL2) and CARD11 genes in primary cold agglutinin disease. *Br J Haematol.* 183(5), 838–842.
10. Malecka, A., Troen, G., Delabie, J. et al. (2021). The mutational landscape of cold agglutinin disease: CARD11 and CXCR4 mutations are correlated with lower hemoglobin levels. *Am J Hematol.* 96(8), E279–E283.
11. Berentsen, S., Barcellini, W., D'Sa, S. et al. (2020). Cold agglutinin disease revisited: a multinational, observational study of 232 patients. *Blood* 136(4), 480–488.12.
12. Luzzatto L, Pandolfi PP. (2015). Causality and chance in the development of cancer. *N Engl J Med.* 373(1), 84–8.
13. Roth, A., Barcellini, W., D'Sa, S. et al. (2021). Sutimlimab in cold agglutinin disease. *N Engl J Med.* 384(14), 1323–1334.
14. Berentsen S. (2025). Diagnosis and management of cold agglutinin disease. *Hematology Am Soc Hematol Educ Program.* 2025(1), 295–304.

Case 26

When It Rains, a Microbe Makes It Pour

Patient Details

Age: 11 *Sex:* M
Ethnic background: Zambia

Reason for Referral

Previously diagnosed as sickle cell disease.

History and Clinical Findings in Brief

The mother reported that this boy had been originally diagnosed as sickle cell disease in their native country, Zambia, at the age of two. Over the last one year, the patient had had one hospital admission for one week. Apart from this, he was rather well; he did well in school, and his steady-state Hb was 7–8 g/dl. On this occasion, the patient was admitted to our hospital because of cough, malaise and chest pain, which had started three days previously. On examination, he was of minute build, with weight and height at the third centile. He was tachypnoeic and mildly icteric, with coarse crepitations and bronchial breathing in the left lower part of the chest. A chest X-ray revealed a left upper lobe consolidation.

Laboratory Findings

The patient had moderate to severe anaemia, slightly microcytic, normochromic (see Table 26.1). The blood film (see Figure 26.1) showed significant auto-agglutination, many target cells, some of which had their central membrane area folded over as if forming an envelope. There were also poikilocytes; some small and dense, but mostly elongated and some with sharp extremities; these do not quite qualify for irreversibly sickled cells because they retain central pallor. True sickle cells were very rare, and some of them appeared to have condensation of their haemoglobin over only one half of the cell (sickle-hemighosts). Also, there were a few microcytic cells that were very hypochromic. In addition, there was polychromasia and an occasional nucleated red cell. Very occasional metamyelocytes and plasmacytoid lymphocytes (Turk cells) could be seen.

Table 26.1 Haematology Data

	Patient	Mother
Hb (g/dl)	7.6	13.4
RBC ($\times 10^{12}$/l)	2.74	4.46
MCV (fl)	77.0	90.6
MCH (pg)	27.7	30.0
MCHC (g/dl)	36.0	33.2
RDW (S.D.)	65.4	45.8
Retic (%)	7.0	–
Retic ($\times 10^9$/l)	191	–
Hb A_2 (%)	2.9	2.6
Hb F (%)	2.7	0.5
G6PD (IU/g Hb)	5.8	2.1
α-globin	α-/αα	-

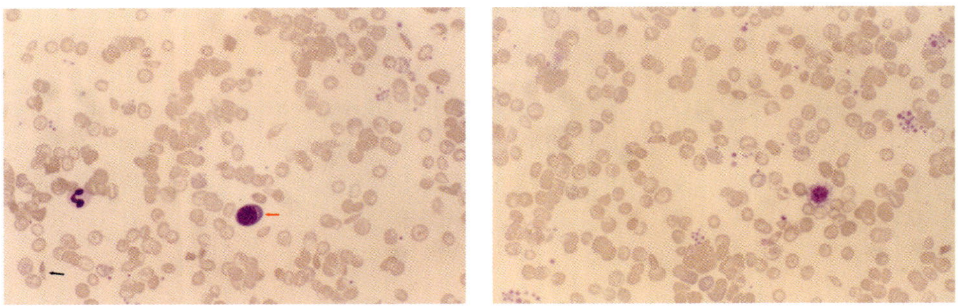

(a) (b)

Figure 26.1 Peripheral blood film; (a) and (b) medium power views. In (a) note sickle-hemighost (black arrow); Turk cell (red arrow).

Initial Assessment

We had no reason to doubt the prior diagnosis of sickle cell disease. The haemoglobin level would be compatible with homozygous Hb S; the many target cells might have suggested Hb S/C disease, but Hb C is common in parts of West Africa, not in Zambia. Hb S/beta thalassaemia would be unlikely, in view of the normal MCH.

Further Investigations

Haemoglobin electrophoresis showed Hb S (94.4%) and Hb A_2 (2.9%) with absence of Hb A. The Hb F level was 2.7%. Agar gel electrophoresis confirmed homozygous Hb S. α-globin gene analysis was consistent with α^+ thal heterozygous state. Assay of G6PD revealed G6PD deficiency, and enzyme electrophoresis confirmed G6PD A–. From these data, the diagnosis of sickle cell anaemia made in Zambia was fully supported. However, the red cell auto-agglutination is not explained by this diagnosis. In view of the respiratory infection, serological investigations were carried out (see Table 26.2).

Comments

The clinical spectrum of sickle cell anaemia is wide: in this patient it has been "mild" with respect to pain crises and hospital admissions, but his physical development was impaired, possibly due to inadequate folic acid supply during growth (his α-thalassaemia trait might have prevented his MCV from becoming high).

Several microorganisms can cause pulmonary complications in patients with sickle cell disease; and the term "acute chest syndrome" (ACS) was introduced by Davies et al. to designate a clinical event that is potentially life-threatening [1]. In a review of nearly 600 episodes

Table 26.2 Additional Studies

DAGT	Weakly positive[a]
Cold agglutinin titre	>1/512[b]
Monospot	Negative
CMV	1/16
Mycoplasma pneumoniae	1/8000

[a] Complement only.
[b] Two weeks later this reduced to 1/64.

of ACS, *Mycoplasma pneumoniae* was involved in 9% of cases [2]. This patient had pulmonary consolidation but he did not qualify for ACS because he had no dyspnoea or oxygen desaturation. Auto-agglutination *in vitro* at room temperature occurring immediately after withdrawal of blood is a striking finding in patients with *M. pneumoniae*: in our case it was noted by our senior registrar, who suggested the diagnosis, which was indeed confirmed by serology. Thus, treatment was promptly instigated, and the pneumonia responded to erythromycin without significant exacerbation of the anaemia. The autoantibody is IgM, and the basis for its anti-I specificity is related to the close chemical relationship between carbohydrate structures on the surface of *M. pneumoniae* and the Ii antigens of human red cells [3].

A G6PD assay was carried out as part of a haemolytic anaemia work-up. A G6PD-deficient hemizygous male would usually have a level below 2 IU/g Hb (normal range 7–10.4), but it is well known that in sickle cell anaemia the level is increased – sometimes even to the extent of being in the normal range – on account of reticulocytosis and a young red cell population [4]. From the data in this old paper and from a recent review [5], we can say there is no major impact of G6PD deficiency on the clinical steady state of sickle cell disease.

This patient with a chronic haemolytic disorder, sickle cell anaemia, had also an additional genetic abnormality of the red cell, G6PD deficiency, which made him susceptible to acute haemolysis [6]; and he suffered from an infection (*M. pneumoniae*) that can also by itself cause acute haemolysis. Thus, compared to his steady state, during this episode he may have had accelerated haemolysis; it is almost surprising that, from clinical and laboratory data, this has not been more conspicuous. G6PD deficiency might have contributed to the morphology of red cells (hemi-ghosts).

Follow-up

Once the infection was cleared, the boy was discharged on regular folic acid (5 mg/day); at several outpatient visits over a period of one and a half years, there were no further complications. We notice that the importance of adequate supply of folic acid in patients with sickle cell disease – especially children – is not sufficiently appreciated. This boy's height and weight came nearly within the normal range, and he continued to do very well at school.

Conclusion

Mycoplasma pneumoniae pulmonary infection in a patient with homozygous sickle cell anaemia, α^+ thalassaemia trait and G6PD deficiency.

Acknowledgements

Dr. Irene Roberts, Department of Haematology, Hammersmith Hospital, London, UK.

References

1. Davies, S.C., Luce, P.J., Win, A.A. et al. (1984). Acute chest syndrome in sickle-cell disease. *Lancet* 1(8367), 36–38.
2. Neumayr, L., Lennette, E., Kelly, D. et al. (2003). *Mycoplasma* disease and acute chest syndrome in sickle cell disease. *Pediatrics* 112(1 Pt 1), 87–95.
3. Loomes, L.M., Uemura, K., Childs, R.A. et al. (1984). Erythrocyte receptors for *Mycoplasma pneumoniae* are sialylated oligosaccharides of Ii antigen type. *Nature* 307, 560–563.
4. Bienzle, U., Sodeinde, O., Effiong, C.E. et al. (1975). Glucose 6-phosphate dehydrogenase deficiency and sickle cell anemia: frequency and features of the association in an African community. *Blood* 46, 591–597.
5. Karafin, M.S., Fu, X., D'Alessandro, A. et al. (2018). The clinical impact of glucose-6-phosphate dehydrogenase deficiency in patients with sickle cell disease. *Curr. Opin. Hematol*. 25, 494–499.
6. Luzzatto, L., Ally, M., and Notaro, R. (2020). Glucose-6-phosphate dehydrogenase deficiency. *Blood* 136, 1225–1240.

See also related Cases 6, 15 and 34.

Case 27

Double Membranes May Prove Ineffective

Patient Details

Age: 38 *Sex:* M
Ethnic background: English

Reason for Referral

Investigation of anaemia and jaundice.

History and Clinical Findings in Brief

The patient, who works in the "Dry-cleaning" business, reported suffering of malaise and mild anaemia for many years. On examination, he was mildly jaundiced and his liver was enlarged to 3 cm below the costal border. The spleen was also similarly enlarged, and there were five spider naevi over the upper sternum.

Laboratory Findings

The patient had a mild macrocytic anaemia (see Table 27.1) with normal white cell and platelet counts. The reticulocyte percentage is increased, but the absolute count is normal. Examination of the blood film (see Figure 27.1) confirmed the slight macrocytosis and also showed poikilocytes, densely contracted cells, occasional polychromatic cells and very rare nucleated red cells.

Additional baseline studies (see Table 27.2) revealed an increased bilirubin, increased ferritin and undetectable haptoglobins, consistent with intravascular haemolysis. By contrast, serum B12 and folate levels were normal. In view of the macrocytic picture, with normal B12 and folate, a diagnostic bone marrow aspirate was indicated (see Figure 27.2).

This was extremely cellular. Myeloid : erythroid ratio was 1 : 5. There was marked erythroid hyperplasia with an excess of mature orthochromic normoblasts, many of which had pycnotic nuclei. The most striking abnormality was the presence of numerous binucleated and multinucleated normoblasts, with frequent karyorrhexis and sometimes with the appearance of "bomb-shell" nuclear fragmentation. Abundant iron was present in the fragments but relatively little in the erythron; these findings, taken together, indicated severe dyserythropoiesis.

Table 27.1 Haematology Data

Hb (g/dl)	11.0
RBC ($\times 10^{12}$/l)	3.05
MCV (fl)	101
MCH (pg)	36.0
MCHC (g/dl)	35.8
RDW (S.D.)	63.1
Retic (%)	2.8
Retic ($\times 10^{9}$/l)	85
WBC ($\times 10^{9}$/l)	6.2
PLT ($\times 10^{9}$/l)	197

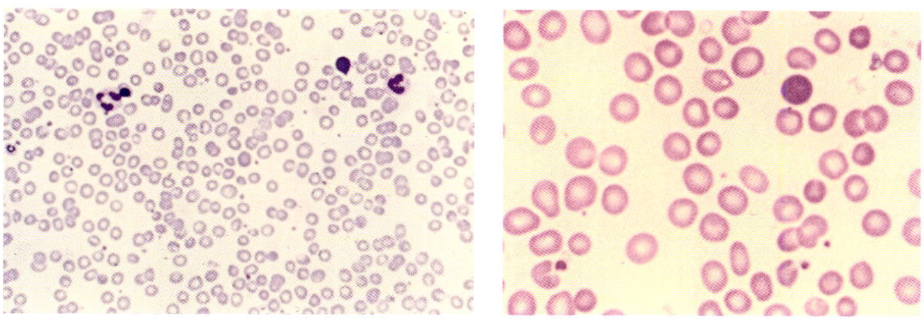

(a) (b)

Figure 27.1 Peripheral blood film: (a) medium power view; (b) high power view.

Table 27.2 Additional Baseline Studies

Bilirubin (μmol/l)	72
AST (IU/l)	56
B12 (ng/l)	410
Serum folate (μg/l)	1.88
Red cell folate (μg/l)	201
Ferritin (μg/l)	1765
Haptoglobins (mg/dl)	Undetected

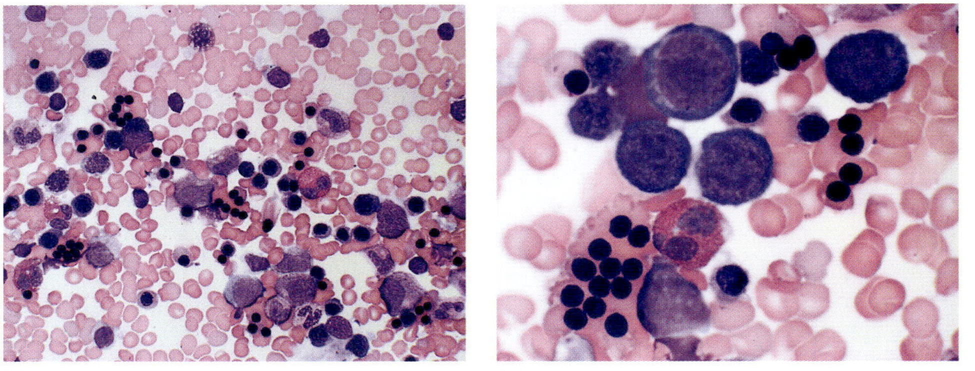

(a) (b)

Figure 27.2 Bone marrow aspirate: (a) low power view; (b) high power view.

Initial Assessment

The patient has a mild macrocytic anaemia, apparently of long standing. The bone marrow findings, particularly binucleated and multinucleated erythroid precursors, were highly suggestive of CDA II, known at the time also by the acronym HEMPAS (*Hereditary Erythroblastic Multinuclearity with Positive Acidified Serum*). The marked erythroid hyperplasia, as against the rather modest reticulocyte output, was consistent with ineffective erythropoiesis, a major pathophysiologic characteristic of CDA.

Further Investigations

Haemoglobin electrophoresis, osmotic fragility and red cell enzyme assays were all normal. Investigations for unstable haemoglobins, the direct antiglobulin test, urinary haemosiderin were all negative. An autohaemolysis test (see Table 27.3) was markedly abnormal, with full correction by glucose. Although we could not find any previous data on the results of this test in CDA, this finding was consistent with an abnormal red cell membrane.

Ferrokinetic studies (see Table 27.4) revealed a very rapid clearance of radiolabelled iron, an approximately sixfold increase in turnover rate and poor utilization, providing definitive confirmation of ineffective erythropoiesis.

As for the acidified serum test, it is based on antibodies that recognize abnormally glycosylated band 3 (the anion-exchanger AE1 that is the most abundant protein in the red cell membrane). These complement-binding IgM antibodies are present in some but not all normal people [1], and they are absent in patients with CDA II. We tested our patient's red cells against ABO-compatible sera from 20 different donors (see Table 27.5). The result was positive with 7 out of 20 sera, and haemolysis ranged from 9 to 27% (Table 27.5). As expected, and unlike in PNH, the result was negative with the patient's own serum.

Another serological finding in CDA II is that the red cells react strongly with anti-i, as though they were from newborn infants (not done in this case).

Red cells from our patient were studied extensively in the laboratory of Michiko Fukuda (La Jolla, California); she found decreased glycosylation of membrane proteins and incompletely processed asparagine-linked oligosaccharides (see Figure 27.3). It was thought at

Table 27.3 Results of Autohaemolysis Test

	% Lysis at 48 hours	
	Without glucose	Addition of glucose
CONTROL	1.9	0.6
PATIENT	23.0	1.7

Table 27.4 Ferrokinetic Data

Plasma Fe. clearance time (T_{50}; min)	32	(N 60–140)
Plasma Fe. turnover (µmol/l/day)	813	(N 100–150)
Red cell Fe. utilization by day 14 (%)	17	(N 70–80)

Table 27.5 Results of Acidified Serum (Ham) Test

	Patient's serum	Donor serum							13 additional donor sera
		A	B	C	D	E	F	G	
% lysis[a]	0	27	14	11	11	25	9	15	<2

[a] Of patient's red cells.

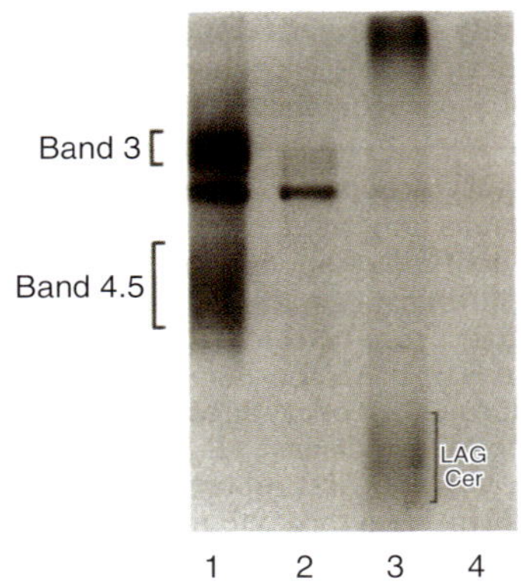

Figure 27.3 Fluorogram of surface-labelled red cell membrane components. Erythrocytes were treated with galactose oxidase followed by $NaB[^3H]_4$. Surface-labelled erythrocytes were incubated with or without endo-β-galactosidase. Erythrocyte membranes were then prepared, dissolved in $NaDodSo_4$ sample buffer and analyzed by $NaDodSo_4$/PAGE followed by fluorography. Fluorograms of normal (lanes 1 and 2) and patient (lanes 3 and 4) membranes have been treated with (lanes 2 and 4) and without (lanes 1 and 3) endo-β-galactosidase. LAG-Cer = polylactosaminylceramides. [2]/with permission of National Academy of Sciences.

the time that the primary lesion might be an enzyme deficiency; in our patient acetylglucosaminyltransferase II activity was normal, whereas alpha-mannosidase II was low, but the results were inconclusive.

In the event, it was not until 2009 that the molecular basis of CDA II was cracked [3]. The gene had been mapped to 20p11.23, and it was now identified as *SEC23B*. Molecular analysis of DNA of our patient performed at Kings College Hospital, London, revealed biallelic mutations of *SEC23B*: one allele had a previously reported missense mutation, c.325G>A p.(Glu109Lys); and the other allele had a novel missense mutation, c.800G>T p.(Gly267Val).

Comments

CDA type II is a rare form of genetically determined anaemia, with a recessive pattern of inheritance. The lifelong anaemia varies from mild to severe, and usually there is associated splenomegaly [4]. The pathogenesis of the anaemia is twofold; decreased production due to ineffective erythropoiesis is probably the major component, but increased peripheral destruction due to the mature red cells being abnormal is not negligible, as attested by the fact that splenectomy may alleviate the anaemia.

The path of investigations in our patient illustrates somehow the history of our understanding of CDA II. Initially the diagnosis was based on the remarkable multi-nuclearity seen in the bone marrow; then came the serological findings, whereby this was the only condition, other than PNH, with a positive Ham test; then came the abnormal glycosylation of red cell membrane proteins; and finally, bi-allelic mutation of *SEC23B*.

SEC23B[1] is a key component of the outer layer of the coat protein complex II (COPII) vesicles, which mediate protein transport from the endoplasmic reticulum (ER) to the Golgi apparatus. *SEC23B* may play a role in the assembly or deconstruction of the mid-body, a structure consisting of microtubules and other proteins that forms during the final stages of cell division; thus, loss of *SEC23B* function might account for the impaired cytokinesis observed in CDA II erythroblasts, and *SEC23B* is also involved in autophagy. Clustering of band 3-associated proteins and lipids may account for the characteristic abnormal structures, including vesicles and autophagic vacuoles, with blebs and clefts, associated with a double membrane, seen by electron microscopy in CDA II [5]. Why the phenotype associated with *SEC23B* mutations is erythroid-specific is still incompletely understood: erythroid-specific cargoes, such as the highly abundant band 3, might require, for appropriate transport, a high level of *SEC23B*, the function of which, in other cells, might be surrogated by the other COPII component *SEC23A*. In the majority of patients, CDA II is caused by missense mutations [6, 7]; and no patient has two nonsense mutations, suggesting that complete inactivation of *SEC23B* might be lethal.

A good animal model of CDA II has not yet been achieved. However, when *SEC23B* was silenced in human erythroleukemia cells, binucleated cells were formed [3]; and short hairpin RNA-mediated suppression of *SEC23B* expression recapitulates the cytokinesis defect. In zebrafish, knockdown of *sec23b* leads to aberrant erythrocyte development.

Although haemosiderosis is seen also in patients with a variety of other anaemias, in some patients with CDA type II it can be particularly severe, leading to liver cirrhosis [8, 9]. Recently it has been suggested that luspatercept, already in use to ameliorate ineffective erythropoiesis in thalassaemia and in MDS, might be useful in CDA II [10].

[1] The term SEC echoes the role of this protein in secretory pathways, but in erythroid cells we are dealing with intracellular protein trafficking rather than secretion. *SEC23B* is a GTPase-activating protein.

Follow-up

Over some 20 years the patient has remained moderately anaemic, but stable, and without evidence of systemic iron overload. At the age of 62, hypothyroidism was diagnosed and the patient was commenced on thyroxine. Subsequently, following an infection, the patient developed acute renal failure and nephrotic syndrome; he was started on a blood transfusion regimen and, for some time, he required 2 units of blood per month plus erythropoietin 8,000 units three times per weeks. Seven months later, a FerriScan revealed iron overload, and the patient was started on deferasirox. Later that year, he underwent a splenectomy. At the most recent clinic appointment (age 73), his counts have remained stable, with haemoglobin of 10.8, neutrophil count of 16 and a platelet count (post-splenectomy) of 425. Clearly CDA II is a serious condition, but we can see from this case history that it is manageable and compatible with active life and a normal life span.

Conclusion

Congenital dyserythropoietic anaemia: CDA type II.

Acknowledgements

Referred by Dr. A. J. P. Willis, Consultant physician, Southend Hospital, Essex, UK.
M.N. Fukuda, La Jolla Cancer Research Foundation, California, USA.
Dr. M.J. Mills, Department of Haematology, Southend Hospital, Essex, UK.
Dr. N. Traub, Department of Haematology, Southend Hospital, Essex, UK.
The Department of Molecular Pathology, Kings College Hospital, London, UK.

References

1. Crookston, J.H., Crookston, M.C., Burnie, K.L. et al. (1969). Hereditary erythroblastic multinuclearity associated with a positive acidified-serum test: a type of congenital dyserythropoietic anaemia. *Br. J. Haematol.* 17(1), 11–26.
2. Fukuda, M.N., Masri, K.A., Dell, A. et al. (1990). Incomplete synthesis of N-glycans in congenital dyserythropoietic anemia type II caused by a defect in the gene encoding alpha-mannosidase II. *Proc. Natl. Acad. Sci. USA*. 87, 7443–7447.
3. Schwarz, K., Iolascon, A., Verissimo, F. et al. (2009). Mutations affecting the secretory COPII coat component SEC23B cause congenital dyserythropoietic anemia type II. *Nat. Genet.* 41, 936–940.

4. Iolascon, A., Andolfo, I., and Russo, R. (2020). Congenital dyserythropoietic anemias. *Blood* 136, 1274–1283.
5. Fresco, R. (1981). Electron microscopy in the diagnosis of the bone marrow disorders of the erythroid series. *Semin. Hematol.* 18, 279–292.
6. Iolascon, A., Heimpel, H., Wahlin, A. et al. (2013). Congenital dyserythropoietic anemias: molecular insights and diagnostic approach. *Blood* 122(13), 2162–2166.
7. Musri, M., Venturi, V., Ferrer-Cortès, X. et al. (2023). New cases and mutations in *SEC23B* gene causing congenital dyserythropoietic anemia type II. *Int. J. Mol. Sci.* 24, 9935.
8. Faruqui, S., Abraham, A., Berenfeld, M.R. et al. (1982). Normal serum ferritin level in a patient with HEMPAS syndrome and iron overload. *Am. J. Clin. Path.* 78, 97–101.
9. Halpern, Z., Rahmani, R., and Levo, Y. (1985). Severe hemochromatosis: the predominant clinical manifestation of congenital dyserythropoietic anaemia type II (CDA II). *Br. J. Haematol.* 50, 35–41.
10. Cazzola, M. (2021). Ineffective erythropoiesis and its treatment. *Blood* 139(16), 2460–2470.

Case 28

Making Less but Being Dominant

Patient Details

Age: 32 *Sex:* M
Ethnic background: Iran
Occupation: Civil engineer

Reason for Referral

Mild persistent jaundice in a patient with β-thalassaemia trait.

History and Clinical Findings in Brief

The patient has enjoyed good health and lives a very active life. He remembers having been admitted to hospital on two occasions, at the age of 10 for jaundice (when he was told he had infective hepatitis) and at the age of 18 for "glandular fever." He is aware that his eyes are always "a bit yellow" and that this discolouration tends to fluctuate in intensity. The Royal Marsden Hospital kindly provided records for this patient since 1968, from which we learned: (i) the patient's haemoglobin at the age of 10 varied between 8.4 and 10.8 g/dl over a four-month period; (ii) the osmotic fragility was markedly *reduced*; (iii) there was an episode of jaundice with a marked increase in transaminase, but this fully reverted to baseline, compatible with an outbreak in the school of what we assume must have been hepatitis A. “Thalassaemia trait” had been traced in his family through three generations. On physical examination, the patient’s general condition was good. He appeared slightly pale and mildly jaundiced. His spleen could not be felt. The rest of the examination was essentially normal.

Laboratory Findings

The patient had a moderate microcytic, hypochromic anaemia (see Figure 28.1). The blood film was quite spectacular (see Figure 28.2), with very numerous poikilocytes and marked anisocytosis: the red cells in general were very microcytic, and some were incredibly tiny in size. We saw teardrop cells, in some of which the projection was longer and thicker than commonly observed (“hand-mirror” cells). Some cells were dense and irregular in shape, whilst others looked like they were on their way to becoming spherocytes; others showed uneven condensation (“puddling”) of haemoglobin; others yet were profoundly

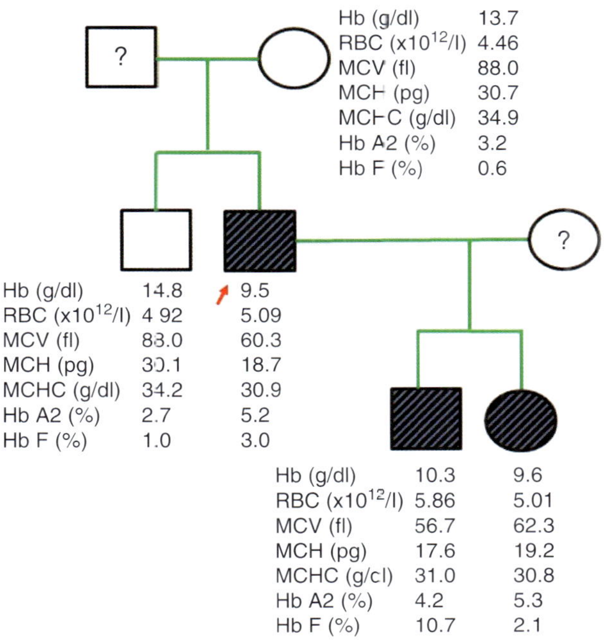

Figure 28.1 Family pedigree. The index case, indicated by the red arrow, had been diagnosed as β-thalassaemia intermedia. His brother and mother had normal red cell parameters, including normal HbA_2. The patient’s partner was unavailable for peripheral blood analysis; his daughter and son also had mild anaemia and thalassaemic indices, implying they had inherited their father’s β-thalassaemia allele. Unlike his father and his sister, the son was found to have raised Hb F level, 10.7%.

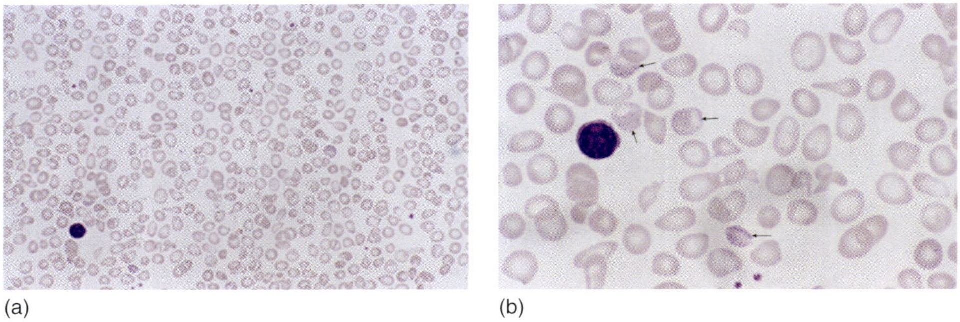

Figure 28.2 Peripheral blood film: (a) low power; (b) high power to show basophilic stippling (arrowed).

Table 28.1 Additional Baseline Studies

Bilirubin (μmol/1)	63.4
Haptoglobin (mg/dl)	<35
P-5′-N (Ratio)[a]	2.8
G-6-PD (IU/g Hb)	19.3

[a] Ratio of absorbances; 280:260.

hypochromic. What appeared to be confined to the more polychromatic cells was quite pronounced basophilic stippling, with coarse granules in some of the cells.

Additional baseline studies (see Table 28.1) revealed an increased bilirubin and decreased level of haptoglobins, consistent with extravascular and mild intravascular haemolysis. In view of the basophilic stippling, we tested for pyrimidine-5′-nucleotidase (P-5′-N), which was normal. G6PD activity was above the top of the reference range.[1]

Initial Assessment

The elevated Hb A_2 was consistent with β thalassaemia trait; of the red cell indices, the MCV and MCH were in keeping with this, but the MCHC is usually normal in β thalassaemia trait. The important additional fact was that the patient had a long-standing mild to moderate anaemia, and we felt

[1] The high G6PD level can be explained by a young red cell population. In addition, it should be borne in mind that calculation based on lysate-haemoglobin measurement will overestimate the enzyme activity per red cell when red cells are small; for this reason, in the past it has been sometimes preferred to express enzyme activity in units per red cell count.

the abnormalities of the red cells were far too florid, the basophilic stippling too pronounced for an "ordinary" β thalassaemia trait.

Further Investigations

An *in vitro* biosynthetic globin-chain analysis yielded a non-α : α ratio of 0.47, consistent with heterozygous β-thalassaemia.

Heat stability of haemoglobin and isopropanol precipitation tests were also normal. In view of the marked morphological abnormalities of the red cells, we considered the possibility of a membrane abnormality (the increased osmotic *resistance* associated with β-thalassaemia trait might have masked this in the osmotic fragility test). However, the analysis of red cell membrane proteins by SDS-PAGE on a gradient gel stained with Coomassie Blue and of the glycoproteins (PAS stain on a 10% acrylamide gel) yielded normal patterns.

A bone marrow aspirate (see Figure 28.3) showed marked erythroid hyperplasia, with karyorrhexis in some of the cells. The bone marrow trephine (see Figure 28.4) showed erythroid hyperplasia with dyserythropoietic features. There was mild focal increase in reticulin (not shown). The karyotype was normal.

A ferrokinetic study showed rapid iron clearance with high plasma iron turnover but low utilization (see Table 28.2). Thus, the patient has an incompletely compensated chronic haemolytic disorder with evidence of ineffective erythropoiesis.

β-thalassaemia is relatively prevalent in Iran: given its geographic location, the β-thalassaemia alleles found among Iranians include both some common in Asia and some common in the Mediterranean. We first tested

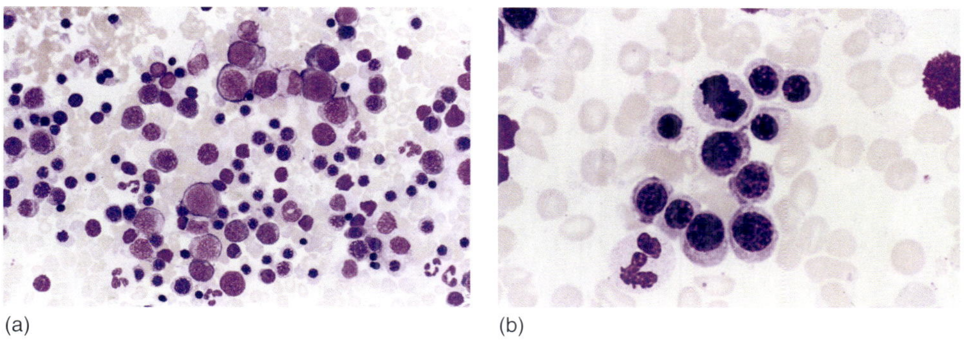

Figure 28.3 Bone marrow aspirate: (a) medium power view; (b) high power view showing dyserythropoietic features.

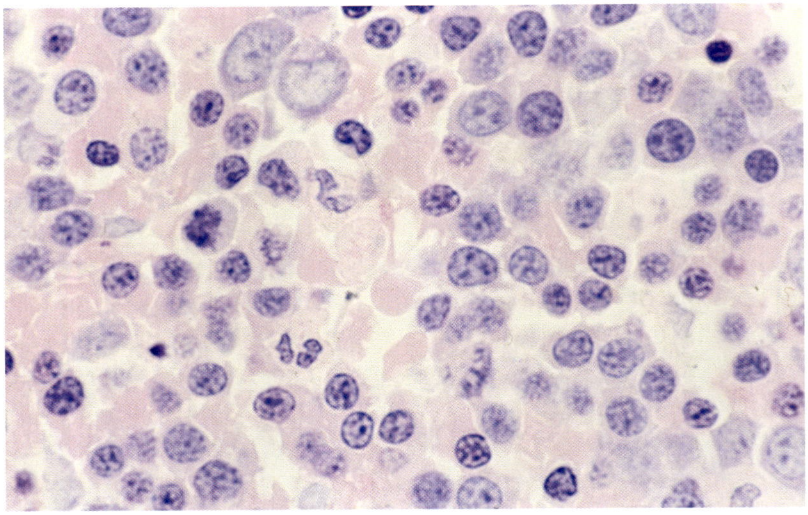

Figure 28.4 Bone marrow trephine: high power view.

Table 28.2 Ferrokinetic Studies

Plasma iron (μmol/1)	9.0	
Transferrin (g/l)	2.08	
TSI (%)	16	
Plasma Fe. clearance time (T_{50}; min)	18	(N 60–140)
Plasma Fe. turnover (μmol/1/day)	345	(N 100–150)
Plasma Fe. utilization[a] (%)	31	(N 70–80)

[a] By day 11.

for these mutations (see Table 28.3), but none of them was found. Southern blot analysis yielded only normal fragments with α, β and γ-globin genomic probes.

Direct sequencing of the PCR-amplified β-globin gene revealed, in addition to a normal allele, a mutant allele that had, at the 5' end of intron 2, an 11 bp insertion and a 2 bp deletion (see Figure 28.5). Sequencing of cDNA reverse transcribed from RNA from the patient's peripheral blood reticulocytes revealed, in addition to the normal mRNA, two species of abnormal mRNA, that must have arisen through activation of alternative (cryptic) splice sites. Based on the size of these mRNA species we can infer translation into two species of abnormally short β-globin chains, with lengths of 101 and 107 amino acids respectively (instead of 146).

Table 28.3 Point Mutations Reported from Iran

IVS 1 nt 1	(G→T)
IVS 1 nt 1	(G→A)
IVS 1 nt 110	(G→A)
IVS 1 nt 5	(G→C)
Codon 39	(C→T)
Frameshift codon 8/9	(+G)

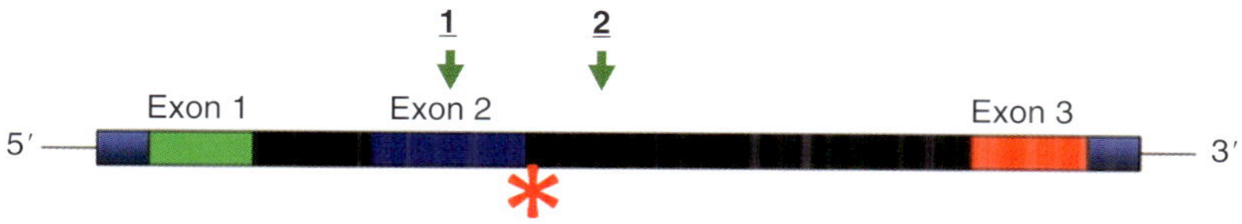

Figure 28.5 Diagram of β-globin gene (*HBB*). In this patient an insertion-deletion at the boundary of exon 2 and intron 2 (red asterisk) destroys the intron 2 splice donor site. As a result, two 'cryptic' splice sites are activated (green arrows), one in exon 2 and one in intron 2.

These globin chains include "illicit" translation of intronic sequences, and are therefore in large part gibberish: they are terminated when a stop codon is encountered.

Comments

The notion that in a heterozygote a gene can be dominant or recessive is one that goes back to Gregor Mendel, the recognized founder of formal genetics. We can now see clearly that this notion must be applied to individual alleles of the same gene. Nearly all of the millions of people with β-thalassemia have one of many *loss of function* mutations, that simply make less or no β-globin chains (in jargon, β^+ or β^0): therefore these alleles are recessive. In this patient, instead, the mutant allele produces abnormal β-globins: thus, this is a gain of function mutation or, from the pathophysiological point of view, a *gain of malfunction* mutation. It has indeed two effects: (i) the mutant allele cannot make normal β-globin; (ii) the mutant allele produces abnormal β-globin chains that form highly unstable αβ dimers and haemoglobin tetramers, or cannot make them at all: therefore the maturation of erythroid cells is damaged. (i) accounts for the decreased non-α/α biosynthetic ratio and for the increased Hb A_2; (ii) accounts for ineffective erythropoiesis.

Since gain of malfunction causes trouble even with only one mutant allele, the clinical manifestations are conspicuous in a heterozygote, and therefore the condition is also referred to as *dominant β-thalassaemia*. This explains in our patient the lifelong anaemia with hyperbilirubinaemia, which may be subject to acute exacerbations during infective episodes, as was the case when he first presented at age 10. Since the patient has never had blood transfusion and his anaemia has been mild to moderate, he can be also regarded as belonging to the heterogeneous group of *thalassaemia intermedia*.

To the best of our knowledge, the mutation found in this patient is unique [1]. There are several groups of mutations causing dominant β-thalassemia: this one belongs to the group with frameshifts or aberrant splicing [1]. The patient and his two affected children have low MCHC values, which may be a consequence of loss of haeme from abnormal haemoglobin molecules (as previously observed in another family [2]. For the two children, who had inherited the paternal mutation, appropriate clinical and haematological monitoring was recommended.

Follow-up

The patient was discharged on folic acid. At the age of 37, the patient had an aplastic crisis attributed to Parvovirus. Imaging studies showed hepatic haemangiomas and an enlarged spleen. At the age of 58, he had elective aortic repair for a dilated aortic root. At the age of 59, a full haematology review gave results very similar to those at the age of 32; a bone scan was normal. The patient stated that he was well in himself and that he had recently switched to a vegan diet.

Conclusion

β-thalassaemia intermedia (also referred to as "dominant β-thalassaemia" or inclusion-body β-thalassaemia trait), due to a single mutant β-globin allele producing abnormal β-chains.

Acknowledgements

Referred by Dr. M. J. Saary, Consultant Haematologist, 81, Harley Street, London, UK.
Dr. M. Reid, International Blood Group Reference Laboratory (IBGRL), Bristol, UK.
The Royal Marsden Hospital, London. UK.

References

1. Thein, S.L. (2001). Structural variants with a β-thalassemia phenotype. In: Steinberg, M.H., Forget, B.G., Higgs, D.R. et al. editor. *Disorders of Hemoglobin*. Vol. 1. Cambridge: Cambridge University Press. pp. 342–355.
2. Stamatoyannopoulos, G., Woodson, R., Papayannopoulou, T. et al. (1974). Inclusion-body beta-thalassemia trait. A form of beta thalassemia producing clinical manifestations in simple heterozygotes. *N. Engl. J. Med*. 290(17), 939–943. https://doi.org/10.1056/NEJM197404252901705. PMID: 4361439.

Case 29

Two Enzymes Down, Still Standing

Patient Details

Age: 18 months *Sex:* F
Ethnic background: Oman

Reason for Referral

Investigation of congenital anaemia.

History and Clinical Findings in Brief

This young girl, the fifth child of her mother, had been born at full term by spontaneous vaginal delivery. Very shortly after birth, she was noted to be jaundiced. Her haemoglobin level at birth was 9.8 g/dl with a reticulocytosis of 21%. Her serum bilirubin was raised at 300 μmol/l. She was given an exchange blood transfusion and subsequently discharged home. Four weeks later, the girl was readmitted to hospital with recurrent anaemia. Further investigations in Oman failed to find the cause of her anaemia. She was therefore started on regular red cell transfusions and required about 300 ml every two months. She grew and developed normally. Family history revealed that her parents were first cousins; she had three siblings, all of whom were alive and well; there had been one stillborn male child.

Upon referral to Hammersmith Hospital, the girl looked well; her height was on the 90th centile, and her weight was on the 50th centile. She had hepatosplenomegaly: the liver was 4 cm and the spleen 3 cm below the costal border.

Laboratory Findings

On a blood count performed some five weeks after her last blood transfusion, the girl had a normal haemoglobin with normal reticulocyte, white cell and platelet counts. Her mean cell haemoglobin concentration was slightly reduced (see Table 29.1). The blood film showed mainly normal red cells, which were probably transfused; however, poikilocytes were rather prominent (not shown). Liver function tests gave normal results.

Bone marrow examination showed increased erythroid activity, but no other abnormalities. The red cell glucose-6-phosphate dehydrogenase (G6PD) activity was 5.4 U/g Hb (normal range 7.2–12.8 U/g Hb), and the red cell pyruvate kinase (PK) activity was also 5.4 U/g Hb (normal range 6.2–14.2 U/g Hb). Haemoglobin electrophoresis on cellulose acetate membrane revealed Hb A and Hb C; the latter quantitated at 31%. This was intriguing because neither of her parents had haemoglobin C.

Initial Assessment

We felt that recent blood transfusion precluded a definitive diagnosis. The red cell enzyme assays were borderline low, but blood transfusion might have masked an enzyme deficiency, and/or the transfused blood might have been itself G6PD deficient, as we knew this abnormality had a

Table 29.1 Haematology Data (Five Weeks Post Blood Transfusion)

Hb (g/dl)	11.7
MCV (fl)	82
MCH (pg)	27.3
MCHC (g/dl)	29
Retic (%)	1.6
WBC ($\times 10^9$/l)	9.4
Plt ($\times 10^9$/l)	358

prevalence of 26% in male donors in Oman [1]. The abnormal haemoglobin band required explaining. The family returned to Oman, where the child continued to receive periodic blood transfusions.

Further Investigations

A year later, the child returned to London for review and further investigations. She had been well in the preceding 11 months, and her growth and development remained normal. Her last red cell transfusion had been three months previously. On examination, she was pale and had hepatosplenomegaly, as previously noted. On this occasion, investigations revealed a severe macrocytic anaemia with elevated reticulocyte count (see Table 29.2).

Her blood film now showed macrocytosis, polychromasia and again spiculated red cells (see Figure 29.1). Repeat haemoglobin electrophoresis showed only Hb A and Hb A_2, confirming that the Hb C band detected previously had originated from transfused red cells. Her serum bilirubin concentration was mildly increased at 27 μmol/l. Her serum ferritin concentration was increased at 467 mg/l. An acidified serum lysis (Ham) test to exclude paroxysmal nocturnal haemoglobinuria gave negative result, and an osmotic fragility test was normal. The autohaemolysis test was positive, giving 6% lysis without additional glucose and 5.5% lysis with glucose (a control patient had 0.9% and 0.1% lysis without and with glucose). This "type II" pattern (no correction by glucose) suggested a glycolytic enzyme abnormality. Repeat assay of G6PD was significantly lower, suggesting homozygous G6PD deficiency; presumably, the earlier value was caused by G6PD-normal transfused red cells. The pyruvate kinase activity was again low (see Table 29.3), in spite of the marked reticulocytosis.

Table 29.2 Haematology Data

Hb (g/dl)	4.7
MCV (fl)	104.8
MCH (pg)	33.7
MCHC (g/dl)	29
Retic (%)	20.0
WBC ($\times 10^9$/l)	9.3
Plt ($\times 10^9$/l)	338

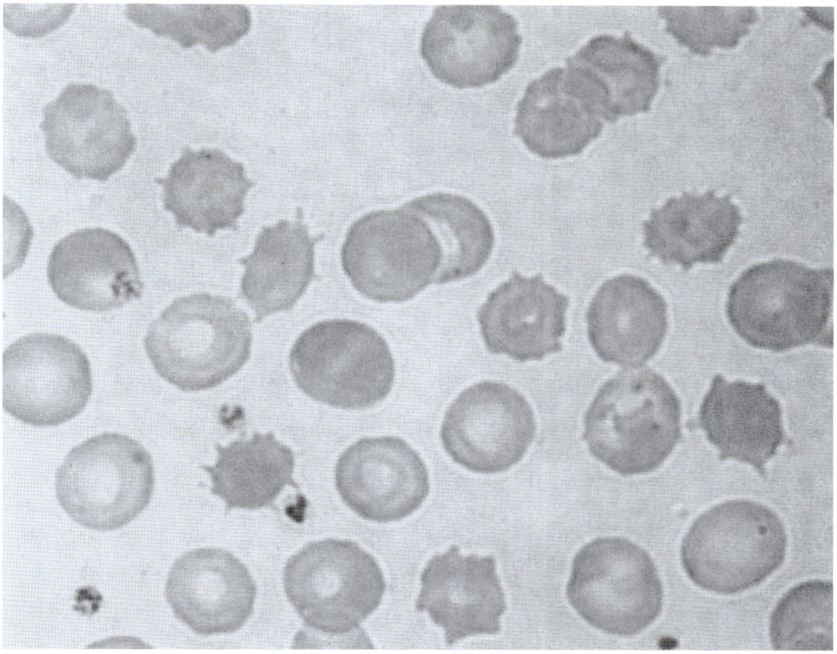

Figure 29.1 Peripheral blood film showing "prickle cells" in a patient with pyruvate kinase deficiency (picture not from this patient, whose blood film was very similar to this).

Table 29.3 Glucose-6-phosphate Dehydrogenase and Pyruvate Kinase Activities of Patient with Haemolytic Anaemia and Reference Ranges

	Initial	Follow-up	Reference range
G6PD (U/gHb)	5.4	0.7	7.2–12.8
PK (U/gHb)	5.4	4.5	6.5–14.2

Study of the patient's immediate family (Figure 29.2) revealed segregation not only for G6PD and PK deficiency, but also for β thalassaemia.

Comments

This patient had both G6PD deficiency and PK deficiency. In principle, her haemolytic anaemia might have resulted from either of the two enzymopathies or from a combination of both; however, DNA analysis showed that her G6PD deficiency was the common Mediterranean type (the most common variant in Oman) [1], and this variant does not cause *chronic* haemolysis, although it can cause acute haemolytic episodes when the patient is exposed to oxidant drugs, infections, or fava beans. This patient

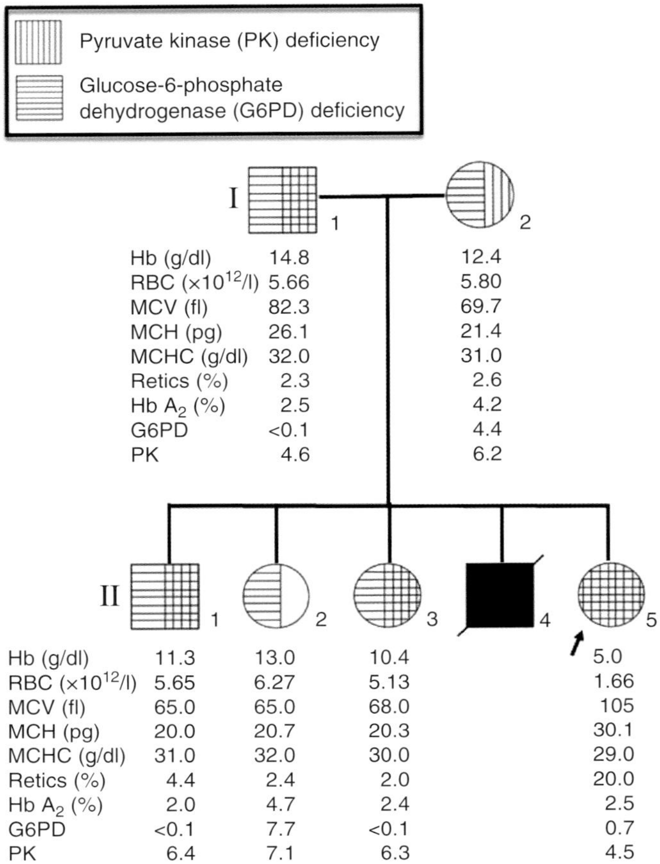

Figure 29.2 Pedigree of patient's family showing segregation of pyruvate kinase (PK), deficiency, glucose-6-phosphate dehydrogenase (G6PD) deficiency and β thalassaemia. Subjects I-1, II-1 are hemizygous for G6PD deficiency and heterozygous for PK deficiency; subject II-3 is homozygous for G6PD deficiency and heterozygous for PK deficiency; subject I-2 is heterozygous for both PK deficiency and G6PD deficiency; subject II-2 is heterozygous only for G6PD deficiency; and our patient, II-5 (arrowed), is homozygous for both G6PD deficiency and PK deficiency. Segregation of β thalassaemia is also seen, based on the high Hb A_2 level in I-2 and II-2 but not in II-1, II-3 and II-5.

also illustrates how multiple potentially pathogenic mutations can coexist, when a rare mutation (in this case in the *PKLR* gene) is present in a person belonging to a population where another mutation (in this case G6PD *Mediterranean*) is prevalent.

PK deficiency was first described in 1961 by Valentine et al. [2]; since then it has emerged as the second most common red cell enzyme defect after G6PD deficiency, and also as the most common cause of congenital chronic non-spherocytic haemolytic anaemia worldwide, with an estimated prevalence of one in 100,000 to one in 300,000 people [3]. PK deficiency results from mutations in the *PKLR* gene [4], which maps to chromosome 1q23; it is transmitted as an autosomal recessive trait, and because of its rarity most affected patients probably have inherited two different mutant allelic genes. However, a consanguineous marriage can result in a true homozygote, as presumably occurred in our patient.

More than 300 *PKLR* mutations causing PK deficiency have been reported (https://databases.lovd.nl/shared/genes/PKLR). These include missense mutations, stop-mutations, mutations that affect splicing, rare large deletions and others [5]. Overall, patients with two non-missense allelic mutations tend to have more severe disease; not surprisingly, since their PK activity in red cells is essentially absent.

Deficient PK activity results in inadequate ATP production: this failure of energy supply impacts on the cation pump, causing dehydration, membrane rigidity and ultimately premature destruction of red cells in the spleen or liver. Reticulocytes, because of their shift of ATP supply from oxidative phosphorylation to glycolysis, are particularly susceptible to dehydration and injury in the splenic environment [6]; as a result, paradoxically, they are sometimes low in PK activity in spite of haemolysis (not in our patient: see Table 29.2). As PK is the terminal enzyme in glycolysis, proximal glycolytic intermediates, including 2,3-bisphosphoglycerate (2,3-BPG) are generally increased. Anaemia is typically severe to moderate (haemoglobin levels ranging from 4.0 to 10.0 g/dl) but may be better tolerated, thanks to the increased 2,3-BPG concentration, which shifts the oxygen dissociation curve to the right, leading to increased oxygen supply to tissues.

The most important recent progress in the management of PK deficiency has been the introduction of mitapivat, a small molecule that is a specific activator of PK. A clinical trial has shown improvement of haemoglobin levels [7], specifically in patients in whom at least one *PKLR* mutation is of the missense type [8]; and mitapivat is now part of guidelines for the management of PK deficiency [3].

Follow-up

We recommended at the time that the patient receives antimalarial prophylaxis: in 2010, Oman has been declared by WHO malaria-free, and therefore this would be no longer necessary in that country. Today it would be indicated to do in this patient *PKLR* mutation analysis and, if appropriate, to introduce mitapivat therapy.

Conclusion

Congenital haemolytic anaemia due to pyruvate kinase deficiency, with coexistent glucose-6-phosphate dehydrogenase deficiency.

A summary of this case has been previously published [9].

Acknowledgement

Dr. Prem Mahendra, Department of Haematology, Hammersmith Hospital, London, UK.

References

1. Daar, S., Vulliamy, T.J., Kaeda, J. et al. (1996). Molecular characterization of G6PD deficiency in Oman. *Hum. Hered*. 46, 172–176.
2. Valentine, W.N., Tanaka, K.R., and Miwa, S. (1961). A specific erythrocyte glycolytic enzyme defect (pyruvate kinase) in three subjects with congenital non-spherocytic hemolytic anemia. *Trans. Assoc. Am. Physicians*. 74, 100–110. PMID: 13924348.
3. Al-Samkari, H., Shehata, N., Lang-Robertson, K., et al. (2024). Diagnosis and management of pyruvate kinase deficiency: international expert guidelines. *Lancet. Haematol*. 11(3), e228–e239.
4. Kanno, H., Fujii, H., Hirono, A. et al. (1991). cDNA cloning of human R-type pyruvate kinase and identification of a single amino acid substitution (Thr384—Met) affecting enzymatic stability in a pyruvate kinase variant (PK Tokyo) associated with hereditary hemolytic anemia. *Proc. Natl. Acad. Sci. USA*. 88 (18), 8218–8221.
5. Bianchi, P., Fermo, E., Lezon-Geyda, K. et al. (2020). Genotype-phenotype correlation and molecular heterogeneity in pyruvate kinase deficiency. *Am. J. Hematol*. 95(5), 472–482.
6. Mentzer, W.C. Jr., Baehner, R.L., Schmidt-Schönbein, H. et al. (1971). Selective reticulocyte destruction in erythrocyte pyruvate kinase deficiency. *J. Clin. Invest*. 50(3), 688–699.
7. van Dijk, M.J., Rab, M.A.E., van Oirschot, B.A. et al. (2023). One-year safety and efficacy of mitapivat in sickle cell disease: follow-up results of a phase 2, open-label study. *Blood Adv*. 7(24), 7539–7550.
8. Grace, R.F., Rose, C., Layton, D.M. et al. (2019). Safety and efficacy of mitapivat in pyruvate kinase deficiency. *N. Engl. J. Med*. 381(10), 933–944.
9. Mahendra, P., Dollery, C.T., Luzzatto, L. et al. (1992). Pyruvate kinase deficiency: association with G6PD deficiency. *Br. Med. J*. 305, 760–762.

Case 30

Sickle Cell Disease at 75

Patient Details

Age: 68 *Sex:* F
Ethnic background: Sierra Leone

Reason for Referral

An experienced GP referred this patient, believed to be a "sickler": but he thought she was too old for that.

History and Clinical Findings in Brief

The patient had been treated intermittently for gastritis. When she was in her late 40s, a sickling test was carried out as part of a routine check-up and was reported as positive. More recently, the patient tended to be fatigued and was thought to be somewhat depressed; she did complain recurrently about pains in her joints, and this was thought to be "rheumatic." On examination, the patient was in good general condition; somewhat overweight, not pale and not clinically jaundiced. The only specific physical finding was a spleen tip.

Laboratory Findings

The patient had a very mild normocytic, normochromic anaemia (see Table 30.1). On the blood film (see Figure 30.1), we could see target cells, in which the central portion was often eccentric and appeared to be pushed to the side of the cell. There were numerous small poikilocytes with a smooth outline, but also "teardrop" poikilocytes with sharp projections, and occasional large polychromatic cells. Highly contracted cells were also seen in small numbers.

Haemoglobin electrophoresis (see Figure 30.2a) revealed a major band of Hb S and minor bands of Hb A (17.4%) and Hb F (11.6%). Quantitation of Hb A_2 yielded a value of 5.1% (see Figure 30.2b).

Table 30.1 Haematology Data

	Patient	Sister
Hb (g/dl)	11.2	13.2
RBC ($\times 10^{12}$/l)	3.97	4.69
MCV (fl)	84.9	83.4
MCH (pg)	28.2	28.1
MCHC (g/dl)	33.2	33.8
RDW (S.D.)	44.0	45.5
Retic (%)	2.31	–
Retic ($\times 10^{9}$/l)	92	–
Hb A_2 (%)	5.1	4.4
Hb F (%)	11.6	3.0
Non-α : α ratio[a]	0.99	–
($\beta^S + \beta^A$): α ratio[a]	0.83	–

[a] Globin chain biosynthetic ratio.

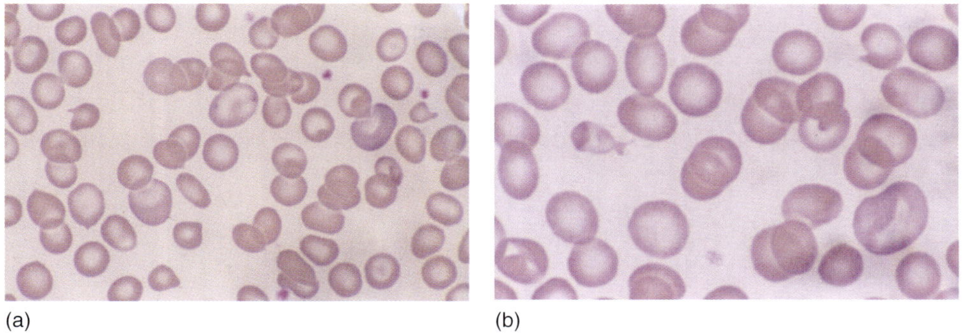

Figure 30.1 Peripheral blood film: (a) high power view; (b) higher magnification.

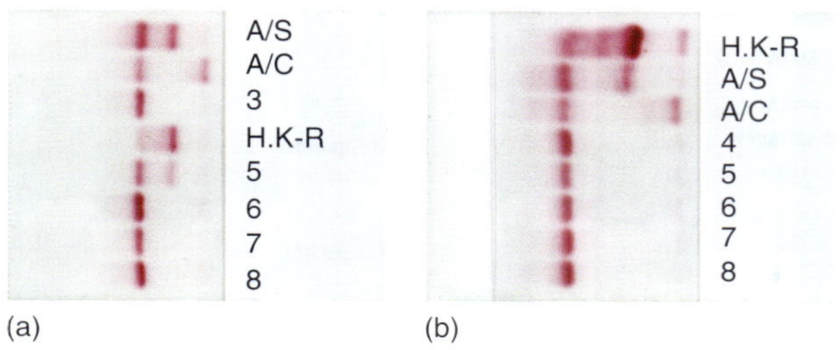

Figure 30.2 (a) Haemoglobin electrophoresis on cellulose acetate membrane; the migration of the haemoglobin fractions is from right to left. An A/S control and A/C control are in lanes 1 and 2, respectively. The patient H.K-R is in lane 4. (b) As (a), but with deliberate sample overloading. The patient H.K-R is in lane 1; the A/S control and A/C control are in lanes 2 and 3, respectively.

Initial Assessment

The patient's relatively mild clinical history, her age and the absence of sickle cells on the blood film were against a diagnosis of homozygous sickle cell anaemia; and this was ruled out by the presence of Hb A that, since she had not received any blood transfusion, must be her own. The most likely diagnosis was S/β^+ thalassaemia, although we were surprised by the patient's normal RBC indices.

Further Investigations

Vitamin B12 and folate levels were normal.

Beta-globin sequence analysis revealed the patient to be heterozygous for the (–)29 A → G mutation (see Figure 30.3). Analysis of the α-globin gene cluster (see Figure 30.4) revealed the patient to be heterozygous for α^+ thalassaemia (i.e. α–/αα). Upon testing the patient's sister, we found that she too had a raised Hb A_2 level, the (–)29 A → G mutation and that she was heterozygous for α^+ thalassaemia (but she did not have Hb S).

Comments

The clinical spectrum of S/β^-thalassaemia is known to be wide, and this patient is at the mild end of the spectrum; she was certainly our first patient with this condition in her age group and with so little complaints. Considering that homozygous sickle cell anaemia is the prototype structural haemoglobinopathy, that homozygous β-thalassaemia is

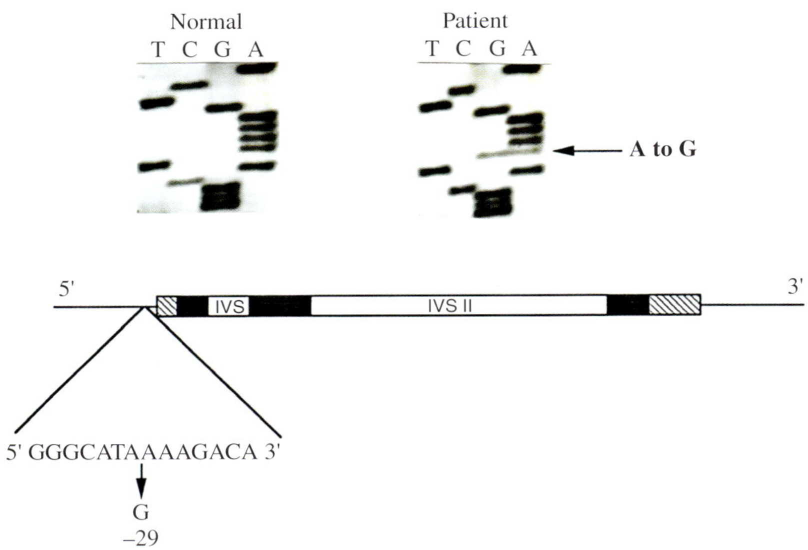

Figure 30.3 Bottom: diagram of the β-globin gene, with exons and introns indicated by black and white boxes, respectively; the shaded areas represent the 5′ and 3′ untranslated regions, and below the former is part of the promoter sequence. Top: direct sequence analysis of PCR products. The arrow at the right points to the mutation A → G, identified at position –29 relative to the CAP site, within the TATA box in the promoter. It is seen that the patient is heterozygous for this mutation.

the prototype quantitative haemoglobinopathy, and that both are serious diseases, it is interesting that the combination is often milder than either. In our patient, the mechanism can be rationalized, at least to an extent.

First, the β-thalassaemia mutation involved is a β^+ mutation that allows for a significant residual β^A chain synthesis: it has been regarded as mild [1]. Second, the patient's Hb S level (66%) was not a lot higher than in an A/S heterozygote; and with Hb F being 12%, we can estimate that the proportion of F cells that are slower to sickle was about 50% [2]. Third, the patient had an α-globin gene deletion: as a result, her non-α/α ratio was 0.99; thus, there was no globin chain imbalance, and we can assume this has largely prevented the ineffective erythropoiesis that is the main pathophysiologic feature of thalassaemia in the bone marrow.

The co-existence of α-thalassaemia may also offer an explanation for the normal MCV and MCH in this patient and in her sister; as this has been previously well documented (e.g. Pirastu et al. [3]; Akerman et al. [4]; Melis et al. [5]).

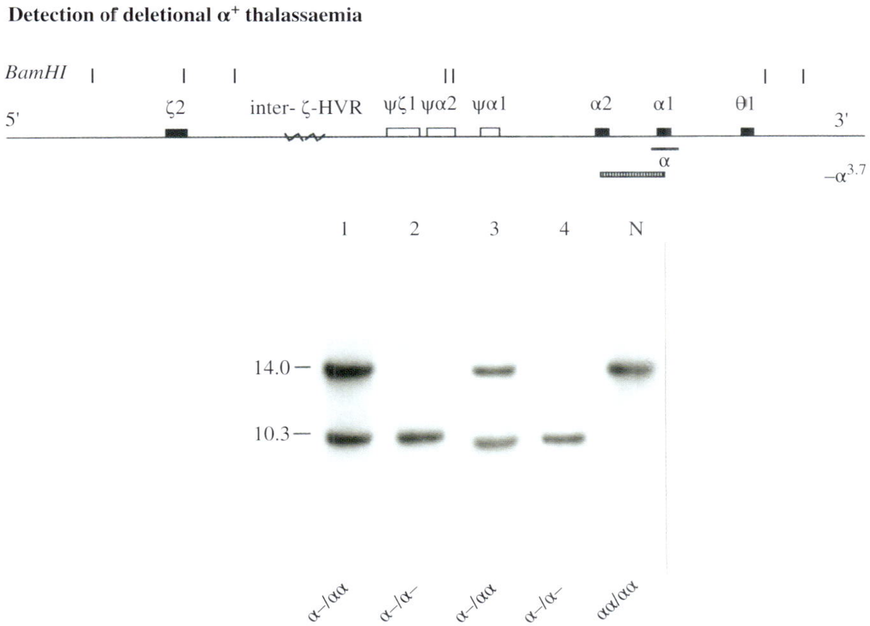

Figure 30.4 α-globin gene analysis. Top: α-globin gene cluster, with *BamHI* restriction sites indicated by short vertical lines. Clear boxes represent pseudogenes, and black boxes represent expressed genes; HVR is the inter-zeta hypervariable region. The black bar represents the position of the genomic α_1-globin gene probe used in hybridization studies; the shaded box indicates the extent of the polymorphic 3.7 Kb deletion. Bottom: Southern blot analysis of *BamHI*-digested genomic DNA samples hybridized to the α_1-globin gene probe. The normal control (N) DNA yielded the expected 14.0 Kb fragment. The patient's DNA (in lane 1) revealed a 10.3 Kb fragment in addition to the 14.0 Kb fragment, consistent with the α-/αα genotype: i.e. the patient is heterozygous for α^+-thalassaemia caused by the 3.7 Kb deletion. The inferred α-globin genotype is shown below each one of the other samples.

Within the wide spectrum of clinical severity of all types of sickle cell disease [6], patients with sickle-β^+ thalassaemia tend to be on the milder side [7]; and this patient reached her seventh decade before the diagnosis was made. Although in many countries the mortality of sickle cell anaemia is still sadly high in children, we can now expect to see an increasing number of patients in their 60s and 70s [8].

Follow-up

Over the next seven years, the patient has remained clinically stable and so have her Hb, MCV and MCH.

Conclusion

Sickle cell/$\beta^{+(-29\ A\rightarrow G)}$ thalassaemia disease with α^+ thalassaemia.

Acknowledgements

Professor Konotey-Ahulu, Cromwell Hospital, London, UK.

References

1. Thein, S.L. (2013). The molecular basis of beta-thalassemia. *Cold Spring Harb. Perspect. Med.* 3(5), a011700.
2. Urio, F., Nkya, S., Rooks, H. et al. (2020). F cell numbers are associated with an X-linked genetic polymorphism and correlate with haematological parameters in patients with sickle cell disease. *Br. J. Haematol.* 191, 888–896.
3. Pirastu, M., Ristaldi, M.S., Loudianos, G. et al. (1990). Molecular analysis of atypical beta-thalassaemia heterozygotes. *Ann. N. Y. Acad. Sci.* 612, 90–97.
4. Akerman, B.R., Fujiwara, T.M., Lancaster, G.A. et al. (1988). Identification of deletion and triple alpha-globin gene haplotypes in the Montreal beta-thalassaemia screening program: implications for genetic medicine. *Am. J. Med. Genet.* 36, 76–84.
5. Melis, M.A., Pirastu, M., Galanello, R. et al. (1983). Phenotypic effect of heterozygous α and β^0-thalassemia interaction. *Blood* 62, 226–229.
6. Serjeant, G.R. (2001). The emerging understanding of sickle cell disease. *Br. J. Haematol.* 112(1), 3–18.
7. Serjeant, G.R. and Serjeant, B.E. (2001). *Sickle Cell Disease*. 2 ed. Oxford: Oxford Medical Publications.
8. Thein, M.S., Igbineweka, N.E., and Thein, S.L. (2017). Sickle cell disease in the older adult. *Pathology* 49(1), 1–9.

Case 31

Strong but Frail

Patient Details

Age: 32 *Sex:* M
Ethnic background: Afro-Caribbean

Reason for Referral

Investigation of haemolysis (blood sample only).

History and Clinical Findings in Brief

The patient reported no prior medical history other than treatment for orchitis four years earlier; apparently no blood tests were performed at that time. He now complained of abdominal pain of eight months' duration. He had noticed that his urine tended to be often dark, particularly in the morning. The patient is very keen on physical training and some seven months previously had taken some "performance-enhancing" anabolic steroids, which had been provided by a friend. He was also on a "high protein diet." He is an occasional smoker and drinks no alcohol. He has two siblings, and his parents are both alive. There is no family history of illness or of any known haemoglobinopathy. He has a four-year-old daughter who is well also. On examination, the only finding was upper abdominal pain, mainly in the epigastrium without associated vomiting or weight loss.

Laboratory Findings

The patient had a moderate normocytic hypochromic anaemia with vigorous reticulocytosis (see Table 31.1). His white cell count was normal, but his platelets were low. On the blood film (see Figure 31.1), there seemed to be two populations of red cells; in one, the cells appeared to be normally haemoglobinized and in the other, they looked quite hypochromic i.e. a dimorphic blood film. There were also hyper-dense cells, some of which had an irregular outline; some appeared to have "bites" taken out of them (degmacytes); others were true spherocytes, and a few, on closer inspection, had an additional area which was free of haemoglobin (hemighosts). Some macro-target cells were present, and polychromatic cells were seen in every field. Occasional nucleated red cell was also seen.

Additional baseline studies revealed an elevated bilirubin, low haptoglobin and haemosiderin in the urinary sediment. The DAGT was negative. Vitamin B12 and folate were within the normal range; the serum ferritin was borderline. Other biochemistry was normal (see Table 31.2). His renal function was reported to be normal.

Initial Assessment

This patient had a haemolytic anaemia with evidence of intravascular haemolysis; and the referring physician suspected that abnormal haematology might have been of long standing. The negative Coombs test was against autoimmune haemolytic anaemia (AIHA); and although the clinical presentation would be compatible with PNH, the red cell morphology seemed far too "florid," and it was reminiscent of oxidative damage.

Table 31.1 Haematology Data

Hb (g/dl)	8.9
RBC ($\times 10^{12}$/l)	3.81
MCV (fl)	87.7
MCH (pg)	23.4
MCHC (g/dl)	26.6
RDW (S.D.)	92.2
Retic (%)	9.3
Retic ($\times 10^9$/l)	345
Hb A_2 (%)	3.3
Hb F (%)	1.5
WBC ($\times 10^9$/l)	7.2
PLT ($\times 10^9$/l)	81

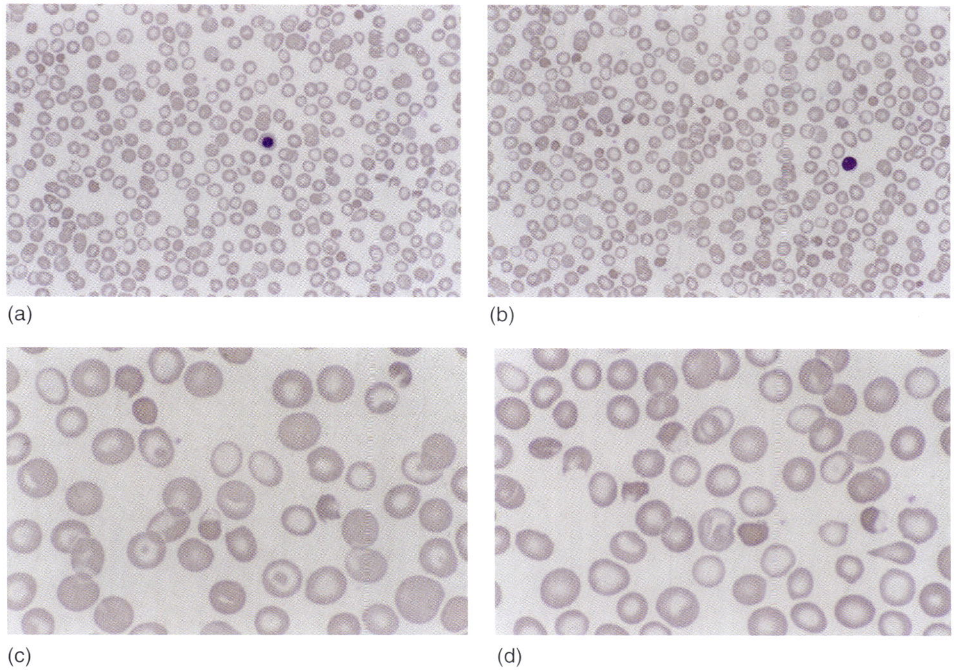

Figure 31.1 Peripheral blood film (a) and (b) medium power view; (c) and (d) high power view.

Table 31.2 Additional Baseline Studies

DAGT	Negative
Bilirubin (μmol/l)	80
Haptoglobin (mg/dl)	<35
Haemosiderin	positive
Ferritin (μg/l)	26
B12 (ng/l)	720
Serum folate (μg/l)	5.5
Red cell folate (μg/l)	735
Alk. Phos. (IU/l)	120
A.L.T. (IU/l)	25
Gamma-G.T. (IU/l)	17

Further Investigations

A G6PD assay yielded an elevated result, in keeping with a young population of erythrocytes. An autohaemolysis test was abnormal, and glucose did not correct, but actually enhanced lysis (Type 2 pattern). This pattern of aggravated lysis is typically seen in pyruvate kinase (PK) deficiency, but PK activity was high (see Table 31.3).

Table 31.3 Further Studies

G6PD (IU/g Hb)		26.0
PK (IU/g Hb)		31.0
Autohaemolysis test:		
—	% Lysis at 48 hours	
—	(−) glucose	(+) glucose
Control	0.8	0.1
Patient	6.4	13.2

The acidified serum (Ham) test was negative. A Heinz body preparation revealed occasional cells (<1%) with a single Heinz body. Hb electrophoresis on cellulose acetate membrane revealed, in addition to the normal bands of Hb A and Hb A_2, a faint, diffuse "band" between the positions of Hb S and Hb C (much closer to Hb S: see Figure 31.2). Upon elution, the abnormal component amounted to 7.3%.[1]

On citrate agar gel electrophoresis, the abnormal component migrated to a position midway between Hb A and Hb S. With alkaline globin chain electrophoresis, only bands in the normal positions of α^A and β^A were seen (we assumed the abnormal "haemoglobin" must be a β-chain variant, because there was no Hb A_2 variant observed on routine cellulose acetate, which of course there would be in the case of an α-chain variant). Heat stability and isopropanol precipitation tests were positive and therefore indicated that the patient had an unstable haemoglobin. A time-course study over a four-hour period revealed progressive instability and precipitation. Quantitation of the unstable haemoglobin by the usual procedure

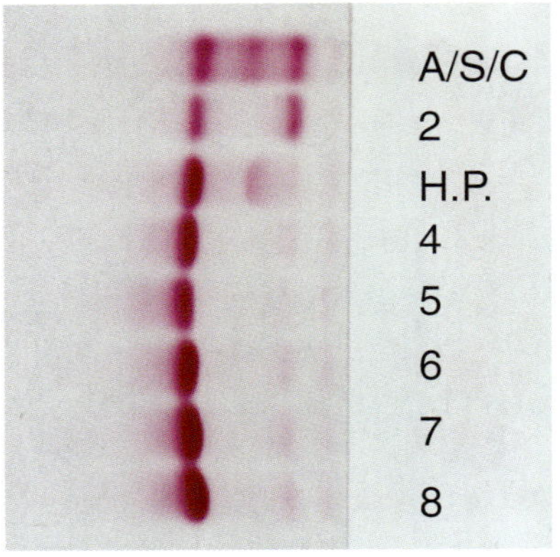

Figure 31.2 Haemoglobin electrophoresis on cellulose acetate membrane; the migration of the haemoglobin fractions is from right to left. A combined A/S/C control is in lane 1. The patient (H.P.) is in lane 3.

[1] Interestingly, a markedly elevated Hb A_2 had been reported from two other laboratories: evidently the abnormal haemoglobin had been missed.

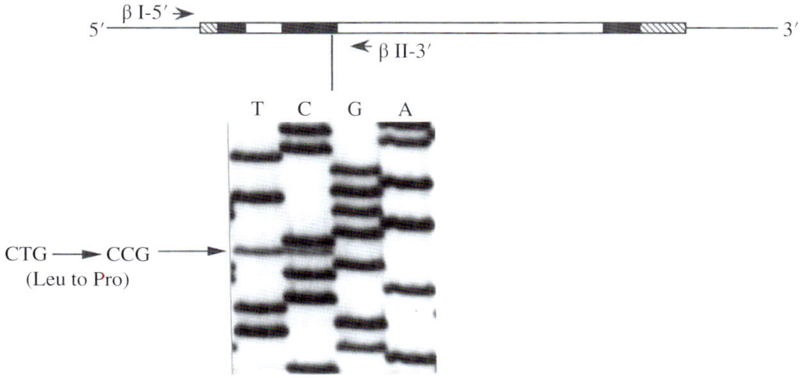

Figure 31.3 The β-globin gene, with exons and introns indicated by black and white boxes, respectively. The shaded areas represent the 5′ and 3′ untranslated regions. Below the diagram, the result of direct sequence analysis of a PCR-amplified product from the patient's DNA. Within codon β91, a band in both T and C tracks is seen (arrow on the left): showing the patient to be heterozygous for a mutation in codon β91.

(cyanmethaemoglobin by Drabkin's conversion) did not reflect the increments in precipitation that were observed macroscopically. We inferred that the haeme group probably became disassociated and remained in solution, while only the globin precipitated.

Next, we proceeded to sequence analysis (see Figure 31.3), which revealed the patient to be heterozygous for a T → C mutation in codon β91, leading to a substitution of Leu by Pro. This mutation has been previously reported in an abnormal haemoglobin called Hb Sabine [1]. Unfortunately, in spite of repeated efforts, we were unable to obtain samples from family members.

Comments

Hb Sabine was one of the first unstable haemoglobins to be discovered, in 1969, by Rose Schneider and colleagues (see patient 1 in Table 31.4) [1], who identified all the salient consequences, including the following: haemolytic anaemia (^{51}Cr red cell survival half-time of four days) of early onset, sometimes requiring blood transfusion; marked abnormalities on the blood smear, such as polychromasia, bizarre poikilocytes and inclusion bodies; excessively rapid heat-denaturation of haemoglobin; and by peptide analysis they identified the Leu → Pro amino acid replacement. Interestingly, in 9 out of the 11 previous cases in the literature (see Table 31.4), Hb Sabine was a *de novo* mutation.

Table 31.4 Reported Cases of Hb Sabine

Subject	Sex	Ancestry	Age at presentation	Age when splenectomized	Benefit	Reference
1	Female	British[a]	10 months	18 months	No	Mills [2][b]
2	Male	Yugoslavian	7	8	Yes	Bogoevski [3]
3	Male	Sardinian	3	9	Yes	Gasperini [4]
4	Female	Irish	8	9	Yes	Hull [5]
5	Male[c]	Irish	3 months	6	Yes	Hull [5]
6	Male[d]	Yugoslavian	2	5	Yes[i]	Pavlovic [6]
7	Female	German[e]	7 months	Na[f]	—	Perez [7]
8	Male	Malaysian	9 months	Na[g]	—	Yasin [8]
9	Male	Chinese	4 months	Na[h]	—	Chen [9]
10	Male	South Asian	4	5	Yes	Jamwal [10]
11	Female	Japanese	15 months	5	Yes	Yamamoto [11]

[a] English/Scotch/German.
[b] Also Schneider [1]; Mills [12]; Mills [13]; Shaeffer [14].
[c] This is the offspring of the patient immediately above.
[d] This is the offspring of Subject 2.
[e] Father German; Mother Spanish.
[f] Receiving folic acid.
[g] Transfused twice during haemolytic episode caused by infection.
[h] Transfused monthly.
[i] Symptom free for three months until thromboembolic complications.

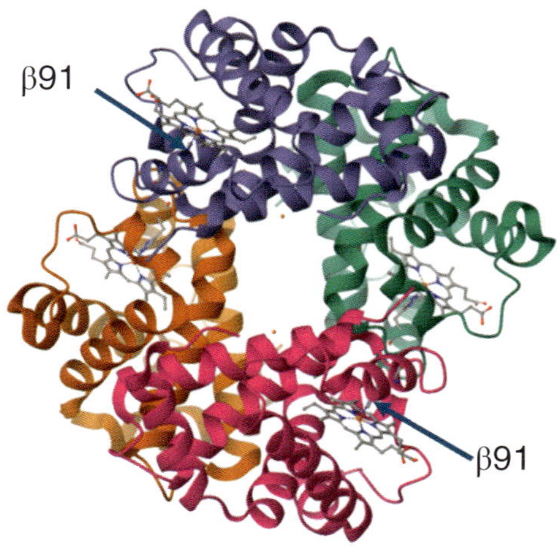

Figure 31.4 Diagram of the α1β1 haemoglobin dimer (downloaded from Protein Data Bank: PDB 3D: 1GZX). Individual amino acid replacements can cause haemoglobin to become unstable through different mechanisms. Amino acid β91, proline replacing leucine in Hb Sabine, is part of the haeme pocket. [15]/ with permission of Elsevier.

Leu91 is residue 7 in the F α-helix of the β chain: proline – that replaces Leu in Hb Sabine – is the only amino acid that strongly disrupts an alpha helical structure, and in this case, disruption is particularly detrimental because the F helix is part of the haeme pocket (see Figure 31.4) [15]. The β91 residue is in close proximity to two critical residues: histidine β92 is the main contact point for the attachment of haeme to globin, and cysteine β93 has an SH group that is important in protecting haeme from oxidation [1]. Instability of Hb Sabine is thus associated with haeme loss and with the production of hemichromes that cause oxidative damage to the red cell and eventually haemolysis. This explains the red cell morphology described above, as well as the reduced MCH and MCHC that are not in line with the MCV: a marked discrepancy among these indices must be regarded as an alarm bell and raise the suspicion of an abnormal haemoglobin.

One would expect a β-chain variant to be about 50% of the total at the time of biosynthesis; however, the abnormal beta-globin is unstable even before the haemoglobin tetramer is formed. The diffuse band that we saw on electrophoresis was difficult to quantitate, but it was certainly much less than 50%, probably on account of instability. Leucine and proline are both uncharged amino acids, but the electrophoretic mobility of haemoglobin can be affected by haeme loss (whereby only the two haeme groups within the α chains are reliably retained [14]) and by the altered tertiary/quaternary structure of the abnormal haemoglobin, which may expose some charges that are normally hidden, and/or conceal others, thus modifying the overall surface charge.

It is remarkable that this patient's blood film, with striking features of oxidative damage, is similar to that of a G6PD-deficient patient. The difference lies in that, in the case of G6PD deficiency, these features are seen only after exposure to a triggering agent (fava beans, or a drug, or infection); with Hb Sabine, instead, oxidative damage is chronic. With other unstable haemoglobins (e.g. Hb Zürich [18, 19], Hb Torino [20], Hb Bushwick [21], Hb Shepherd's Bush [22]), haemolytic crises accelerated by fever or by certain drugs have been reported.

Splenectomy has been regarded as beneficial in some patients of unstable haemoglobin but not in others: clearly the spleen is a site of haemolysis, but haemolysis is in part intravascular. Thrombocytopenia, possibly secondary to hypersplenism, has been noted in some patients (e.g. Hutchison et al. [16]; Paradise et al. [17]; this patient, and case 9).

Of the one hundred or more unstable haemoglobins known, about 80% are β-chain variants. There is no plausible reason to suggest that the β-globin gene is more prone to mutation; it seems more likely that, thanks to the duplication of the α-globin locus, when one α-gene is mutated only one-quarter of haemoglobin molecules will be affected; unless the consequences are severe, they may pass unnoticed.

Although "unstable haemoglobin disease" is a legitimate diagnosis, the spectrum of clinical severity is quite broad: this is not surprising, considering that more than one hundred different mutations can underlie this condition. Therefore, strictly speaking, there is no such thing as "unstable haemoglobin disease." Indeed, a molecular disease is defined by an individual molecule that has its own pathophysiologic consequences; thus, to name only those observed in cases in this book, there is a Hb Sabine disease, a Hb Köln disease and a Hb Bushwick disease.

Follow-up

Over the next three years, the patient remained stable clinically and haematologically. His reticulocytosis indicates that his marrow is active, but it cannot quite compensate for the rate of haemolysis. However, the patient seems to bear rather stoically his persistent anaemia, and we felt we did not have enough compelling evidence to recommend splenectomy.

Conclusion

Heterozygous Haemoglobin Sabine.

Acknowledgements

Referred by Dr. Ann Hunter, Department of Haematology, Nottingham City Hospital, Nottingham, UK.

Dr. A.P. Haynes, Department of Haematology, Nottingham City Hospital, Nottingham, UK.

Dr. Irene Roberts, Department of Haematology, Hammersmith Hospital, London, UK.

References

1. Schneider, R.G., Ueda, S., Alperin, J.B. et al. (1969). Haemoglobin Sabine Beta 91 (F7) Leu → Pro. An unstable variant causing severe anaemia with inclusion bodies. *N. Engl. J. Med*. 280, 739–745.
2. Mills, G.C., Levin, W.C., and Alperin, J.B. (1968). Hemolytic anemia associated with low erythrocyte ATP. *Blood* 32, 15–32.
3. Bogoevski, P., Efremov, G.D., Kezic, J. et al. (1983). Hb Sabine or $\alpha_2\beta_2$ 91 (F7) Leu → Pro in a Yugoslavian boy. *Hemoglobin* 7, 195–200.
4. Gasperini, D., Galanello, R., Melis, M. et al. (1992). Hemoglobin Sabine [β91 (F7) Leu → Pro]: occurrence in a Sardinian individual with hemolytic anemia and inclusion bodies. *Haematologica* 77, 381–383.

5. Hull, D., Winter, P.C., McHale, C.M. et al. (1998). Familial hemolytic anemia due to Hb Sabine [β91 (F7)Leu → Pro] identified by polymerase chain reaction. *Hemoglobin* 22, 263–266.
6. Pavlovic, S., Kuzmanovic, M., Urosevic, J. et al. (2004). Severe central nervous system thrombotic events in hemoglobin Sabine patient. *Eur. J. Haematol.* 72(1), 67–70.
7. Perez, S., Bragós, I., Raviola, M. et al. (2015). Severe hemolytic anemia due to de novo hemoglobin Sabine in an Argentinian newborn. First case in South America. *Int. Blood Res. Rev.* 3(4), 166–170.
8. Yasin, N.M., Yusoff, Y.M., Esa, E. et al. (2018). De novo haemoglobin Sabine presented with chronic haemolytic anaemia: a case report. *Asian J. Med. Biomed.* (12). Available from:
9. Chen, X., Hu, J., Zhu, J. et al. (2019). Severe hemolytic anemia due to combined α thalassemia and de novo Hemoglobin Sabine. *Ann. Hematol.* 98, 783–785 (2019).
10. Jamwal, M., Kaur, J., Chhabra, S. et al. (2020). De novo haemoglobin sabine masquerading as double heterozygosity for HbQ-India and β-thalassemia trait: first report from South Asia. *J. Clin. Pathol.* 73(4), 236–238.
11. Yamamoto, K., Nakamura, K., Shiozawa, R. et al. (2022). First report of familial hemolytic anemia due to hemoglobin Sabine in *Asia. Pediatr. Int.* 64, e15081.
12. Mills, G.C., Alperin, J.B., Hill, F.L. et al. (1971). Unstable hemoglobin hemolytic anemia: *in vitro* incubation studies on erythrocytes with hemoglobin Sabine. *Biochem-Med.* 5, 212–226.
13. Mills, G.C., Alperin, J.B., Hill, F.L. et al. (1972). Additional biochemical studies on erythrocytes containing hemoglobin Sabine. *Biochem. Med.* 6, 355–365.
14. Shaeffer, J.R. (1973). Structure and synthesis of the unstable hemoglobin Sabin (α2β2-91 Leu → pro). *J. Biol. Chem.* 248, 7473–7480.
15. Thom, C.S., Dickson, C.F., Olson, J.S. et al. (2015). Normal and abnormal hemoglobins. In: Orkin, S.H., Fischer, D.E., Ginsburg, D. et al., editor. *Nathan and Osli's Hematology and Oncology of Infancy and Childhood.* 1 ed. Philadelphia, PA: Elsevier Saunders. pp. 630–672.
16. Hutchison, H.E., Pinkerton, P.H., Waters, P. et al. (1964). Hereditary Heinz-body anaemia, thrombocytopenia and haemoglobinopathy (Hb Koln) in a Glasgow family. *Br. Med. J.* 2, 1099–1103.
17. Paradise, S.L., Estep, L., Olson, J. et al. (2014). First North American case of Hemoglobin Shepherds Bush (β74 [E18] Gly → Asp) in a central Pennsylvania family. *BMC Clin. Pathol.* 14(1), 4.
18. Frick, P.G., Hitzig, W.H., and Betke, K. (1962). Hemoglobin Zurich. I. A new hemoglobin anomaly associated with acute hemolytic episodes with inclusion bodies after sulfonamide therapy. *Blood* 20, 261–271. PMID: 13895148.
19. Bachmann, F. and Marti, H.R. (1962). Hemoglobin Zurich. II. Physicochemical properties of the abnormal hemoglobin. *Blood* 20, 272–286. PMID: 13863728.
20. Sansone, G., Sciarratta, G.V., Lang, A. et al. (1976). A drug-induced haemolytic anaemia due to Hb Torino (alpha43(CD1) Phe replaced by Val). second finding in an Italian family. *Acta Haematol.* 56(4), 225–233.

21. Rieder, R.F., Wolf, D.J., Clegg, J.B. et al. (1975). Rapid postsynthetic destruction of unstable haemoglobin Bushwick. *Nature* 254(5502), 725–727
22. White, J.M., Brain, M.C., Lorkin, P.A. et al. (1970). Mild "unstable haemoglobin haemolytic anaemia" caused by Haemoglobin Shepherds Bush (B74 (E18) Gly → Asp). *Nature* 225, 939–941.

See related Case 9.

Case 32

Troublesome Symbiotic Relationship

Patient Details

Age: 7 months *Sex:* M
Ethnic background: Greece (Athens)

Reason for Referral

Investigation of severe anaemia.

History and Clinical Findings in Brief

The patient was the firstborn (full-term) child of unrelated parents. At the age of six months, he was noted to have severe pallor. When he was investigated in Athens, where a Hb level of 3.3 had been recorded, a diagnosis of congenital pure red cell aplasia (PRCA: Diamond–Blackfan syndrome) was made and a blood transfusion was given. The infant's general condition was otherwise good and he was well nourished. On examination, the child was indeed very pale, and he was noticed to have wide-spaced nipples, a flat chest and a high arched palate.

Laboratory Findings

The patient had a very severe, normochromic normocytic anaemia with leukopaenia, thrombocytopaenia and reticulocytopaenia (see Table 32.1). On the blood film (see Figure 32.1), there was mild anisocytosis and poikilocytosis; some cells had small horn-like projections, while a small number were very dense, and in these, the central area of pallor was either totally lacking or appeared to be pushed to one pole. An occasional small hypochromic cell was also seen.

Table 32.1 Haematology Data

WBC ($\times 10^9$/l)	2.3
Plt ($\times 10^9$/l)	5
Hb (g/dl)	4.8
RBC ($\times 10^{12}$/l)	1.65
MCV (fl)	93.3
MCH (pg)	29.1
MCHC (g/dl)	31.2
RDW (S.D.)	49.5
Retic (%)	0.1
Retic ($\times 10^9$/l)	2

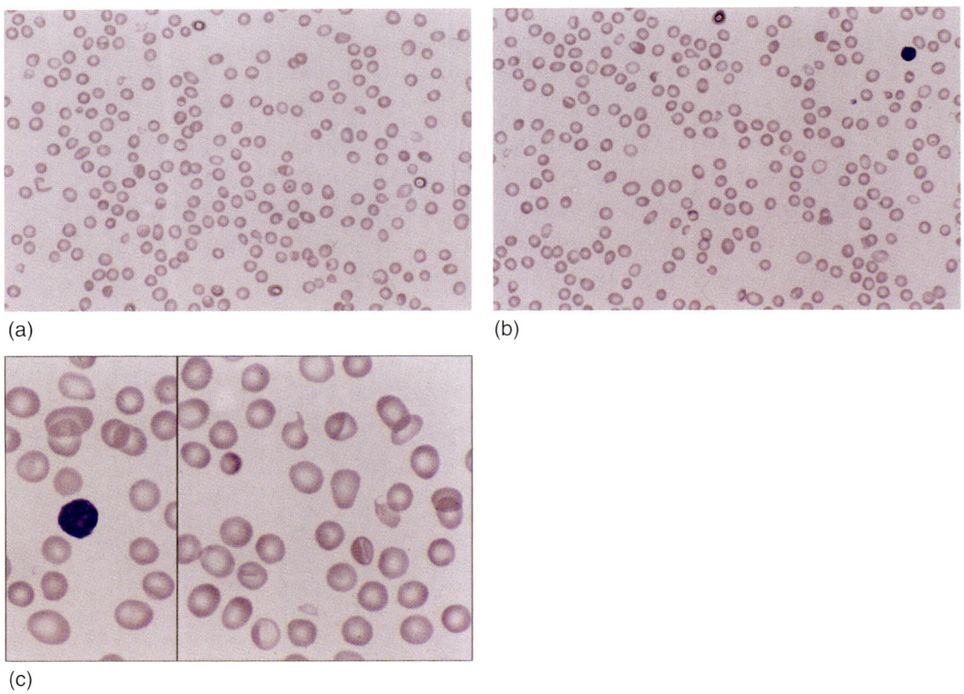

Figure 32.1 Peripheral blood film: (a) and (b) medium power view; (c) high power view (composite).

Table 32.2 Baseline Studies

Hb. electrophoresis	Normal
Serum iron (μmol/l)[a]	43
Transferrin (g/l)[b]	2.0
Tfn. Saturation (%)[c]	81

[a] Range for age = 7–18 (μmol/l).
[b] Range for age = 1.5–3.0 (g/l).
[c] Range for age = 20–45 (%).

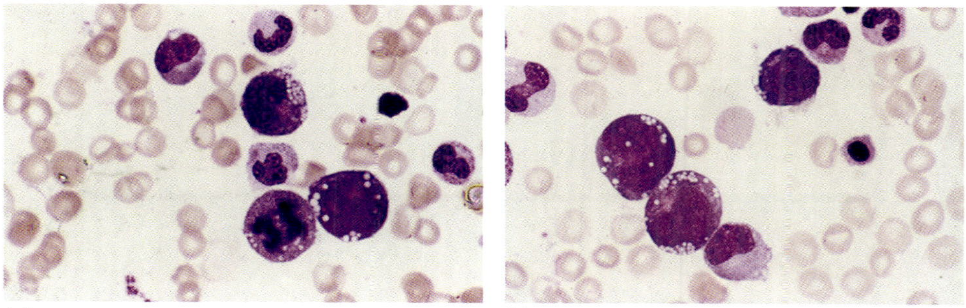

(a) (b)

Figure 32.2 Bone marrow aspirate: (a) and (b) high power view.

Additional studies revealed only normal haemoglobins by cellulose acetate electrophoresis. The serum iron was high, with a high saturation of transferrin (see Table 32.2). Haematological tests on the parents were normal.

A bone marrow aspirate was easy to obtain, and it showed normocellular fragments and trails. However, erythropoiesis was markedly depressed (see Figure 32.2). The most striking feature was vacuolation of the early erythroblasts and also of the early myeloid precursors. The majority of the erythroblasts were ringed sideroblasts (see Figure 32.3), and hemosiderin was prominent in the fragments.

Initial Assessment

Clearly, this child's anaemia was due to decreased red cell production, and it was part of pancytopenia. While the spectrum of differential diagnoses in this situation would have been quite broad (including Diamond–Blackfan, as originally diagnosed), the high prevalence of ringed sideroblasts helped to restrict the spectrum (see Table 32.3). Given the age of the child, one would of course be inclined to consider the congenital group first.

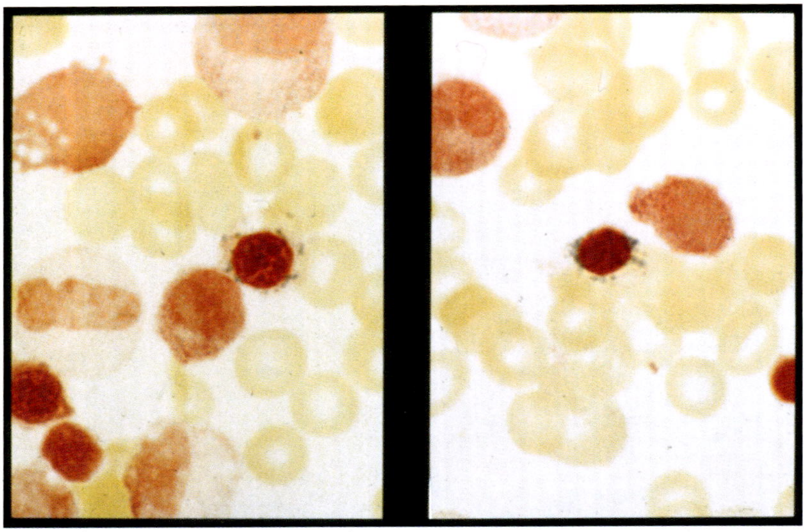

Figure 32.3 Bone marrow iron stain showing ring sideroblasts.

Table 32.3 Classification of the Sideroblastic Anaemias

I Congenital
Isolated, inherited
Associated with mitochondrial myopathy (Pearson's syndrome)
II Acquired
Associated with myelodysplasia, haematological malignancies
Myeloproliferative disorders
Reversible – associated with
Alcoholism
Certain drugs (isoniazid, chloramphenicol)
Copper deficiency (nutritional, zinc toxicity)
Hypothermia
Idiopathic

Within the framework of severe pancytopenia in an infant, and with the conspicuous vacuoles in the erythroid cells, we had to suspect strongly Pearson's syndrome.

Further Investigations

Since congenital sideroblastic anaemia due to ALAS deficiency may respond to pyridoxine, in the meantime the patient was started on treatment with pyridoxine, 50 mg/day. Cytogenetic analysis of bone marrow

Table 32.4 Additional Studies

Lactate (mmol/l)	2.2	(N 0.6–1.8)
Amylase (IU/l)	25	(N 0–70)
Trypsin (μg/l)	21	(N <10)
Faecal fat[a] (g/day)	3.5	(N <2.0)

[a] Collected over a period of 72 hours.

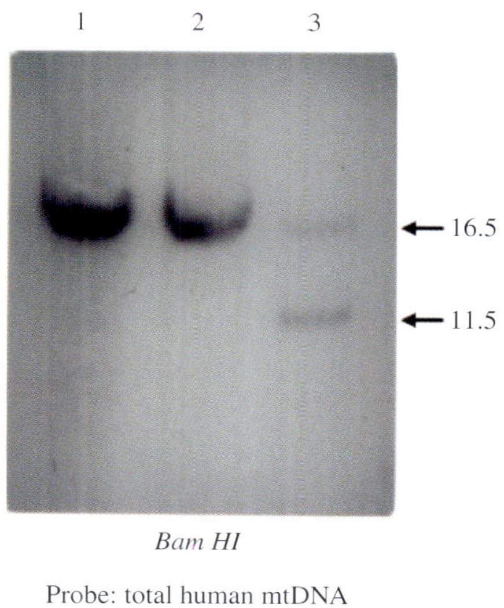

Figure 32.4 Deletion in mitochondrial DNA (mtDNA). The autoradiograph shows the hybridization of a total mtDNA probe to a *Bam HI* digest of DNA from the mother (lane 1) and father (lane 2) of the affected baby (lane 3). Only the normal fragment at 16.5 Kb is seen in both parents; but in the patient, a smaller band at 11.5 Kb is also seen, representing about 60% of the total signal in this track.

cells came back normal. Colony culture studies yielded no growth of BFU-E, and CFU-GM at the lower limit of normal, indicating bone marrow insufficiency in spite of apparently normal cellularity. Additional studies showed increased faecal fat, although clinically there was nothing to suggest malabsorption; this and other findings (see Table 32.4) suggested instead pancreatic insufficiency.

We next analyzed the patient's mitochondrial DNA (mtDNA). Peripheral blood mononuclear cells from the patient showed two types of mtDNA: about 40% was normal in size, whereas about 60% had a deletion of approximately 5 Kb (see Figure 32.4). This deletion was similar in size and in map position to that previously demonstrated in other patients with Pearson's syndrome [1].

Comments

Features of Pearson's syndrome include; (i) onset in infancy; (ii) both sexes affected; (iii) parents haematologically normal; (iv) severe transfusion dependent anaemia and reticulocytopaenia; (v) neutropaenia and thrombocytopaenia of variable degree; (vi) bone marrow of normal cellularity with ringed sideroblasts, vacuoles in erythroid and myeloid precursors, haemosiderosis; (vii) pancreatic exocrine dysfunction. Our patient had all of these features. With respect to differential diagnosis, it is not the first time that an initial diagnosis of Blackfan–Diamond has to be revised to Pearson's [2]. The bone marrow was the giveaway in this case.

With respect to aetiology, the specificity of the syndrome originally described by Pearson was vindicated when Rotig et al. [1] discovered that it originated from deletions within mtDNA, and it is therefore a multi-system mitochondrial cytopathy. The deletion identified in our patient is almost certainly identical to that found in several others [3] (see also Figure 32.5); it is presumed that occurrence of this deletion is favoured by the presence of a 13 bp DNA repeat sequence normally present at both of its ends.

The mitochondria present in our cells are a marvel of evolution. Many lines of evidence concur in supporting the notion that an anaerobic eukaryotic cell – thriving at the time when there was little oxygen in the atmosphere, perhaps 2 billion years ago – has incorporated as an endosymbiont a prokaryotic cell (a small bacterium) capable of using oxygen to produce energy through oxidative phosphorylation (OXPHOS). Thus, still today mtDNA is a small (16 Kb) molecule, circular like in bacteria, present in 2–10 copies in each mitochondrion; and still today the main energy supply in most animal cells is the OXPHOS apparatus in mitochondria. In the course of evolution most of the OXPHOS proteins have become encoded by nuclear genes; but a few are still encoded by mtDNA.

As usual in biology, there is nothing like a genetic change to remind us that mtDNA, though very small, is important: the relationship between the eukaryotic cell and the symbiotic prokaryote may become compromised. Indeed, deletions and even point mutations in mtDNA can be highly detrimental, since they reduce energy production, as in Pearson's syndrome. The enzymes of the haeme biosynthetic pathway are encoded by nuclear genes, but some of that pathway takes place in mitochondria, and evidently it becomes impaired in the defective mitochondria of patients with this syndrome.

Since mitochondria are present in the oocyte but not in the sperm cell (except in its tail, that is left out during the process of fertilization), all our mitochondria are of maternal origin. A mitochondrial disease, such as Pearson's, originates when the fertilized oocyte has a mtDNA mutation. If a deletion such as the one in our patient were in every molecule, it would be incompatible with life: but it is instead "heteroplasmic," i.e. present only in some proportion of molecules: about 60% in our case. Since there are 5–10 molecules of mtDNA in each mitochondrion, with hundreds of

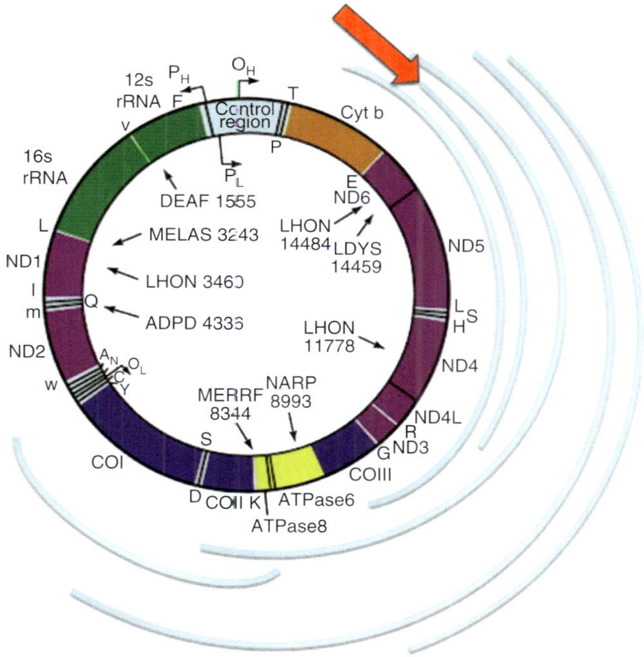

Figure 32.5 Schematic map of the circular mtDNA molecule. Regions encoding different functional complexes (indicated by acronyms outside map) are in different colours (for instance, the genes for the NAD dehydrogenase complex are in pink). Acronyms inside the map are for various syndromes associated with mtDNA mutations (e.g. LHON for Leber's hereditary optic neuropathy). Blue arches outside the map indicate the span of mtDNA deletions found in different patients with Pearson's syndrome. The red arrow indicates the 4977 bp deletion found in our patient that affects genes involved in OXPHOS. [4]/with permission of Elsevier.

mitochondria in each cell, and since we can presume the deletion originally occurred in just one mtDNA molecule, it is still not clear how a heteroplasmy of 60% can be reached. Recently, it has been found in cultures of induced pluripotent stem cells that the rate of heteroplasmy may increase; as though, up to a point, it conferred a growth advantage [5]. Therefore, heteroplasmy has dynamic features, whereby the proportion of mutant DNA may change during oogenesis, in the embryo and after birth. This may account for why in individual patients there may be more impact on the bone marrow or the pancreas, and why Pearson's syndrome may evolve [6], particularly into the so-called Kearns-Sayre syndrome (KSS), defined by progressive external ophthalmoplegia, retinal degeneration and cardiac conduction defects.

The prognosis of Pearson's syndrome is unfortunately rather bleak, mainly due to its nature with multi-system involvement. Bone marrow transplantation can be expected to correct at least bone marrow failure: it has been carried out in a few cases but there have been several complications, including malignancy [7].

Follow-up

The patient received supportive management with blood transfusions and iron chelation at the Department of Paediatrics of Athens University. At the age of 5 he was started on vitamin E (50 mg/day; later increased to 100 mg/day). His blood counts have improved and he no longer required blood transfusion. At the age of 6 his growth was within the normal range and his mental development was regarded as normal-high. Since mtDNA comes only from the mother, Pearson's syndrome and all mtDNA diseases are non-Mendelian; but genetic counselling is appropriate. A good thing we can discuss with the parents is that, given the pathogenesis outlined above, the risk of recurrence is very low [8].

Conclusion

Bone marrow-pancreas Pearson's syndrome.

Acknowledgements

Referred by Professor C. Kattamis, Department of Paediatrics, Athens University Children's Hospital, Athens, Greece.

Dr. Mary Chapple, Haematology Department, Hammersmith Hospital, London, UK.

References

1. Rotig, A., Cormier, V., Blanche, S. et al. (1990). Pearson's marrow-pancreas syndrome. A multisystem mitochondrial disorder in infancy. *J. Clin. Invest.* 86, 1601–1608.
2. Alter, B.P. (2014). Pearson syndrome in a Diamond-Blackfan anemia cohort. *Blood* 124, 312–313.
3. Rotig, A., Bourgeron, T., Chretein, D. et al. (1995). Spectrum of mitochondrial DNA rearrangements in the Pearson marrow-pancreas syndrome. *Hum. Mol. Genet.* 4, 1327–1330.

4. Bessler, M., Mason, P.J., Link, D.C. et al. (2015). Inherited bone marrow failure syndromes. In: Orkin, S.H., Fischer, D.E., Ginsburg, D. et al., editor. *Nathan and Oski's Hematology and Oncology of Infancy and Childhood*. Vol. 1. Philadelphia, PA: Elsevier Saunders. pp. 182–253.
5. Russell, O.M., Fruh, I., Rai, P.K. et al. (2018). Preferential amplification of a human mitochondrial DNA deletion in vitro and in vivo. *Sci. Rep.* 8, 1799.
6. Farruggia, P., Di Marco, F., and Dufour, C. (2018). Pearson syndrome. *Expert Rev. Hematol.* 11, 239–246.
7. Tumino, M., Meli, C., Farruggia, P. et al. (2011). Clinical manifestations and management of four children with Pearson syndrome. *Am. J. Med. Genet. A* 155A, 3063–3066.
8. Bernardino Gomes, T.M., Ng, Y.S., Pickett, S.J. et al. (2021). Mitochondrial DNA disorders: from pathogenic variants to preventing transmission. *Hum Mol Genet* 30, R245–R253.

Case 33

Not Letting Go

Patient Details

Age: 18 *Sex:* F
Ethnic background: English (Berkshire)

Reason for Referral

Identification of abnormal haemoglobin (blood sample only).

History and Clinical Findings in Brief

There was no significant medical history in this patient apart from reports of heavy menstrual blood loss in the past, for which reason she was now on iron treatment. She is also on oral contraceptives. The patient reported that when she was an infant her mother and her grandfather had been found to have an "abnormal haemoglobin."

Laboratory Findings

The patient had an elevated haemoglobin level, with normal red cell indices (see Table 33.1). The reticulocyte count was slightly increased. On the blood film (see Figure 33.1), the red cell morphology looked normal.

Table 33.1 Haematology Data

Hb (g/dl)	16.5
RBC ($\times 10^{12}$/l)	4.95
MCV (fl)	95.6
MCH (pg)	33.3
MCHC (g/dl)	34.9
RDW (S.D.)	44.8
Retic (%)	2.4
Retic ($\times 10^{9}$/l)	118.8
WBC ($\times 10^{9}$/l)	6.8
PLT ($\times 10^{9}$/l)	204
Hb A_2 (%)	2.5

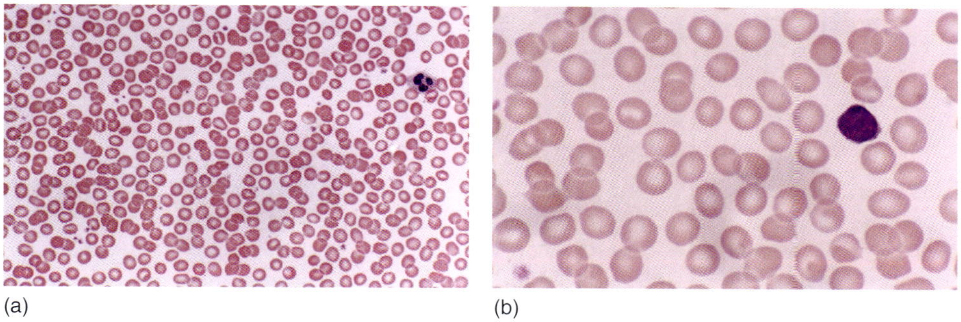

Figure 33.1 Peripheral blood film: (a) medium power view; (b) high power view.

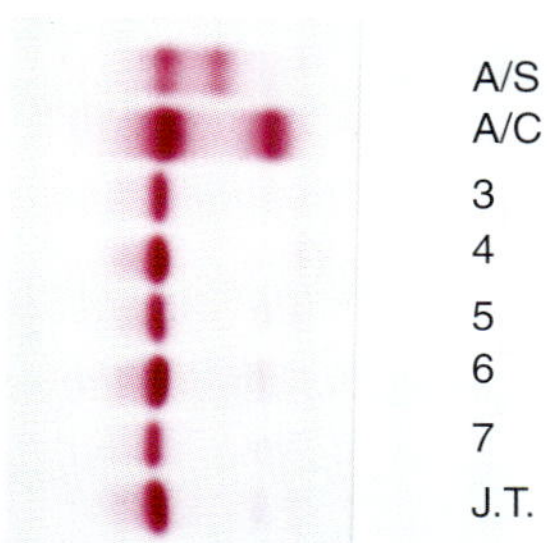

Figure 33.2 Haemoglobin electrophoresis on cellulose acetate membrane; the migration of the haemoglobin fractions is from right to left. An A/S control and A/C control are in lanes 1 and 2, respectively. The patient (J.T.) is in lane 8.

Cellulose acetate electrophoresis revealed bands in the normal positions of Hb A and Hb A_2 only (see Figure 33.2).

Initial Assessment

The patient's haemoglobin level was just above the top of the reference range, and she had a normal WBC and platelet count; thus, there was no suggestion of polycythaemia rubra vera (PRV). With the benefit of the family history the patient gave us, it was tempting to surmise that her erythrocytosis might be secondary to a high oxygen affinity haemoglobin. The normal result of Hb electrophoresis was not against this hypothesis, because in about one-half of cases the electrophoretic mobility of high-affinity haemoglobins is the same as that of Hb A.

Further Investigations

An oxygen dissociation study revealed a marked left shift in the curve with a P_{50} value of only 9.5 mm Hg (see Figure 33.3). β-globin gene sequence revealed the patient to be heterozygous for nucleotides C and G at the third position of codon β103, leading to a substitution of Phe by Leu (see Figure 33.4). This amino acid replacement has been previously reported in an abnormal haemoglobin called Hb Heathrow [1–3].

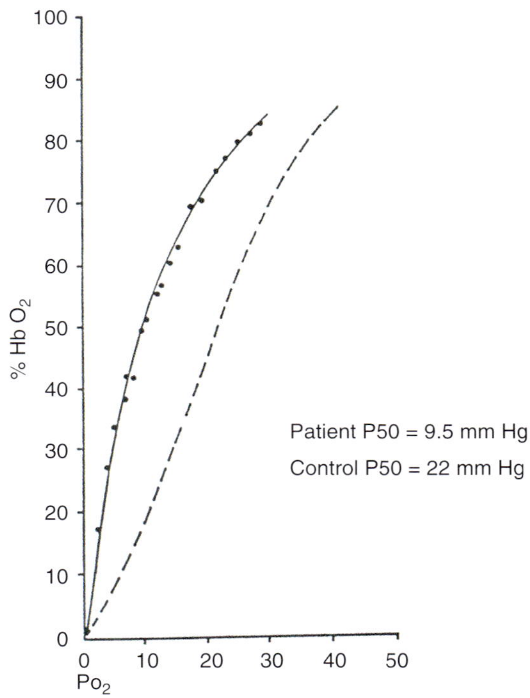

Figure 33.3 Oxygen dissociation curve of patient (•——•) and control (----).

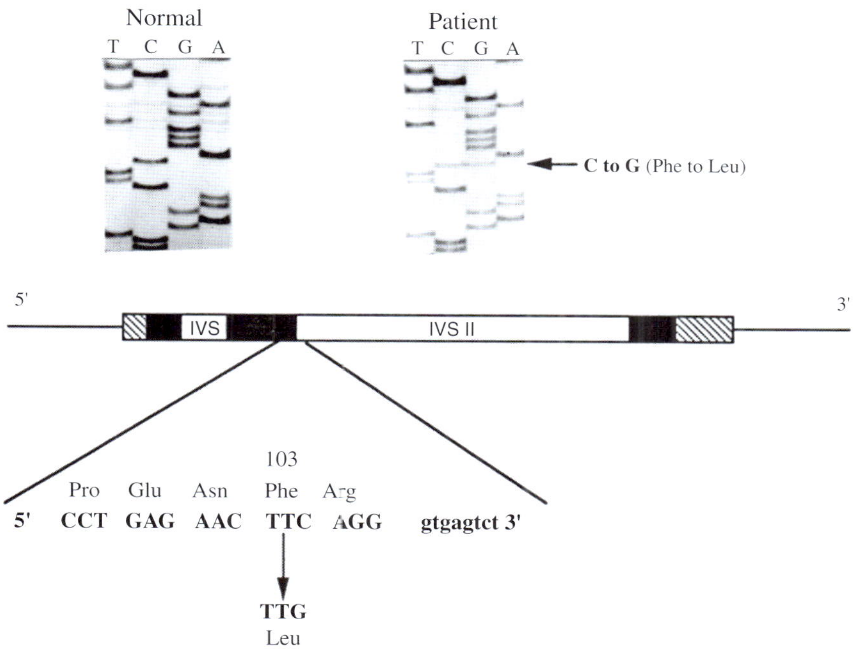

Figure 33.4 Analysis of the β-globin gene by Sanger sequencing. Auto-radiographs of original gels, displaying for each sample the four lanes corresponding to the 4 bases in DNA. In the patient's DNA, at the third position of codon β103, a band in both C and G tracks is seen (highlighted by the arrow on the right), showing the patient to be heterozygous for a mutation in codon β103. The diagram below represents the β-globin gene, with exons in black and introns in white; the shaded areas represent the 5′ and 3′ untranslated regions.

Comments

In a young woman who does not smoke, and with heavy menses, an Hb level of 16.5 g/dl is rather suspicious; and the family history she volunteered was more than helpful.

A shift to the left in the Hb–O_2 dissociation curve in the blood of a person with a high-affinity haemoglobin causes a significant decrease in oxygen supply to tissues, entailing an erythropoietin response by the O_2 sensor in the kidney, resulting in an increased red cell mass, as already previously observed in other patients with Hb Heathrow (see Table 33.2).

The main mechanisms whereby specific amino acid replacements can cause increased O_2 affinity of haemoglobin are either stabilization of the so-called T (or *tense*) state or decreased binding of the allosteric regulator BPG [7]. Changes in subunit interactions will affect particularly the former

Table 33.2 Haematological Findings in Patients with Hb Heathrow

Sex	White et al. [2]	Beard et al. [4]		Marsh et al. [5]	Shin et al. [6]
		Case I	Case II		
	Male	Male	Male	Male	Male
Hb (g/dl)	21.0	18.0	17.7[b]	21.7	20.4
PCV	0.66	0.53[a]	0.51	0.63	0.58
RBC Vol. (ml/kg)	55.0	35.3	35.0	57.0	–
Plasma Vol. (ml/kg)	42.0	34.9	42.0	42.0	–
P_{50} (mm Hg)	9.5	17.0	12.0	12.0	14.3

[a] A PCV as high as 0.62 has been noted in the past.
[b] Haemoglobin levels as high as 20 g/dl have been noted in the past.

Table 33.3 Codon Usage

Phe-codon	Leu-codon[a]	Leu-codon found in patients			
		1	2	3	4
TTC[b]	TTG	TTG	TTG	TTG	TTG
TTC	TTA	–	–	–	–
TTC	CTC	–	–	–	–

[a] Potentially arising by point mutations from Phe-codons.
[b] Codon at position β103.

mechanism, and it happens that the phenylalanine 103 residue is very close to the $\alpha_1 \beta_1$ interface; however, exactly how the change to leucine in Hb Heathrow affects oxygen binding has not yet been elucidated.

Upon further investigation of records, we found that it was in this very patient's family that the presence of Hb Heathrow had been originally described, at the Hammersmith, by Professor J. White et al. [3]. Our patient's mother, grandfather, aunt and two cousins also have the same abnormal haemoglobin.

In the genetic code, there are six codons for leucine; therefore, a replacement of Leu for Phe could theoretically take place in six different ways; however, since the Phe codon at position 103 in the normal β -globin gene is TTC, this could change to a Leu codon in only three different ways (see Table 33.3). There were only three other known instances of Hb Heathrow in the world, and through the courtesy of colleagues we were able to test two of them, one from New Zealand (Beard et al.) [4] and one from Middlesex, England (Marsh et al.) [5]; they all had the same base change as our patient. One wonders whether the patient in Berkshire, the one in Middlesex, and the two in New Zealand share a common ancestor.

Follow-up

In the management of PRV, a moderate degree of iron deficiency associated with repeated phlebotomies, although controversial, may be desirable within limits [8]. In patients with a high-affinity haemoglobin, on the other hand, tolerance to anaemia is low, and therefore a decrease in Hb is not desirable. Our patient was advised to use iron supplementation only when iron deficient; she has continued to do well, just like her mother and her grandfather.

Conclusion

Patient heterozygous for the high O_2 affinity haemoglobin Heathrow.

Acknowledgements

Dr. Chris Hatton, Department of Haematology, Wexham Park Hospital, Slough, UK.
Dr. P. H. Mackie, Department of Haematology, Wexham Park Hospital, Slough, UK.

References

1. Gillies, I.D., Lehmann, H., Lorkin, P.A. et al. (1973). Haemoglobin Heathrow--a new high affinity haemoglobin. *J. Physiol.* 231(2), 85P–87P. PMID: 4720961.
2. White, J.M., Szur, L., Roberts, P. et al. (1973). Hb Heathrow: beta G5 103 phenylalanine-leucine: a new high affinity haemoglobin. *Br. J. Haematol.* 25(2), 284. PMID: 4726919.
3. White, J.M., Szur, L., Gillies, I.D. et al. (1973). Familial polycythaemia caused by a new haemoglobin variant: Hb Heathrow, beta 103 (G5) phenylalanine leads to leucine. *Br. Med. J.* 3(5882), 665–667.
4. Beard, M.E., Hamer, J.W., Brennan, S.O. et al. (1979). Familial relative polycythaemia due to haemoglobin Heathrow. *Aust. N. Z. J. Med.* 9, 297–301.
5. Marsh, G., Marino, G., Pucci, P. et al. (1991). A third instance of the high oxygen affinity variant, Hb Heathrow [beta 103 (G5) phenylalanine → leucine]: identification of the mutation by mass spectrometry and by DNA analysis. *Hemoglobin* 15, 43–51.

6. Shin, S.Y., Kim, H.Y., Kim, H.J. et al. (2017). Hb Heathrow [β103 (G5)Phe → Leu], a first report in an Asian patient with erythrocytosis. *Yonsei Med. J.* 58(3), 665–667.
7. Thom, C.S., Dickson, C.F., Olson, J.S. et al. (2015). Normal and abnormal hemoglobins. In: Orkin, S.H., Fischer, D.E., Ginsburg, D. et al. editor. *Nathan and Osli's Hematology and Oncology of Infancy and Childhood*. 1 ed. Philadelphia, PA: Elsevier Saunders. pp. 630–672.
8. Spivak, J.L. (2002). Polycythemia vera: myths, mechanisms, and management. *Blood* 100(13), 4272–4290.

Case 34

Hellenic Class A

Patient Details

Age: 3 *Sex:* M
Ethnic background: Greece

Reason for Referral

Investigation of chronic haemolytic anaemia.

History and Clinical Findings in Brief

This young boy from Thessaloniki had originally presented in the neonatal period with severe anaemia and jaundice: an exchange transfusion was performed at three hours, followed by phototherapy. The jaundice cleared within eight days. A blood test revealed that he was G6PD deficient. The patient's anaemia persisted, and he required blood transfusion at approximately two-month interval. The mother observed that exacerbation of the child's anaemia often followed illness and fever. On one occasion, after a high temperature (39 °C) there was a precipitous fall in the child's haemoglobin to a level of 3.9 g/dl. Both parents are well. The mother reported having had one early abortion and two stillborn children. By the time the patient was referred to the Hammersmith

Hospital, he had been already transfused on 17 occasions. On examination, the child's general condition was good, although he was on the small side; weight 14.6 kg (25th percentile) and height 93 cm (10th percentile). There was herpes labialis. The only other significant physical findings were marked enlargement of the spleen (8 cm below the coastal border) and of the liver (5 cm below the coastal border). A chest X-ray was normal. Abdominal X-ray was normal except for hepatomegaly, and skull X-ray showed no expansion of the diploe.

Laboratory Findings

The patient had a moderate macrocytic, normochromic anaemia (see Table 34.1). The red cell morphology (see Figure 34.1) showed considerable anisocytosis (contributed in some part by the transfused red cells), macrocytosis, polychromasia, occasional spherocytes and occasional nucleated red cells, some of which had megaloblastic features (not shown). Examination of the parents' blood film did not show any obvious abnormalities.

A biochemical profile was normal except for a slight increase in bilirubin. Additional studies revealed normal osmotic fragility and haemoglobin electrophoresis; a globin-chain biosynthetic study did not suggest any form of thalassaemia. A Heinz body preparation was negative. A review of a previous bone marrow revealed marked erythroid hyperplasia without much evidence of dyserythropoiesis.

Table 34.1 Laboratory Findings

	Patient	Mother	Father
Hb (g/dl)	8.2	13.0	15.0
RBC ($\times 10^{12}$/l)	2.49	3.99	5.28
MCV (fl)	103	94	86
MCH (pg)	32.9	32.6	28.5
MCHC (g/dl)	32.0	34.7	33.3
Retic (%)	28.8	–	–
Retic ($\times 10^{9}$/l)	717	–	–
Hb A_2 (%)	2.4	2.3	2.2
Hb F (%)	2.3	0.9	0.6
β:α ratio[a]	0.96	–	–
G6PD (IU/gHb)	2.7	7.8	8.9
Bilirubin (μmol/l)	43	22	15

[a] Globin chain biosynthetic ratio.

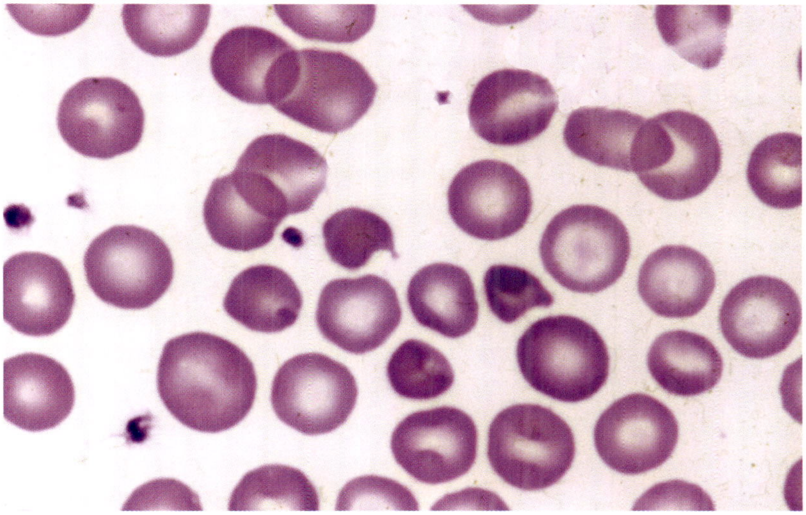

Figure 34.1 Peripheral blood film.

Initial Assessment

This boy clearly had a relatively severe chronic haemolytic anaemia. From red cell morphology, he did not appear to have HS or HE. We knew that he was G6PD deficient, but so are about 5% of males in Thessaloniki.

Further Investigations

The autohaemolysis test was abnormal, with only partial correction by glucose (see Table 34.2). Next, we set out to find out whether the patient had an unusual variant of G6PD.

Table 34.2 Results of Autohaemolysis Test[a]

	% Lysis at 48 hours	
	Without glucose	Addition of glucose
Control	1.5	0.3
Patient	5.0	1.7
Mother	0.9	0.3
Father	1.0	0.2
G6PD A–	1.4	0.7
G6PD Med	1.1	0.5

[a] Including representative figures from a small series of patients with G6PD A– and G6PD Mediterranean deficiencies.

Table 34.3 Characterization of Enzyme

	Cell type	G6PD activity[a]	Electrophoretic mobility[b]	K_m^{G6P} (μM)
Patient	Erythrocytes	2.7[c]	100	80
	Fibroblasts	0.6[d]	94	90
Mother	Erythrocytes	7.8[c]	100	–
	Fibroblasts	66.4[d]	100	–
Control	Erythrocytes	9.5[c]	100	50–80
	Fibroblasts	75–110[d]	100	150

[a] With the normal substrate G6P.
[b] As % of normal G6PD B.
[c] International units (IU)/g haemoglobin.
[d] mIU/mg protein.

A G6PD assay on the patient's leucocytes gave a level of about 3% of normal: it is usually 20–30% with G6PD-Mediterranean, suggesting in this patient a different variant with more severe deficiency. In view of the transfusion history, it was impossible to characterize the patient's G6PD from red cells. Instead, we grew primary fibroblasts from a skin biopsy (as has been done in other similar cases [1]) and used those as source of the variant enzyme [2]. Quantitative assay revealed extreme deficiency also in these cells (see Table 34.3); the K_m^{G6P} was about 40% lower than normal, and activity with the substrate analogue 2dG6P was undetectable.

These findings confirmed severe G6PD deficiency in this boy and ruled out G6PD Mediterranean. By DNA analysis [3], the only difference from the sequence of normal DNA was a T → G substitution at nucleotide position 648 in exon 7, which predicts a substitution of leucine for phenylalanine at amino acid position 216. This new variant has been named G6PD Harilaou (a section of Thessaloniki).

Comments

G6PD deficiency is one of the most common inherited abnormalities of red cells, estimated to be present in at least 500 million people [4]; it is mostly asymptomatic, and it is caused by one of a number of mutations; polymorphic in many populations, referred to as class B mutations [5]. In contrast, chronic non-spherocytic haemolytic anaemia (CNSHA[1]) caused

[1] Although occasional spherocytes can be seen in this condition, the term CNSHA is time-honoured: it is meant to differentiate it from the more common hereditary spherocytosis.

by G6PD deficiency is a very rare disease; it results from a distinct set of rare mutations, referred to as class A mutations [5]. Within this rare group there is a spectrum of clinical severity, depending on individual mutations: our patient unfortunately has rather severe disease. Indeed, his steady-state Hb level qualified for moderate to severe anaemia; in addition, he has suffered exacerbations of his anaemia, and he has required blood transfusion recurrently, to the extent that he had to be regarded as transfusion-dependent (see Figure 34.3). This patient illustrates that the distinction between class A and class B mutations is clinically very important. Although in CNSHA due to G6PD deficiency, the spleen does not play the specific role that it plays in the pathophysiology of HS, it is a major site of red cell destruction, and splenectomy can be highly beneficial (see below).

On account of gradual loss during red cell ageing, in general any enzyme deficiency is more marked in erythrocytes than in nucleated cells: since the G6PD activity in this patient's fibroblasts is about 1% of normal, we infer that its deficiency in erythrocytes must be extreme; thus, we have no doubt it is responsible for the patient's CNSHA and for its severity.

Enzymatically active G6PD exists in red cells in the form of both a dimer and a tetramer of a single subunit that is 515 amino acids long: G6PD mutations can cause deficiency because of protein instability, low catalytic activity, abnormal kinetics, or any combination of the above. Many of the class A mutations are in exon 10, and they affect the dimer–dimer interface, and therefore the stability of the tetramer. The mutation of G6PD Harilaou (see Figure 34.2) is instead in exon 7; we are not yet sure whether its severe enzymatic deficiency is due to instability or to drastically impaired catalytic activity, or both.

Since G6PD deficiency is X-linked, and in view of the fact that the mother is clinically and haematologically normal, one might have thought that G6PD-Harilaou had arisen in this boy through a *de novo* mutation. However, analysis of the mother's fibroblasts revealed mosaicism, and DNA analysis confirmed that she is heterozygous for this mutation. This must mean that marked somatic cell selection has occurred in her haematopoietic cells, favouring those with the normal G6PD allele on the active X-chromosome. The same phenomenon has been observed in heterozygotes for other class A mutations [8].

A newborn child with G6PD-Harilaou (related to our patient) has been reported [9], who suffered intrauterine haemolysis before birth and meconium aspiration: in spite of appropriate intensive care, the baby passed away 39 hours after birth. Whereas common (class B) G6PD deficiency,

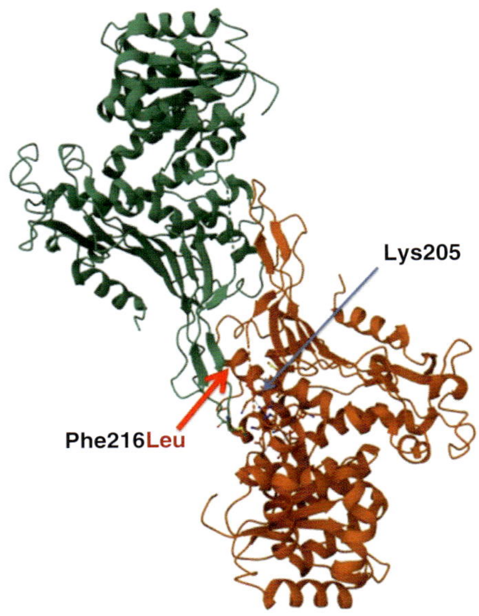

Figure 34.2 Structure of the G6PD dimer (downloaded from Protein Data Bank: PDB ID 7SNF). The 3D structure of the molecule was solved in the year 2000 [6]. The mutation in this patient, at amino acid 216 (red arrow) is rather near the lysine 205 residue (blue arrow) that is essential for catalytic activity. [7]/with permission of Elsevier.

affecting millions, requires attention only as a risk factor for haemolysis, each class A variant is a disease with its own pattern of severity: it requires appropriate management, including genetic counselling.

Follow-up

Since there was no evidence of ineffective erythropoiesis or of excessive expansion of marrow spaces, the patient continued on folic acid and on blood transfusion management, aiming to maintain a comfortable level of haemoglobin (7–9 g/dl), rather than aiming to suppress erythropoiesis (as is recommended in thalassaemia). At the age of eight, splenectomy and cholecystectomy were performed (see Figure 34.3).[2] There were no postoperative complications, and the child was commenced on penicillin prophylaxis. On subsequent blood tests, the patient has maintained a level of haemoglobin of about 11 g/dl with a retic count of about 6%. In the following three years, he has not required any blood transfusion.

[2] The spleen was large, hard and covered with white spots; it weighed 375 g and measured 15×11×5 cm. There was a reduction of the white pulp and thickening of the fibrous strands. There were no foci of extramedullary erythropoiesis seen. The gall bladder appeared swollen and inflamed; it measured 5 × 1 cm and contained small polygonal stones of 0.2–0.4 cm in diameter.

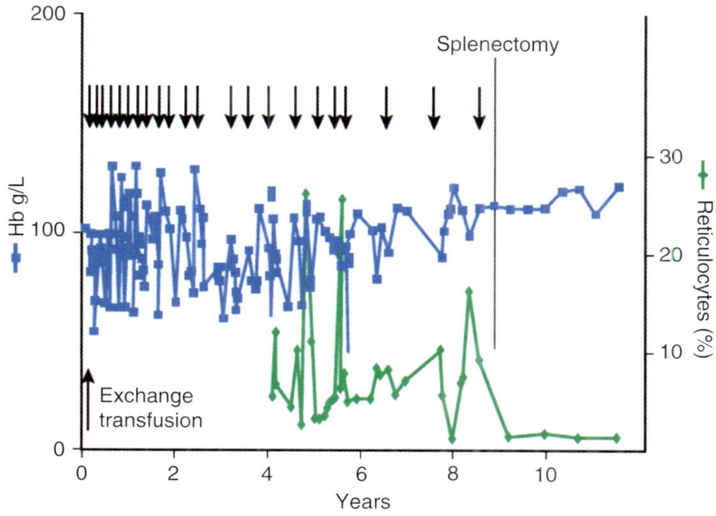

Figure 34.3 Chart showing clinical follow-up.

Further Follow-up

The patient, now aged 42, has continued to be generally well; his steady-state haemoglobin is about 10 g/dl, but he is intermittently transfused. He has graduated from school and has then taken part in a master chef competition. However, he has had thrombosis affecting both of his eyes, and also an episode of pulmonary embolism, for which he had placement of an "umbrella" device in his inferior vena cava; he is receiving anticoagulant treatment.[3]

Conclusion

CNSHA due to G6PD Harilaou (a new class A variant).

Acknowledgements

Dr. Miranda Athanassiou-Metaxa, Paediatric Haematology Department, University of Thessaloniki, Hippokration General Hospital, Thessaloniki, Greece.
Dr. Maria Papaioannou, Paediatric Haematology Department, University of Thessaloniki, Hippokration General Hospital, Thessaloniki, Greece.

[3] With the common variants of G6PD deficiency (class B), thrombosis has been very rarely encountered [10]; and in a deliberate study it was found in Sardinia that G6PD-deficient patients have a significantly decreased risk of developing retinal vein occlusion [11]. Therefore, we cannot say whether the serious thrombotic complications experienced by our patient may be related to this particular class A variant, G6PD-Harilaou, or whether there is some other risk factor.

References

1. Junien, C., Kaplan, J.C., Heienhofer, H.C. et al. (1974). G6PD-Baudelocque: a new unstable variant characterized in cultured fibroblasts. *Enzyme* 18, 48–40.
2. Town, M., Athanasiou Metaxa, M., and Luzzatto, L. (1990). Intragenic interspecific complementation of glucose-6-phosphate dehydrogenase in human-hamster cell hybrids. *Somat. Cell Mol. Genet.* 16, 97–108.
3. Poggi, V., Town, M., Foulkes, N.S. et al. (1990). Identification of a single base change in the G6PD gene by PCR amplification of the entire coding region from genomic DNA. *Biochem. J.* 271, 157–160.
4. Luzzatto, L., Ally, M., and Notaro, R. (2020). Glucose-6-phosphate dehydrogenase deficiency. *Blood* 136(11), 1225–1240.
5. Luzzatto, L., Bancone, G., Dugue, P.A. et al. (2024). New WHO classification of genetic variants causing G6PD deficiency. *Bull. World Health Organ.* 102(8), 615–617.
6. Au, S.W., Gover, S., Lam, V.M. et al. (2000). Human glucose-6-phosphate dehydrogenase: the crystal structure reveals a structural NADP(+) molecule and provides insights into enzyme deficiency. *Structure* 8(3), 293–303.
7. Bautista, J.M., Mason, P.J., and Luzzatto, L. (1995). Human glucose-6-phosphate dehydrogenase. Lysine 205 is dispensable for substrate binding but essential for catalysis. *FEBS Lett.* 366, 61–64.
8. Filosa, S., Giacometti, N., Wangwei, C. et al. (1996). Somatic cell selection is a major determinant of the blood cell phenotype in heterozygotes for glucose 6-phosphate dehydrogenase mutations causing severe enzyme deficiency. *Am. J. Hum. Genet.* 59, 887–895.
9. Athanasiadou, K.I., Amarantidou, M., Drogouti, E. et al. (2021). G6PD deficiency and Harilaou variant in a newborn: intrauterine haemolysis and meconium aspiration syndrome. *J. Mother Child.* 25(1), 61–64.
10. Albertsen, J., Ommen, H.B., Wandler, A. et al. (2014). Fatal haemolytic crisis with microvascular pulmonary obstruction mimicking a pulmonary embolism in a young African man with glucose-6-phosphate dehydrogenase deficiency. *BMJ Case Rep.* 2014, bcr2013201432.
11. Pinna, A., Carru, C., Solinas, G. et al. (2007). Glucose-6-phosphate dehydrogenase deficiency in retinal vein occlusion. *Invest. Ophthalmol. Vis. Sci.* 48(6), 2747–2752.

Case 35

When the Sickle Stabs the Kidney

Patient Details

Age: 27 *Sex:* M
Ethnic background: Nigerian
Occupation: Social Science Graduate

Reason for Referral

Management, jointly with nephrology, of patient with sickle cell anaemia.

History and Clinical Findings in Brief

At the age of 2, the patient had been diagnosed as having sickle cell anaemia in Nigeria, where he was born. Until the age of 24, he had a relatively mild clinical course: he recalls not more than one painful crisis every two years requiring hospital treatment. Recently, the patient complained of feeling generally more tired, with episodes of breathlessness; he said his exercise tolerance had decreased over the last six to seven months, although he felt otherwise well. He had received blood transfusions only for surgery, specifically because, in 1987 and in 1988, he had two craniotomies for clipping of intracranial aneurysms. In the past two years, the patient has had more frequent crises requiring hospital admissions (2–3 per year). Investigations revealed renal failure and proteinuria, and he was referred to the Renal Medicine unit at the Hammersmith Hospital in November 1991. A renal biopsy showed no evidence of glomerulonephritis; however, it revealed segmental sclerosis of the glomeruli with associated tubular atrophy and a moderate inflammatory cell infiltrate with mononuclear cells. The patient's renal failure was thought to be due to "ischaemic changes secondary to repeated sickle cell crises." On examination, the patient was in fair general condition, although pale and jaundiced. His abdomen was not tender, but there was a palpable firm liver edge. The spleen could not be felt.

Laboratory Findings

The patient had a very severe anaemia (see Table 35.1). The mild increase in MCV was probably attributable to his marked reticulocytosis. On the blood film (see Figure 35.1), we saw numerous irreversibly sickled cells (ISC) that were so thin and hyperdense they looked as though they might readily snap in two; others were canoe-shaped with minimal central pallor as if on their way to becoming ISCs. Several cells exhibited "puddling" of haemoglobin; an occasional cell appeared as a hemighost, while some were homogeneously dense. A few target cells and many polychromatic cells were also seen. An ISC was seen even among reticulocytes (Figure 35.2). The extreme anisocytosis was reflected in the markedly elevated RDW value (see Figure 35.3).

Initial Assessment

There was no question that the patient had homozygous sickle cell anaemia. Although the patient had a full-time job and was in fact planning a trip around the world, his level of haemoglobin was much less than is encountered in the majority of patients with this condition in the steady state. The

Table 35.1 Haematology Data

Hb (g/dl)	4.7
RBC ($\times 10^{12}$/l)	1.22
MCV (fl)	100.0
MCH (pg)	38.5
MCHC (g/dl)	38.5
RDW (S.D.)	93.2
Retic (%)	18.0
Retic ($\times 10^{9}$/l)	220
Hb F (%)	4.4

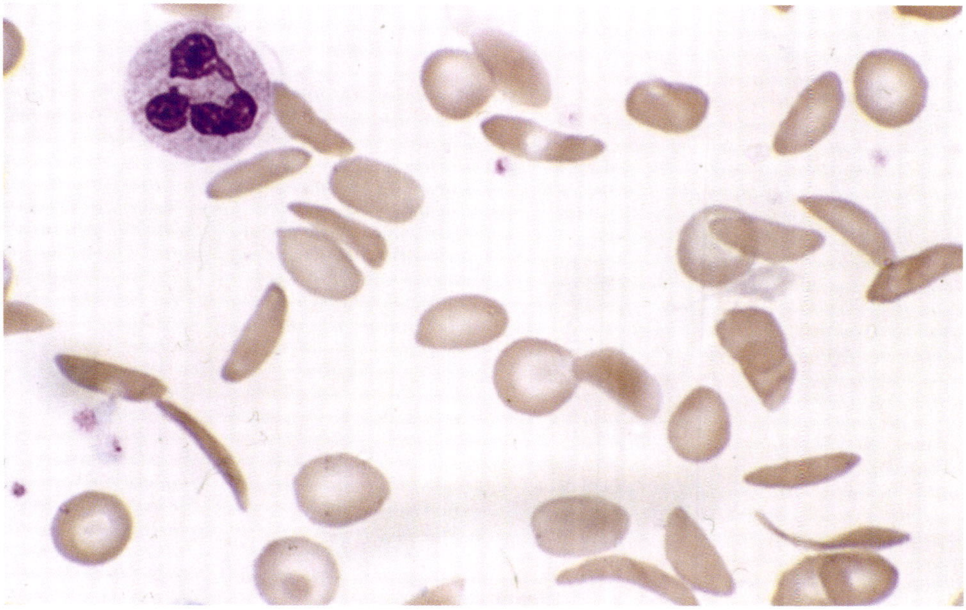

Figure 35.1 Peripheral blood film.

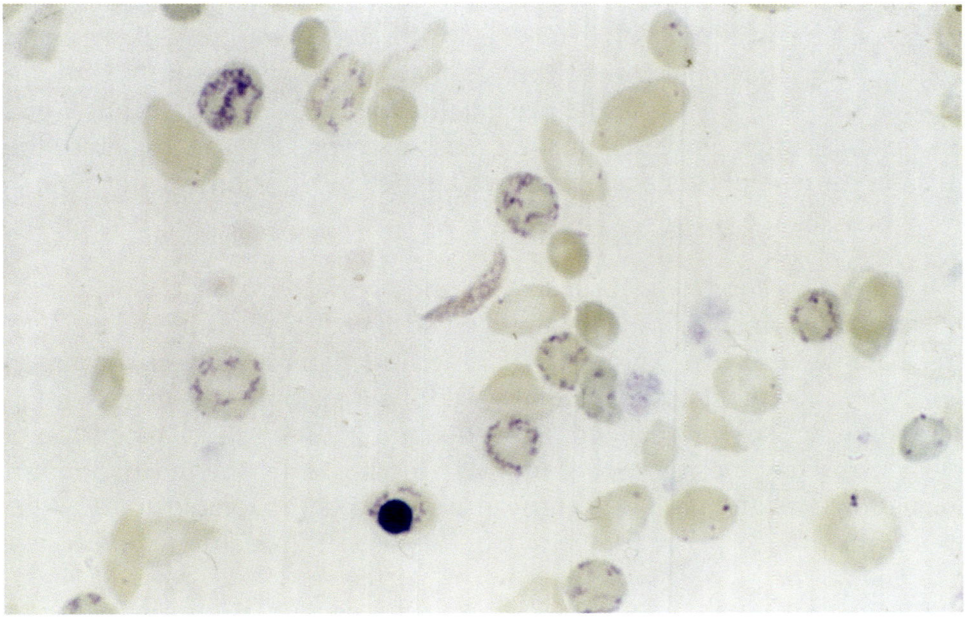

Figure 35.2 Reticulocyte preparation. It is rare to see an irreversibly sickled reticulocyte.

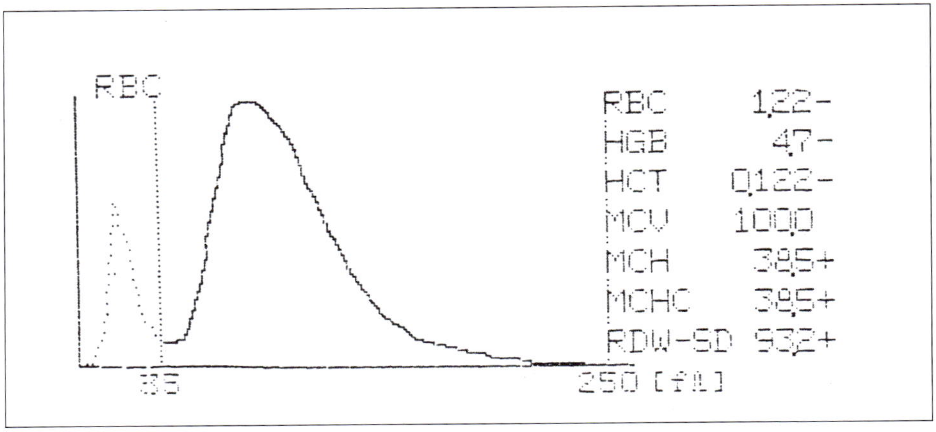

Figure 35.3 Red cell histogram showing markedly raised RDW.

most likely cause for this was chronic renal failure. In addition, although large numbers of ISC will cause an elevation in the MCHC, the value seen here was simply *too* high.

Further Investigations

Although several artefactual causes (including hyperlipidaemia) can cause a spuriously high MCHC [1], in this case, the most likely cause was probably haemoglobin in the plasma. When we centrifuged an aliquot of the patient's blood, the plasma did not appear lipaemic, but it was an opaque coffee-brown colour. By measuring plasma haemoglobin, the intra-erythrocytic haemoglobin was calculated by the following formula:

$$\text{True Hb} = \text{Whole blood Hb} - [(1 - \text{PCV}) \times \text{Plasma Hb}].$$

This gave a corrected Hb level of 4.2 and a corrected MCHC of 35.0 g/dl. Spectroscopic analysis of the patient's plasma confirmed the presence of free haemoglobin (see Figure 35.4a). Thus, the high MCHC was accounted for by true haemoglobin, but some of the haemoglobin was extracellular. The colour was reminiscent of methaemalbumin; this again was confirmed by spectroscopy (positive Schümm's test: Figure 35.4b). Methaemalbumin formation is a landmark of significant intravascular haemolysis (IVH), as it is formed once plasma haptoglobin has been fully saturated with free haemoglobin.

The serum LDH level was about 10× the upper limit of normal, consistent with IVH. A G6PD assay revealed a low enzyme level with a fast electrophoretic mobility, compatible with G6PD A– (see Table 35.2), the

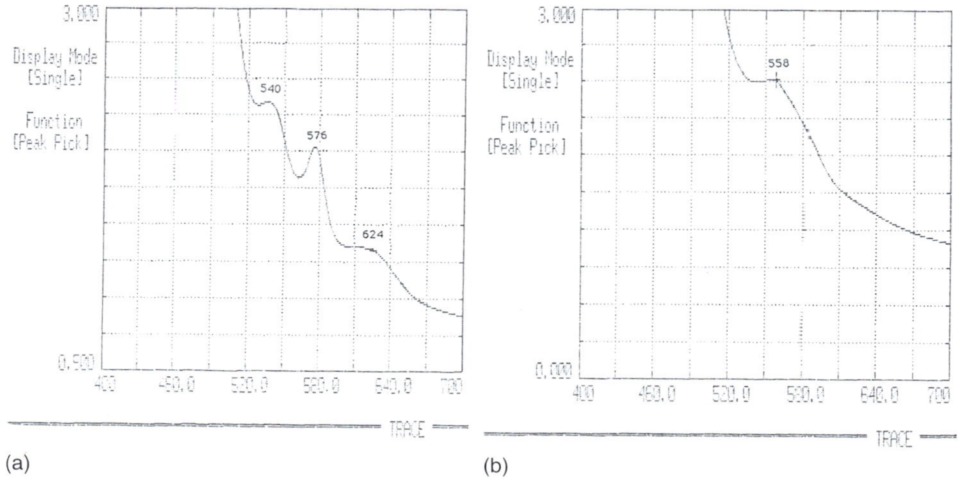

Figure 35.4 Schümm's test; spectral scans of plasma sample showing (a) neat plasma peaks of oxyhaemoglobin (540 nm and 576 nm) and a third peak at 624 nm. (b) After the addition of yellow ammonium sulphide, revealing a single peak at 558 nm, which is characteristic of methaemalbumin.

Table 35.2 Additional Studies

LDH (IU/l)	4375
G6PD (IU/g Hb)	1.8
G6PD E/P	A−
Schumm's test	positive
Heinz body film	positive
Urea (mmol/l)	15.8
Creatinine (μmol/l)	254
Urine haemosiderin	positive
Erythropoietin (milli u/ml)	105
2,3-BPG (μmol/g Hb)	15.4
Bicarbonate (mmol/l)	17

commonest G6PD deficiency variant in Africa and in people of African descent. A Heinz body preparation was positive, with 5% of the red cells exhibiting a single inclusion body. The 2,3-BPG level was at the upper limit of the reference range and may have helped the patient to tolerate his very severe anaemia.

Urea and creatinine (Table 35.2) showed that the patient was in renal failure; venous bicarbonate level was low. Examination of a urinary sediment revealed cells or cellular fragments that were not easy to classify, and occasional hyaline or granular casts; an iron stain showed massive

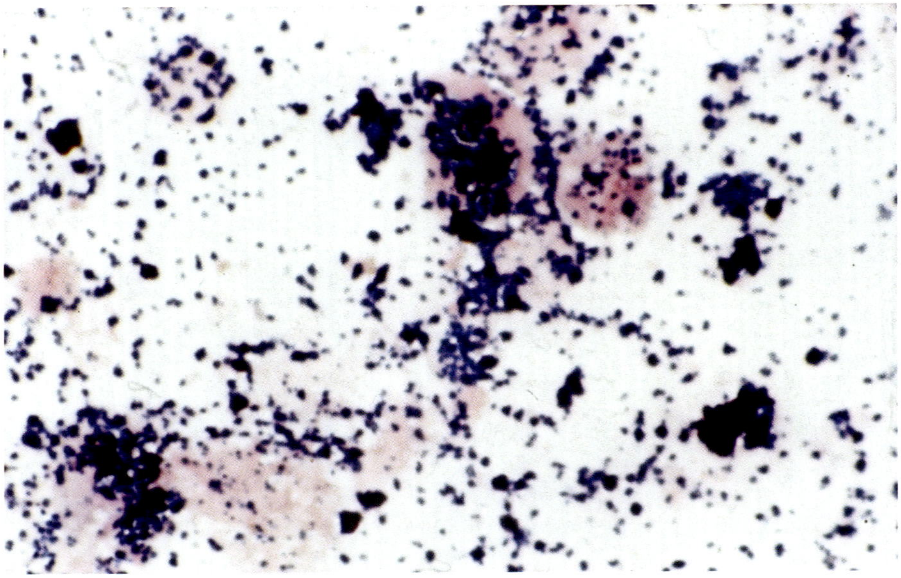

Figure 35.5 Urinary haemosiderin +++.

haemosiderinuria (Figure 35.5). Renal imaging by MRI showed no evidence of papillary necrosis. An assay for erythropoietin (EPO) gave a relatively high value, in spite of renal failure.

Comments

Chronic renal disease (CKD) is not uncommon in patients with sickle cell disease (SCD) [2]; however, most of them do not have severe CKD at age 27. It has been estimated that the annual rate of incidence of CKD is two-to three-fold higher in SCD compared to the general population [3]: when it occurs it is important, since it may account for 16–18% of mortality in this condition [4]. Like for many other serious manifestations of SCD, often we don't know exactly why CKD develops in one patient and not in another: papillary necrosis is a classical manifestation of a vaso-occlusive event in the kidney; however, in this patient the findings were those of segmental glomerulosclerosis, which has been attributed to sickling in the glomerular capillary bed [5]. On the other hand, one of the associations observed with CKD has been with a high LDH level [6], and this is characteristic of IVH.

The shortened red cell life span in patients with sickle cell anaemia is due to both *extravascular haemolysis* (EVH) and IVH [7, 8]; the former is probably predominant in most cases, but the ratio between the two is variable. In this patient, IVH was documented by definitive tests: on grounds of very high LDH and the presence of methaemalbuminaemia, it must have been rather intense, and on grounds of conspicuous haemosiderinuria, it must have been chronic. IVH has emerged, particularly in recent years, as an important factor in the pathophysiology of SCD: it can cause painful attacks from smooth muscle dystonia consequent on nitric oxide depletion, and it may contribute to several serious complications, including CKD and pulmonary hypertension [9–12]. The association of SCD and G6PD deficiency is not uncommon, since there are several parts of the world, including Nigeria, where both are relatively frequent [13]. In the steady state, the coexistence of G6PD deficiency has little impact on the clinical course of SCD, although it tends to lower slightly the steady-state haemoglobin level [14, 15]. In the absence of a trigger, G6PD deficiency of the A– type does not on its own cause IVH; but we cannot exclude that in some way it may have contributed. That the anaemia was predominantly haemolytic is supported by the sustained high reticulocyte count that, however, is not as high as it might be with in the face of a haemoglobin level of 4.2. The marrow remains active, but perhaps erythropoiesis was affected by renal failure.

Follow-up

The patient was given an exchange blood transfusion and was then started on treatment with subcutaneous exogenous EPO. This treatment was "off label" at the time, because unlike exchange transfusion, it would increase the level of Hb S rather than Hb A; however, many subsequent studies have shown benefits [16]. In the event, in spite of escalating EPO to a dose of 15,000 units three times per week (representing a dose of 650 units per kg per week), the patient's haemoglobin level failed to improve and hence this treatment was stopped. The patient was enrolled into a "hyper-transfusion programme"; however, over the next three years his renal function gradually declined: when his urea was 30.8, his creatinine 583, and his estimated glomerular filtration was 13, he had to be regarded as in end-stage renal disease, and he was started on haemodialysis.

Conclusion

Renal failure and G6PD deficiency in a patient with homozygous sickle cell anaemia who had conspicuous IVH.

Acknowledgements

Dr. E. Clutterbuck, Renal Medicine, Hammersmith Hospital, London, UK.
Dr. David Kerr, Renal Medicine, Hammersmith Hospital, London, UK.
Dr. M. F. McMullin, Department of Haematology, Royal Victoria Hospital, Belfast, Ireland.

References

1. Berda-Haddad, Y., Faure, C., Boubaya, M. et al. (2017). Increased mean corpuscular haemoglobin concentration: artefact or pathological condition? *Int. J. Lab. Hematol.* 39(1), 32–41.
2. Wigfall, D.R., Ware, R.E., Burchinal, M.R. et al. (2000). Prevalence and clinical correlates of glomerulopathy in children with sickle cell disease. *J. Pediatr.* 136, 749–753.
3. Yeruva, S.L., Paul, Y., Oneal, P. et al. (2016). Renal failure in sickle cell disease: prevalence, predictors of disease, mortality and effect on length of hospital stay. *Hemoglobin* 40(5), 295–299.
4. Nath, K.A. and Hebbel, R.P. (2015). Sickle cell disease: renal manifestations and mechanisms. *Nat. Rev. Nephrol.* 11(3), 161–171.
5. Bhathena, D.B. and Sondheimer, J.H. (1991). The glomerulopathy of homozygous sickle hemoglobin (SS) disease: morphology and pathogenesis. *J. Am. Soc. Nephrol.* 1, 1241–1252.
6. Parker, M.M., Damrauer, S.M., Tcheandjieu, C. et al. (2021). Association of the transthyretin variant V122I with polyneuropathy among individuals of African ancestry. *Sci. Rep.* 11(1), 11645.
7. Crosby, W.H. (1955). The metabolism of hemoglobin and bile pigment in hemolytic disease. *Am. J. Med.* 18(1), 112–122.
8. Bensinger, T.A. and Gillette, P.N. (1974). Hemolysis in sickle cell disease. *Arch. Intern. Med.* 133(4), 624–631.
9. Gladwin, M.T. (2006). Role of the red blood cell in nitric oxide homeostasis and hypoxic vasodilation. *Adv. Exp. Med. Biol.* 588, 189–205.
10. Kato, G.J., Steinberg, M.H., and Gladwin, M.T. (2017). Intravascular hemolysis and the pathophysiology of sickle cell disease. *J. Clin. Invest.* 127(3), 750–760.
11. Nader, E., Romana, M., and Connes, P. (2020). The red blood cell-inflammation vicious circle in sickle cell disease. *Front. Immunol.* 11, 454.
12. Rother, R.P., Bell, L., Hillmen, P. et al. (2005). The clinical sequelae of intravascular hemolysis and extracellular plasma hemoglobin: a novel mechanism of human disease. *JAMA* 293(13), 1653–1662.
13. Livingstone, F.B. (1971). Malaria and human polymorphisms. *Ann. Rev. Gene.* 5, 33–64.

14. Bienzle, U., Sodeinde, O., Effiong, C.E. et al. (1975). Glucose 6-phosphate dehydrogenase deficiency and sickle cell anemia: frequency and features of the association in an African community. *Blood* 46, 591–597.

15. Nouraie, M., Reading, N.S., Campbell, A. et al. (2010). Association of G6PD with lower haemoglobin concentration but not increased haemolysis in patients with sickle cell anaemia. *Br. J. Haematol.* 150(2), 218–225.

16. Ferreira, F.A., Benites, B.D., Costa, F.F. et al. (2019). Recombinant erythropoietin as alternative to red cell transfusion in sickle cell disease. *Vox Sang.* 114(2), 178–181.

Case 36

Dry Cells, Fake Potassium, Real Iron

Patient Details

Age: 36 *Sex:* M
Ethnic background: Portuguese

Reason for Referral

Investigation of a haemolytic state and associated iron overload.

History and Clinical Findings in Brief

When first seen at the Hammersmith Hospital, the patient looked very fit. There was a slight grey tinge to the skin but he was not pale or jaundiced. There were some small lymph nodes in the left axilla. His liver was palpable 6 cm below the costal margin. The history was very well outlined in the referral letter. Briefly, at the age of 19 (in 1967), after a bout of tonsillitis, the patient was noticed to be jaundiced. Physical examination at that time revealed hepatosplenomegaly. A liver biopsy demonstrated excess iron. Two years later, a diagnosis of spherocytosis was made; splenectomy was recommended, but at that time the patient declined; instead, he was treated with vitamin supplements and oral iron. In 1981, he had an episode of abdominal pain; an oral cholecystogram was negative. Haematological investigations were in keeping with compensated haemolysis. Bone marrow examination revealed erythroid hyperplasia.

Between 1984 and 1986 he had several episodes of abdominal pain ascribed to gallstones; and in 1987 he underwent splenectomy. The spleen was not reported as having excess iron; but a liver biopsy taken at operation showed grade 3–4 haemosiderosis. In January 1988, an intensive programme of phlebotomy was commenced; this was followed by significant reduction in the size of the liver and in the level of serum ferritin.

The family history was quite informative. The patient belongs to a sibship of nine (Figure 36.2). Two brothers and two sisters are also said to show evidence of haemolysis and iron overload. In the next generation, there are 14 children, of whom 4 also show similar manifestations (one being the son of this patient). The patient's father died aged 67 with diabetes, cirrhosis and heart problems (haematological status not known).

Laboratory Findings

Although the patient had a normal haemoglobin (see Table 36.1), his red cell count was low; his MCV was mildly elevated; his MCH and MCHC were very high. The overall appearance of the blood film was hyperchromic (see Figure 36.1). There were many poikilocytes, target cells and rare cells that, instead of having a central area of pallor, appeared to have a slit-like mouth or stoma (stomatocytes). A few cells contained a Howell–Jolly body, and the platelet count was also elevated; these last findings could be attributed to the patient's splenectomized status.

An osmotic fragility test showed increased *resistance*; this finding clearly was against hereditary spherocytosis (HS), and thalassaemia could be ruled out on red cell indices alone. Additional baseline studies (see Table 36.2)

Table 36.1 Haematology Data

	Patient	Son
Hb (g/dl)	13.2	15.1
RBC ($\times 10^{12}$/l)	3.57	4.28
MCV (fl)	99.7	95.1
MCH (pg)	37.0	35.6
MCHC (g/dl)	37.9	37.8
Retic (%)	6.0	8.0
Retic ($\times 10^9$/l)	214	342
WBC ($\times 10^9$/l)	9.2	8.3
PLT ($\times 10^9$/l)	764	241

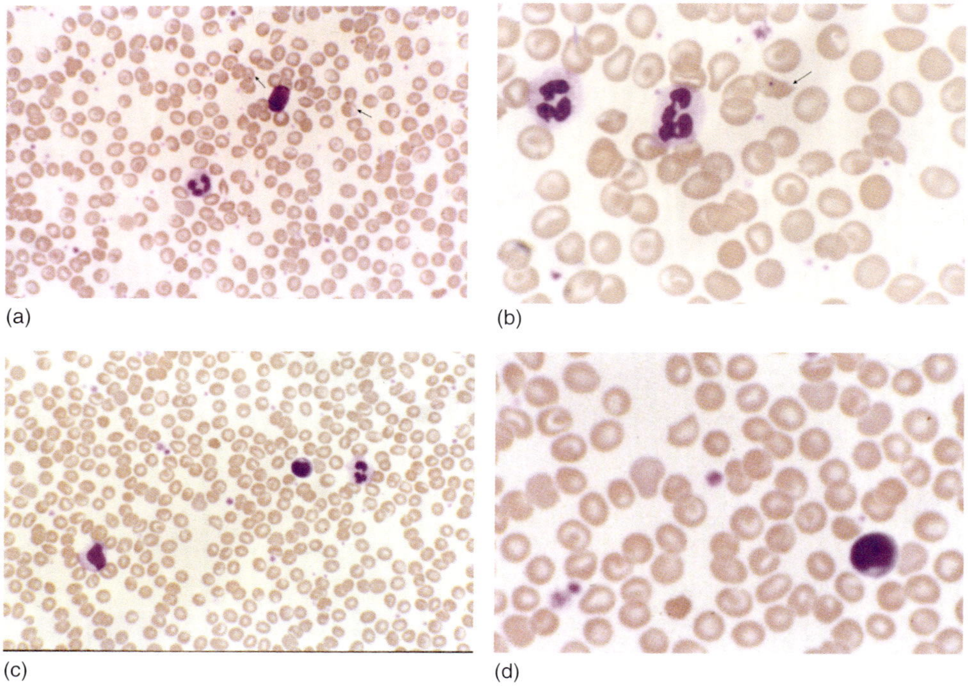

Figure 36.1 Peripheral blood films: patient: (a) medium power view (Howell–Jolly bodies arrowed); (b) high power view (Howell–Jolly body arrowed); son: (c) medium power view; (d) high power view.

Table 36.2 Additional Baseline Studies

	Patient	Son
Potassium (mmol/l)	5.6	6.2
Urea (mmol/l)	8.7	9.1
Bilirubin (μmol/l)	68	74
Haptoglobin (mg/dl)	50	<35
Ferritin (μg/dl)	282	20
Hb E/P	Normal	Normal

showed an increased bilirubin, reduced haptoglobin and increased urea and potassium. A repeat bone marrow aspirate showed erythroid hyperplasia, with mild megaloblastic changes. Marrow iron was not increased, and there were no sideroblasts.

Initial Assessment

Based on the history and blood findings, particularly the significant absolute reticulocytosis, it seemed likely that the patient had indeed a life-long, compensated haemolytic disorder. The family history (see

Figure 36.2) suggested a genetic basis, with autosomal dominant inheritance. Despite the high MCHC, the red cell morphology was not that of HS. In this area, "*the combination of macrocytic cells that are dehydrated (high MCHC and resistance to osmotic lysis) should strongly suggest the diagnosis of hereditary xerocytosis (HX)*": this is a quote from [1]. The coexistence of histological evidence of iron overload in the liver, in the absence of a blood transfusion history also seemed to fit with HX, sometimes also described as dehydrated stomatocytosis (DHS).

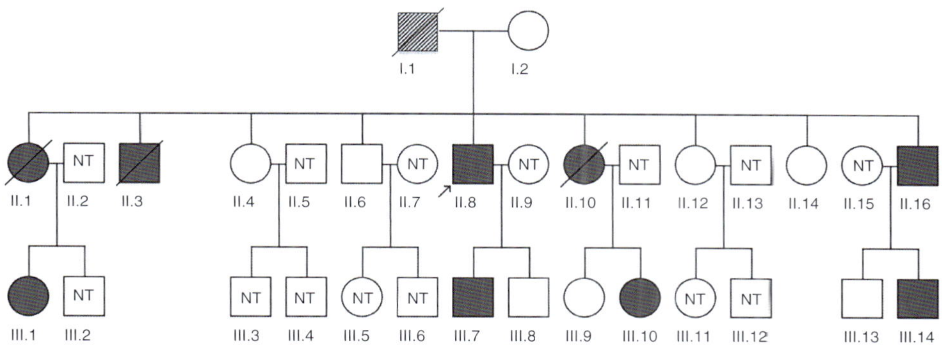

Figure 36.2 Family pedigree and table of results. Patient is indicated by the arrow; the dark symbols correspond to family members with a raised ferritin level, abnormal red cell morphology and signs of haemolysis. NT = not tested. In the table, N stands for normal ferritin level.

Member	Age	Hb	Haemolysis	Red cell morphology	Ferritin
I 2	–	14.1	–	–	—
II 1	51	11.6	+	+	340
II 3	50	13.3	+	+	2260
II 4	46	13.4	–	–	N
II 6	42	17.1	–	–	N
II 8	38	12.4	+	+	505
II 10	36	13.8	+	+	1500
II 12	34	13.8	–	–	N
II 14	31	14.3	–	–	N
II 16	30	14.0	+	+	970
III 1	20	11.6	+	+	181
III 7	18	14.5	+	+	258
III 8	22	15.9	–	–	N
III 9	17	12.0	–	–	N
III 10	27	10.4	+	+	381
III 13	11	13.1	–	–	N
III 14	17	15.6	+	+	358

Further Investigations

Haemoglobin electrophoresis was normal, as were assays for G6PD and pyruvate kinase. The Ham test was negative. An auto-haemolysis test was abnormal, with full correction by added glucose (see Table 36.3).

The high plasma potassium level was not matched by any ECG abnormality, and therefore we suspected it might be an artefact; indeed, when further samples were taken and centrifuged *immediately* after collection, the K^+ levels were normal. However, when blood from the patient, from his son and from a normal control were incubated at 37 °C, during the first three hours there was a fall in plasma K^+ (due to uptake by red cells, a normal expected finding); but subsequently, there was a much greater increase in the plasma K^+ in the patient and son compared to the control (see Figure 36.3); this was associated with increased glucose consumption (not shown). Thus, although the hyperkalaemia observed in our patient, and previously reported in other patients with HX, is qualified by the prefix

Table 36.3 Results of Autohaemolysis Test

	% lysis at 48 hours	
	Without glucose	Addition of glucose
Control	1.2	0.4
Patient	8.7	0.6
Son	15.6	0.4

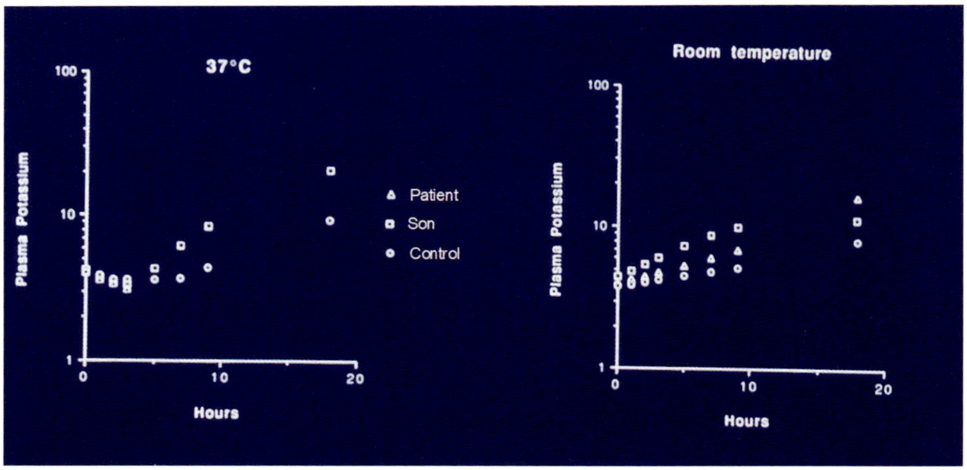

Figure 36.3 Plasma potassium levels during storage of whole blood samples. Left panel, at 37 °C; right panel, at room temperature.

Table 36.4 Studies on Membrane Sodium Pump

	Control	Patient	Son
Na K pump	2.11	5.45	4.82
Na K Cl cotransport	0.72	0.80	0.62
K Cl cotransport	0.02	0.21	0.05
Leak	0.28	0.40	0.22

pseudo-, it does truly reflect potassium leakage, pointing to a serious defect in cation transport.

Special studies on electrolyte transport performed by Dr. Clive Ellory in Oxford revealed very high Na^+ pump activity with a significant volume sensitive K^+/Cl^- flux (see Table 36.4). The inward sodium leak seems to parallel the outward K^+ leak.

SDS-PAGE on a 7.5–10.0% gradient gel revealed a slight increase in the mobility of Band 3 and a reduced ratio of protein 4.1 to protein 4.2. Similar findings have been reported in other patients with HX [2].

With respect to iron overload, a desferal study (10 mg/kg subcutaneous infusion over 12 hours) produced an iron excretion of 70.9 mmol/24 hr (over a baseline excretion of 3.4 mmol/24 hr). This clearly indicates a large excess of iron that can be mobilized by desferal. Molecular analysis for haemochromatosis mutations revealed that both the patient and his son were heterozygous for the p.H63D mutation in the HLA-linked *HFE* gene.

Some years after we carried out these studies, our colleagues at the Institute for Molecular and Cell Biology of the University of Porto found by DNA analysis that the index case in this family has the *PIEZO1* mutation c.7367G>A, p.Arg2456His, already found previously in several HX patients [3].

Comments

In our patient, family history and red cell morphology were highly suggestive of what eventually turned out to be the correct diagnosis. Although the autohaemolysis test (±glucose) is unlikely to be carried out nowadays, it is remarkable that, time and time again, as abundantly exemplified in this book, it is consistently able to discriminate enzymopathies *versus* membranopathies (including channelopathies).

Xerocytosis means *rigid cells*: the red cells in HX are rigid because they are dehydrated, and they are dehydrated because they lose both potassium and water, due to a serious defect in cation transport [4]. Increasing rigidity (or loss of deformability) of red cells normally occurs as they age in circulation [5]; and it is a major factor in causing extravascular haemolysis by erythrophagocytosis [6]. In our patient, red cell rigidity can be presumed to increase prematurely as a result of dehydration, and this is probably the primary mechanism of his chronic haemolysis. Recently, it has been found that in HX altered interplay between *PIEZO1* and the calcium-activated phospholipid scramblase TMEM16F results in increased phosphatidylserine exposure on the outer surface of the red cell membrane; this can contribute to accelerated haemolysis [7].

PIEZO1 is a rather extraordinary membrane protein (Figure 36.4), that can be described as a mechano-sensory transduction channel. In endothelial cells, when *PIEZO1* is activated by fluid shear stress, it allows influx of calcium; this, in turn, triggers downstream signalling pathways that regulate the vascular tone. As for red cells, each time they have to squeeze through a capillary, the mechanical stress will activate *PIEZO1*. Influx of

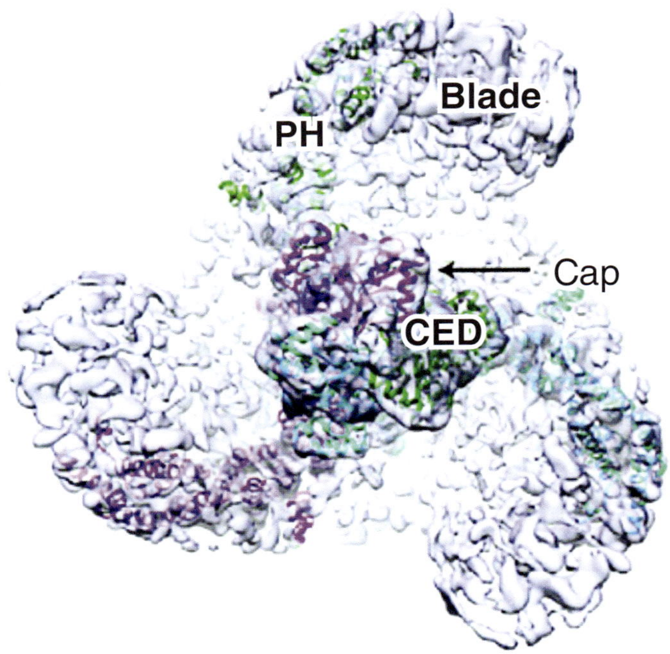

Figure 36.4 *PIEZO1*, a very large membrane protein, is a homotrimer of a 2521 amino acid subunit; its shape is reminiscent of a propeller. *PIEZO1* is embedded in the membrane via 34 transmembrane helical domains; the first 20 of which form each blade of the propeller (PH is one of several peripheral helices). CAP caps the cation channel, or pore; below the pore, there is a regulatory C-terminal domain (CED), which is connected to the blade. The blades confer to the protein its mechano-sensitive properties. The Arg2456His amino acid replacement, present in our patient, is in the pore region. [9]/with permission of John Wiley & Sons.

calcium will activate the protein known for decades as the "Gardos channel" [8]; this will cause loss of K^+ and water, and the decreased volume will facilitate the red cell's passage through the capillary. With normal *PIEZO1*, once the red cell has passage into a venule, these changes will be reversed.

It is not surprising that this sophisticated mechano-sensory mechanism can be critically disturbed by even small structural alterations; indeed, most *PIEZO1* mutations in HX are missense mutations causing single amino acid replacements [3, 10]. A further confirmation of the mechanism outlined above comes from the fact that rarely patients with a haematologic phenotype of HX have a mutation not in *PIEZO1*, but in the gene *KCNN4*, that encodes the Gardos channel [11].

Why a genetic disorder has a dominant inheritance pattern – i.e. it is expressed in heterozygotes – is not a trivial question. In first approximation, if a gene encodes a channel, and if the one-half channel molecules encoded by the mutant gene are leaky, this may cause disease, even though the one-half channel molecules produced by the normal allele are not leaky: thus, explaining dominance. In the case of *PIEZO1*, we can be more specific; since the protein is a homotrimer, if we assume that each trimer is assembled by random sampling of normal and mutant subunits (presumed to be available in equal numbers), only 1/8 of trimers will consist of three normal subunits, whereas 7/8 will include at least one abnormal subunit.[1]

Compared to other genetically determined haemolytic disorders, HX has two somewhat unusual features, both of them conspicuous in our patient: (i) in spite of a high rate of haemolysis, there is often little or no anaemia; (ii) there is often evidence of iron overload: this may occur of course also in other non-transfusion-dependent patients with a chronic haemolytic anaemia, but in HX, it is the rule rather than the exception (as in our patient and in some members of his family). In chronic haemolytic disorders, the rate of erythropoiesis is always increased; but (i) must mean that in HX this is even more true. A likely explanation was offered in one of the first papers on HX (then called DHS), from which we quote [12]: "*The low level of 2,3 diphosphoglycerate will result in a left shift in the oxygen dissociation curve, poor tissue oxygenation and hence increased red cell production. This sequence of events may explain the relatively high hemoglobin levels seen*

[1] "Loss of function" (LOF) mutations are usually recessive, because the un-mutated allele may be sufficient to provide the needed function; in the case of *PIEZO1*, biallelic LOF mutations may cause lymphatic dysplasia and over-hydrated stomatocytosis [15]. The dominant *PIEZO1* mutations that cause HX are instead referred to as "gain of function" (GOF): from the patients' point of view "gain of *mal*function" would seem more appropriate.

in this condition." The low level of 2,3-BPG in HX was recently confirmed in a metabolomics study [13]. As for (ii), a GOF mutation in mouse causes suppression of hepcidin [14]: this and other possible mechanisms of iron overload in HX patients have been extensively discussed [15]. Certainly in our patient's family, like in others, iron overload is associated with DHS; more so than in other chronic haemolytic anaemias, and out of proportion with the severity of haemolysis. Thus, it is likely that (i) and (ii) are not unrelated; the very marked erythroid hyperplasia in the bone marrow, contingent on (i), will produce excessive erythroferrone, with consequent suppression of hepcidin production by the liver; iron overload (ii) will be caused by increased iron absorption through this and/or other mechanisms (reviewed in [16]). In our patient, the p.H63D mutation in *HFE* may have further favoured iron overload.

Splenectomy always increases the risk of thrombosis, at least in part on account of increased platelet counts. In HX, splenectomy is regarded as contraindicated, because the risk of thrombosis is high, and it can occur even after several years; in one retrospective analysis, postsplenectomy thrombosis occurred in 8/8 patients with *PIEZO1* mutations (one of them with the same mutation as our patient); but, interestingly, in none of four patients with *KCNN4* mutations [17]. In our patient, although there was no objective benefit from splenectomy, fortunately there have been no complications.

Follow-up

At the age of 76, and four decades since diagnosis, our patient is still reporting a good quality of life. This can be attributed in good part to the excellent care received from our colleagues at the referring institution in Porto; they have rightly taken advantage of the rather unique feature of HX, whereby the rate of haemolysis is high, but there is no anaemia; thus, they were able to implement a regular and intensive phlebotomy regimen. In the meantime, a diagnosis of HX was confirmed in one of the patient's brothers (II-16 in Figure 36.2) and in his son (III-7 in Figure 36.2), and a similar phlebotomy regimen was instituted.

Conclusion

Hereditary xerocytosis due to a *PIEZO1* mutation, with haemochromatosis.

Acknowledgements

Referred by Dr. Jorge Coutinho, Hospital St. Antonio, Portugal.
Dr. Clive Ellory, University Laboratory of Physiology, Oxford, UK.
Dr. Khedouja Nafa, Department of Human Genetics, Memorial Sloan Kettering Cancer Center, New York, USA.
Dr. Graça Porto, The Institute of Biomedical Sciences Abel Salaza, University of Porto, Portugal.
Dr. Marion Reed, Biochemical Reference Manager, BGRL, Oxford, UK.

References

1. Lux, S.E. (2015). Disorders of the red cell membrane. In: Orkin, S.H., Fisher, D.E., Ginsburg, D.L. et al., editor. *Nathan and Oski's Hematology and Oncology of Infancy and Childhood*. Vol. 1. Philadelphia, PA: Elsevier/Saunders. pp. 515–579.
2. Sauberman, N., Fortier, N.L., Fairbanks, G. et al. (1979). Red cell membrane in haemolytic disease. Studies on variables affecting electrophoretic analysis. *Biochem. Biophys. Acta*. 556, 292–313.
3. Picard, V., Guitton, C., Thuret, I. et al. (2019). Clinical and biological features in PIEZO1-hereditary xerocytosis and Gardos channelopathy: a retrospective series of 126 patients. *Haematologica* 104(8), 1554–1564.
4. Stewart, G.W., Gibson, J.S., and Rees, D.C. (2023). The cation-leaky hereditary stomatocytosis syndromes: a tale of six proteins. *Br. J. Haematol*. 203(4), 509–522.
5. Fortier, N., Snyder, L.M., Garver, F. et al. (1988). The relationship between in vitro generated hemoglobin skeletal protein complex and increased red cell membrane rigidity. *Blood* 71, 1427–1431.
6. Sosale, N.G., Rouhiparkouhi, T., Bradshaw, A.M. et al. (2015). Cell rigidity and shape override CD47's "self"-signaling in phagocytosis by hyperactivating myosin-II. *Blood* 125(3), 542–552.
7. Liang, P., Zhang, Y., Wan, Y.C.S. et al. (2024). Deciphering and disrupting PIEZO1-TMEM16F interplay in hereditary xerocytosis. *Blood* 143(4), 357–369.
8. Gardos, G. (1958). The function of calcium in the potassium permeability of human erythrocytes. *Biochim. Biophys. Acta* 30, 653–654.
9. Wang, Y. and Xiao, B. (2018). The mechanosensitive Piezo1 channel: structural features and molecular bases underlying its ion permeation and mechanotransduction. *J. Physiol*. 596(6), 969–978.
10. Andolfo, I., Russo, R., Rosato, B.E. et al. (2018). Genotype-phenotype correlation and risk stratification in a cohort of 123 hereditary stomatocytosis patients. *Am. J. Hematol*. 93(12), 1509–1517.
11. Glogowska, E., Lezon-Geyda, K., Maksimova, Y. et al. (2015). Mutations in the Gardos channel (KCNN4) are associated with hereditary xerocytosis. *Blood* 126(11), 1281–1284.
12. McGrath, K.M., Collecutt, M.F., Gordon, A. et al. (1984). Dehydrated hereditary stomatocytosis–a report of two families and a review of the literature. *Pathology* 16(2), 146–150.

13. Kiger, L., Oliveira, L., Guitton, C. et al. (2021). Piezo1-xerocytosis red cell metabolome shows impaired glycolysis and increased hemoglobin oxygen affinity. *Blood Adv.* 5(1), 84–88.

14. Ma, S., Dubin, A.E., Zhang, Y. et al. (2021). A role of PIEZO1 in iron metabolism in mice and humans. *Cell* 184(4), 969–982.e13.

15. Andolfo, I., Iolascon, A., and Russo, R. (2025). The evolving landscape of hereditary stomatocytosis. *Blood* 145(26), 3089–3100.

16. Camaschella, C., Nai, A., and Silvestri, L. (2020). Iron metabolism and iron disorders revisited in the hepcidin era. *Haematologica* 105(2), 260–272.

17. Picard, V., Guitton, C., Thuret, I. et al. (2019). Clinical and biological features in PIEZO1-hereditary xerocytosis and Gardos channelopathy: a retrospective series of 126 patients. *Haematologica* 104, 1554–1564.

Case 37

Hb on Target

Patient Details

Age: 29 *Sex:* F
Ethnic background: Ghana

Reason for Referral

Preoperative blood count.

History and Clinical Findings in Brief

There was no significant medical history and no family history of illness. The patient was quite healthy, but she was due to have a termination of pregnancy (TOP) upon her request.

Laboratory Findings

The blood count (see Table 37.1) revealed a normal haemoglobin level, with microcytosis and an elevated MCHC. The blood film (see Figure 37.1) showed numerous target cells, contracted cells and also spherocytes. Some cells appeared to have been folded over in their long axis so as to produce "boat-shaped" forms.

Table 37.1 Haematology Data

Hb (g/dl)	13.9
RBC ($\times 10^{12}$/l)	5.29
MCV (fl)	72.6
MCH (pg)	26.3
MCHC (g/dl)	36.2
RDW (S.D.)	39.7
Retic (%)	4.5
Retic ($\times 10^9$/l)	238
Hb C[a] (%)	75.8
Hb F (%)	24.2

[a] Includes Hb A_2, which cannot be resolved on cellulose acetate.

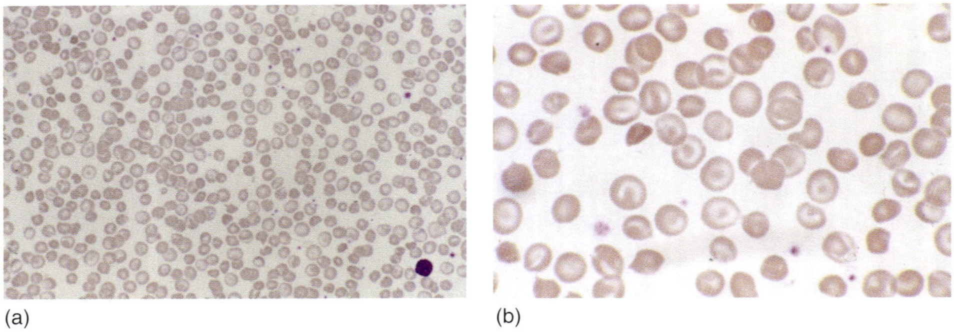

Figure 37.1 Peripheral blood film: (a) medium power view; (b) high power view.

Figure 37.2 Haemoglobin electrophoresis on cellulose acetate membrane; the migration of the haemoglobin fractions is from right to left. An A/S control and A/C control are in lanes 1 and 2, respectively. The patient (R.A.) is in lane 3.

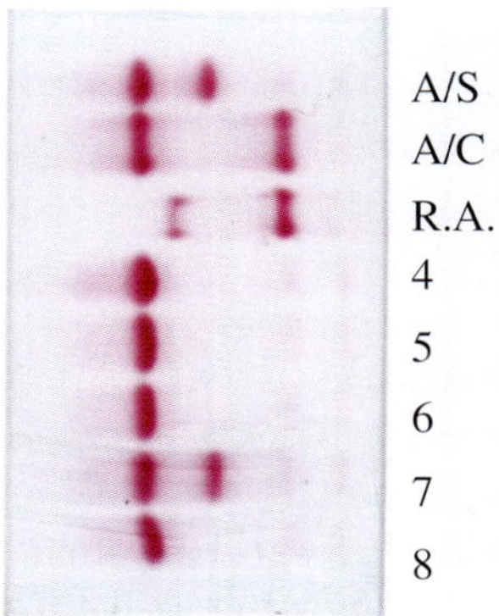

Because this patient was going to have an elective operation under general anaesthesia, haemoglobin electrophoresis was performed (see Figure 37.2). This revealed two haemoglobin bands: one in the position of Hb C (76%) and the other in the position of Hb F (24%).

Initial Assessment

The patient has no clinical symptoms and is not anaemic. However, her red cell morphology is markedly abnormal, and her reticulocytosis is consistent with compensated haemolysis. The large number of target cells on the blood film is compatible with the Hb C seen on electrophoresis. The Hb F level was too high for homozygous Hb C disease; but she could not be an AC heterozygote, since no Hb A was detectable.

Further Investigations

There seemed to be few alternatives in differential diagnosis: C/β^0 thalassaemia, C/$\delta\beta$ thalassaemia, or C/HPFH. In the absence of anaemia and in view of the nearly normal MCH, we favoured the last possibility. Hb A_2 could not be measured in the usual way, since it migrates like Hb C on cellulose acetate membrane.

Agar gel electrophoresis at pH 6.0 confirmed the presence of Hb C and Hb F only (not shown). On globin chain (alkaline) electrophoresis (see Figure 37.3), three bands were seen: one was in the position of α^A, one in the position of β^A and the third was in the exact same position as the β^C of the control sample. The band in the β^A position was of very low intensity compared to the other two bands, which were of equal intensity. Because Hb A was not present in the sample, this had to be γ.

The staining of target cells in the Kleihauer test was of course weaker than in a cord blood, with normal cells, but the distribution of Hb F was clearly pancellular. Southern blot analysis after hybridization to a β-globin probe revealed only normal fragments. After hybridization to a γ-globin probe, we

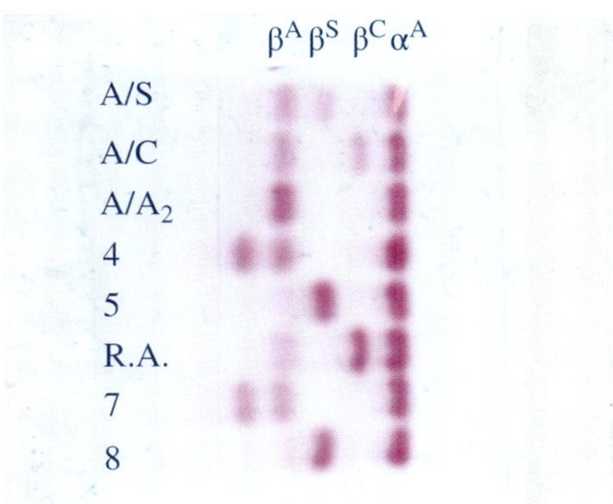

Figure 37.3 Globin chain (alkaline) electrophoresis on cellulose acetate membrane; the migration of the globin chains is from left to right. An A/S, A/C and A/A_2 control are in lanes 1, 2 and 3 respectively. The patient (R.A.) is in lane 6.

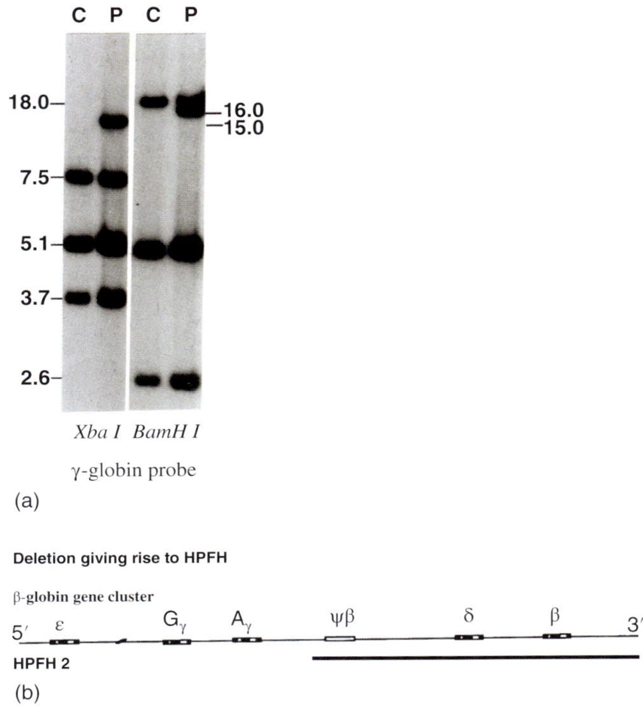

Figure 37.4 (a) Southern blot analysis of patient's DNA, hybridized to a γ-globin probe. Both normal size fragments (indicated in Kb on the left) and abnormal size fragments (indicated in Kb on the right) were seen after digestion with two different restriction enzymes. The abnormal fragments are consistent with the patient being heterozygous for the deletion known as HPFH 2; P: patient; C: normal control. (b) Schematic representation of the β-globin gene cluster (exons are in black boxes and introns in white), and of the HPFH 2 deletion, previously observed among individuals of African origin. The deletion removes the ψβ, δ and β-globin genes.

saw instead both normal and abnormal fragments (see Figure 37.4a and b). This was compatible with a deletion such as would be expected in a heterozygote for HPFH-2.

In view of the low MCV and MCH, we proceeded to analysis of the α-globin gene cluster, which revealed that the patient was heterozygous for α^+ thalassaemia (i.e. α –/ αα).

Comments

Heterozygosity for either Hb C or HPFH is clinically silent; the combination of the two traits in patients with C/HPFH does not generally produce anaemia, but compensated haemolysis [1]. The frequency of haemoglobin C heterozygotes in Ghana is estimated to be as high as 14% [2], and some of the first reports of HPFH have been from Ghana [3].

In patients with homozygous Hb C disease, target cells may be 90% or even more; and target cells were very numerous on this young woman's blood film, in keeping with her 76% Hb C. The spherocytes and contracted cells probably are a consequence of potassium and water loss, secondary to an electrostatic interaction between the positively charged Hb C and the cytoplasmic surface of a negatively charged membrane protein, possibly band 3 [4]. This phenomenon may also explain the patient's high MCHC, reduced red cell deformability and hence their reduced life span. Haemoglobin C crystals, classically seen in Hb C homozygotes, were not seen in this patient.

The MCV has been said to be reduced in AC heterozygotes [5]; however, given that in the area of the Hb C gene HBB^{E6K} (see Figure 37.5), α^{+} thalassaemia is also common, this finding may have been due to association with the latter trait. In a small series from our laboratory, Hb C heterozygotes

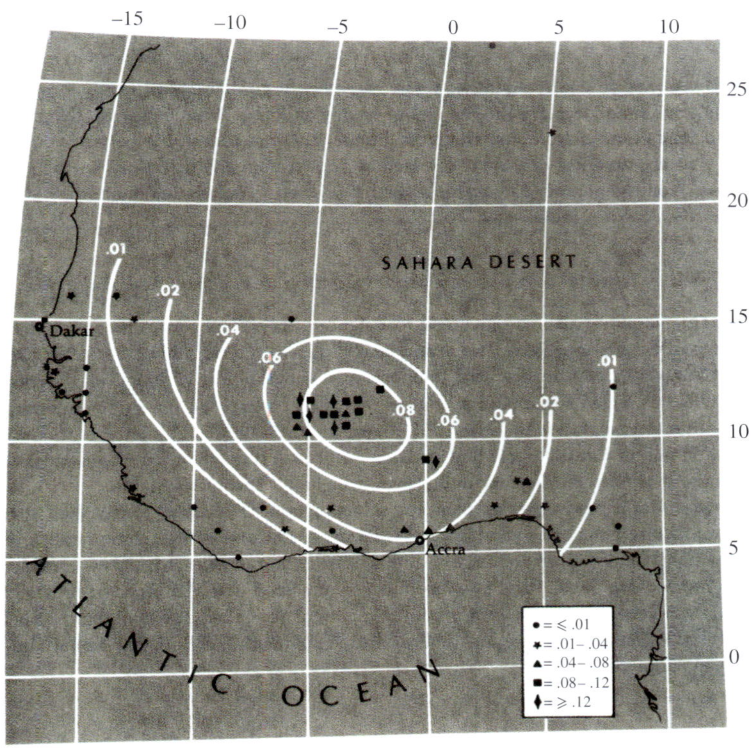

Figure 37.5 Geographical distribution of Hb C gene in West Africa. The numbers 0.01–0.12 are frequencies of the Hb C gene. Reproduced with permission of [6]/W.H. Freeman.

with α-thal trait had a mean MCV of 79.4 fl; but in Hb C heterozygotes with normal α-globin genes and normal iron status, the mean MCV was 83.3 fl (A. Hann, personal communication).

It is interesting that, while we took our usual stepwise approach to reach a definitive diagnosis, in fact it had been already given away by the initial single test of haemoglobin electrophoresis (Figure 37.2), that perhaps today might be bypassed. On the other hand, these days, haemoglobinopathy screening is generally performed by HPLC or capillary electrophoresis. Hb A_2 can be now quantitated even in the presence of Hb C by HPLC (see Figure 37.6).

Both Hb C and Hb S confer protection against mortality from *Plasmodium falciparum* malaria; however, compared to that of Hb S, the geographic distribution of Hb C is much more restricted, with its epicentre in Burkina Faso (Figure 37.5), where presumably the mutation has occurred in an ancestral population. There is a genetic explanation for this. With the Hb S gene, the protection is in heterozygotes; therefore, the gene will be selected for and spread wherever malaria is endemic. With the Hb C gene, the protection may be even greater than in AS heterozygotes, but it is in CC homozygotes [7, 8]; therefore, Darwinian selection operates only where the Hb C gene frequency is high enough to produce a significant number of homozygotes. The protective mechanism is probably also different. In AS heterozygotes,

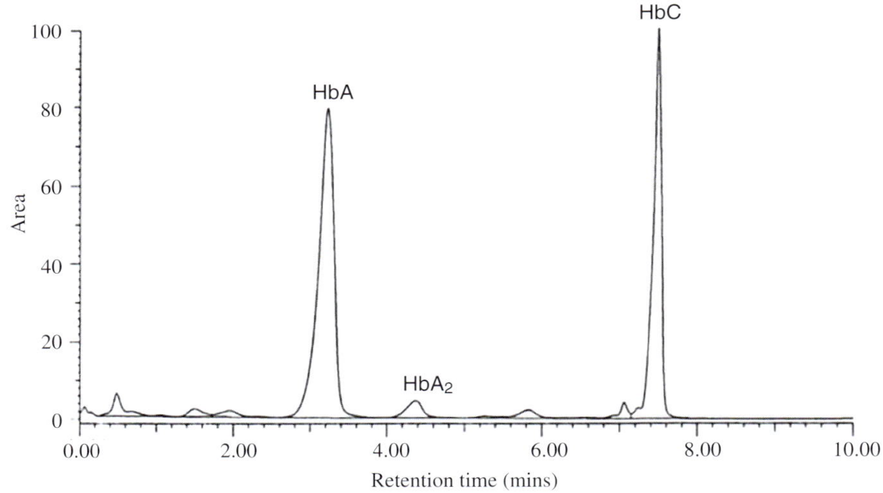

Figure 37.6 HPLC chromatogram from a patient with Hb C trait. The horizontal axis shows the retention (elution) time and [10]/with permission of W.H. Freeman for each haemoglobin. The main peaks identified are (reading from left to right) Hb A, Hb A_2 and Hb C.

parasitization favours sickling, with consequent removal of parasitized red cells by phagocytosis [9]. In CC homozygotes, abnormal actin remodelling specifically interferes with parasite development [10].

Follow-up

The patient had an uneventful TOP. Haemoglobinopathy screening of her partner and her siblings was recommended. Contraceptive advice was offered and follow-up at an appropriate clinic was arranged.

Conclusion

Haemoglobin C/HPFH and α^+ thalassaemia.

Acknowledgements

Amanda Hann (1996), for data on MCV values in Hb C heterozygotes.

References

1. Dacie, J.V. (1985). The Hereditary Haemolytic anaemias. In: Dacie, J.V., editor. *The Haemolytic Anaemias II*. London: Churchill Livingstone. pp. 285–296.
2. Piel, F.B., Howes, R.E., Patil, A.P. et al. (2013). The distribution of haemoglobin C and its prevalence in newborns in Africa. *Sci. Rep*. 3, 1671.
3. Bethlenfalvay, N.C., Motulsky, A.G., Ringelhann, B. et al. (1975). Hereditary persistence of fetal hemoglobin, beta thalassemia, and the hemoglobin delta-beta locus: further family data and genetic interpretations. *Am. J. Hum. Genet*. 27, 140–154.
4. Reiss, G., Ranney, H.M., and Shaklai, N. (1982). The association of haemoglobin C with red cell ghosts. *J. Clin. Invest*. 70, 946.
5. Huisman, T.H. (1977). Trimodality in the percentage of β-chain variants in heterozygotes, the effect of the number of active Hb_α structural loci. *Hemoglobin* 1, 349–382.
6. Bodmer, W.F. and Cavalli-Sforza, L.L. (1976). *Genetics, Evolution, and Man*. San Francisco, CA: W.H. Freeman & Company.
7. Modiano, D., Bancone, G., Ciminelli, B.M. et al. (2008). Haemoglobin S and haemoglobin C: 'quick but costly' versus 'slow but gratis' genetic adaptations to *Plasmodium falciparum* malaria. *Hum. Mol. Genet*. 17, 789–799.
8. Mangano, V.D., Kabore, Y., Bougouma, E.C. et al. (2015). Novel insights into the protective role of hemoglobin S and C against *Plasmodium falciparum* parasitemia. *J. Infect. Dis*. 212, 626–634.

9. Luzzatto, L. (2012). Sickle cell anaemia and malaria. *Mediterr. J. Hematol. Infect. Dis.* 4, e2012065.
10. Cyrklaff, M., Sanchez, C.P., Kilian, N. et al. (2011). Hemoglobins S and C interfere with actin remodeling in *Plasmodium falciparum*-infected erythrocytes. *Science* 334, 1283–1286.

Case 38

Too Little Beta and Too Little Alpha

Patient Details

Age: 23 *Sex:* F
Ethnic background: South East Asia

Reason for Referral

Investigation of thalassaemia (blood sample only).

History and Clinical Findings in Brief

There was no significant medical history; and unfortunately we could not obtain a reliable family history. On a routine antenatal booking at her local hospital, the patient was found to be clinically well, although a little pale.

Laboratory Findings

The patient had a mild anaemia that was severely microcytic, and hypochromic (see Table 38.1). On the blood film (see Figure 38.1), all the red cells were smaller than normal; some were so tiny that their diameter did not exceed the size of a platelet. The hypochromasia was also quite striking. Some red cells had only a thin rim of haemoglobin;

Table 38.1 Haematology Data

Hb (g/dl)	9.9
RBC ($\times 10^{12}$/l)	6.04
MCV (fl)	53.9
MCH (pg)	16.4
MCHC (g/dl)	30.4
RDW (S.D.)	42.1
Retic (%)	1.1
Retic ($\times 10^{9}$/l)	66
Hb A_2 (%)	4.6
Hb F (%)	1.1

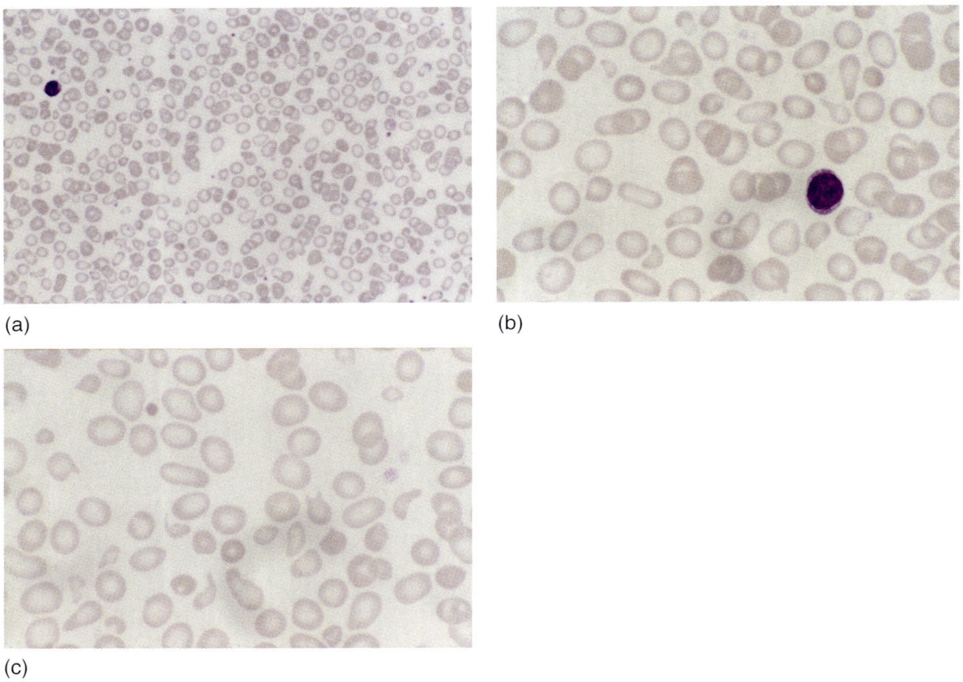

Figure 38.1 Peripheral blood film: (a) medium power view; (b) and (c) high power view.

others, however, seemed so fully haemoglobinized that they looked like microspherocytes. The anisocytosis, very evident on the film, was not reflected in the RDW reported by the analyzer; however, if we make an adjustment for the low MCV, the "corrected" RDW was markedly increased: ["corrected" RDW = analyzer RDW $\times$ (92 $\div$ 53.9) = 71.9]. The platelet profile on the other hand, was significantly affected by the overlap with microcytic red cells; therefore, the count reported is probably an overestimate (see Figure 38.2).

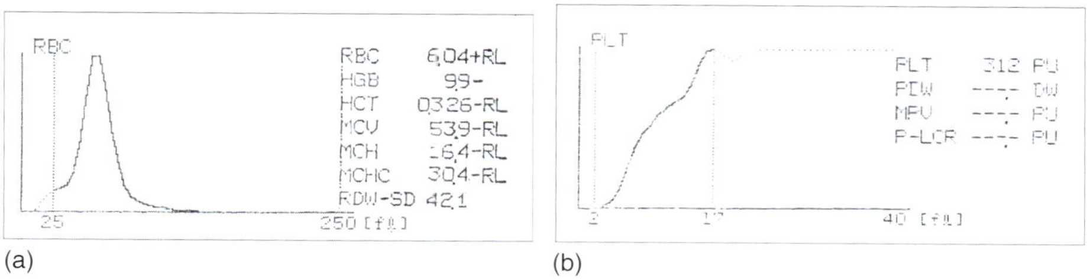

Figure 38.2 (a) Red cell profile and (b) platelet profile.

The referring haematologist had begun investigating this pregnant woman for both β-and α-thalassaemia.

Initial Assessment

The elevated Hb A_2 indicated β-thalassaemia trait. However, we thought the red cell morphology was rather extreme for a simple β-thal trait, and the red cell indices were too abnormal for this to be the complete answer.

Further Investigations

Haemoglobin electrophoresis by both cellulose acetate, and citrate agar gel, revealed normal components only. A normal ferritin level (54 µg/l) did not suggest (although it cannot exclude) iron deficiency. When compared to a group of female patients with β-thalassaemia trait (and normal ferritin levels), previously assessed in our department (see Figure 38.3), the patient's MCV, MCH and Hb were at the lowest end of the spectrum, whereas her "corrected" RDW was much higher.

The Amplification Refractory Mutation System (ARMS) screen[1] for beta thalassaemia point mutations [1] (performed by the National Haemoglobinopathy Reference Lab) yielded a positive result for IVSII-654, a known $β^0$-thalassaemia mutation.

Staining of red cells with new methylene blue solution revealed the presence of Hb H bodies; although they were seen in only a few cells, these had the classic "golf-ball" appearance (see Figure 38.4). Since

[1] This method is used for the detection of point mutations. If there is a mismatch between the target DNA sequence and the 3' end of an oligonucleotide used to prime a PCR reaction, no product will be obtained. Using primers with a normal or mutant base at the 3' end in different PCR reactions, the presence or absence of a product can be therefore used to determine the genotype of an individual.

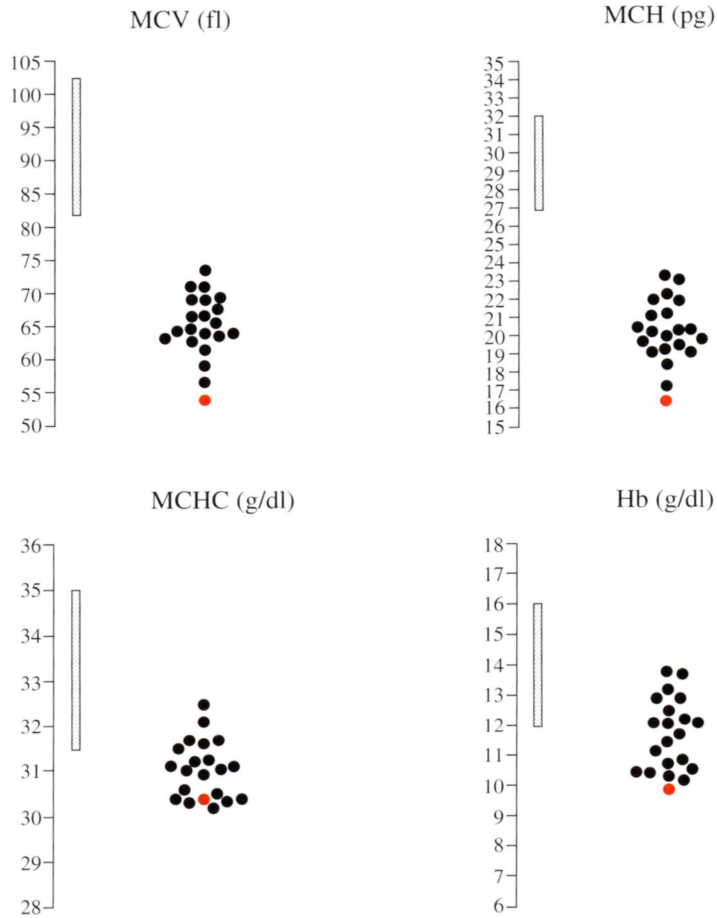

Figure 38.3 Scattergram of red cell indices in a group of females with β-thalassaemia trait and normal ferritin levels (•), and the patient (•). The sidebar represents the laboratory's reference range.

the patient has β-thalassaemia trait, and H bodies are precipitates of β_4 tetramers, their presence indicated, surprisingly, an excess of β-chains.[2] It became imperative to investigate the α-globin genes as well. By DNA analysis, we found restriction fragments compatible with the patient having biallelic mutations; she was a compound heterozygote for the Southeast Asian α^0-thalassaemia gene and the 3.7 Kb α^+-thalassaemia

[2] We note that in this respect, there is an asymmetry in the behaviour of the two globin subunits: there is no α-chain equivalent of Hb H because α-chains without their β partners simply precipitate out of solution. β-globin chains instead, are surprisingly able to bind haem and to form the β_4 tetramerric molecule, which however, is quite abnormal in oxygen affinity and solubility.

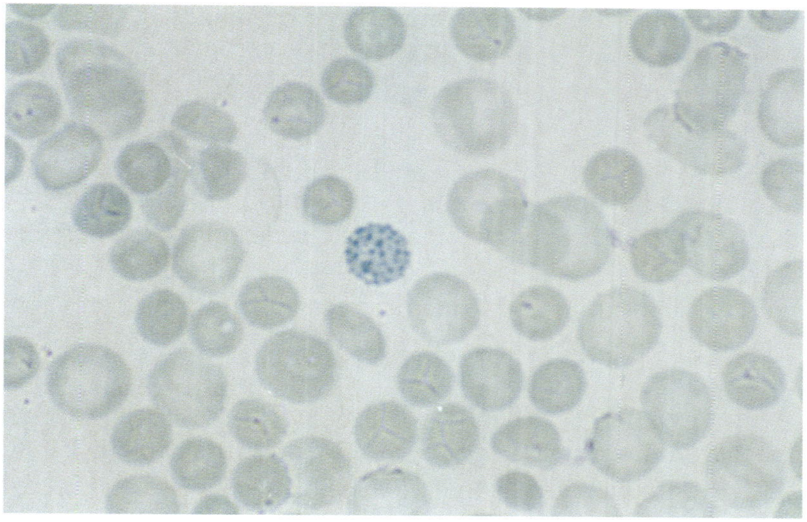

Figure 38.4 Hb H inclusion bodies in a "golf ball" red cell.

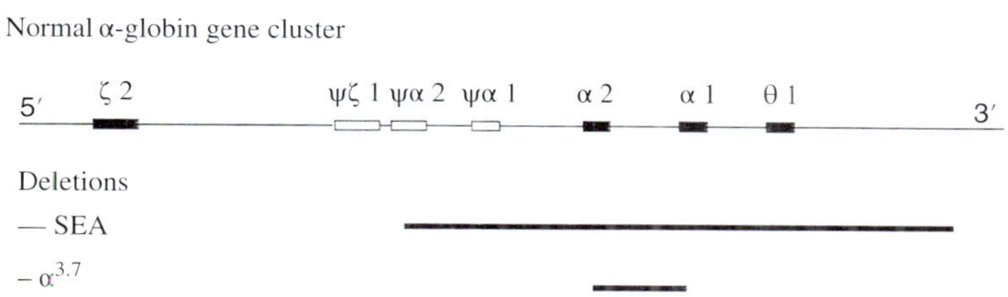

Figure 38.5 Diagram of the α-globin gene cluster and surrounding genes on the telomeric end of chromosome 16p showing deletions giving rise to α^0 and α^+ thalassaemia in this patient. Functional genes are in black. The α-thalassaemia deletions are shown as black bars indicating their lengths and positions.

deletion gene (i.e. $—^{SEA}/–^{3.7}\ \alpha$) (see Figure 38.5). This is the genotype of patients with classic "Hb H disease:" although, even on reinspection of our original electrophoretic strip, we could see no trace of any fast-moving haemoglobin, such as Hb H.

Comments

The molecular basis of α-thalassaemia has been extensively investigated [2]; and the clinical manifestations of haemoglobin H disease are remarkably variable. Some patients are almost as severely affected as patients with transfusion-dependent β-thalassaemia major, while many have a much milder course [3]: even though they may have lifelong anaemia, splenomegaly and bone changes. In this patient, at the age of 23, the diagnostic workup was prompted by a regular antenatal visit; whereas red cell morphology and indices were prominently abnormal, she clearly had a rather mild disease. When we considered that she has only 1 out of four α-globin genes, and only one functional β-globin gene out of two, we thought on one hand that nature has been generous with most of us; on the other hand, that red cells show remarkable resilience.

In fact, there are two major factors involved in the molecular pathophysiology of haemoglobin H disease: (i) the absolute shortage of α chains, (ii) the imbalance between available α and non-α chains. Item (i) causes a shortage of haemoglobin, and therefore small red cells; but (ii) causes positive damage by the formation of nonfunctional β_4 tetramers (Hb H); therefore, we submit that the thalassaemia gene in our patient, by reducing the imbalance, was beneficial. In terms of laboratory findings, the reduced imbalance may also explain why we did not find Hb H on electrophoresis; staining for Hb H inclusion bodies is a much more sensitive technique.

The association between a triple α-gene deletion and β-thalassaemia has been previously documented in the literature [4–7]. Our patient immigrated to Britain from a part of the world where each one of the three genes we have identified (β IVSII-654, $—^{SEA}$, $-^{3.7}\alpha$) are all present at polymorphic frequencies; therefore, it is not too surprising that they can coexist by coincidence in the same person. In a recent study of Hb H disease in Thailand [8] (with $n = 1170$, probably the largest ever published on this condition), one patient had exactly the same genotypic combination as ours, and a very similar haematologic phenotype.

Follow-up

The patient's partner was fully investigated: his red cell indices, Hb electrophoresis and Hb A_2 level were all normal.

Conclusion

Thalassaemia intermedia due to interaction of β-thalassaemia trait (IVSII-654) and biallelic alpha thalassaemia ($—^{SEA}/-^{3.7}\alpha$).

Acknowledgements

Referred by Dr. J. Keidan, Department of Haematology, The Queen Elizabeth Hospital, Norfolk, UK.

Dr. J. Old, National Haemoglobinopathy Reference Lab., Institute of Molecular Medicine, John Radcliffe Hospital, Oxford, UK.

Dr. T. J. Vulliamy, Haematology Department, Hammersmith Hospital, London, UK.

References

1. Wallace, R.B., Shaffer, J., Murphy, R.F. et al. (1979). Hybridization of synthetic oligodeoxyribonucleotides to phi chi 174 DNA: the effect of single base pair mismatch. *Nucl. Acids Res.* 6, 3543–3557.
2. Higgs, D.R. (2013). The molecular basis of alpha-thalassemia. *Cold Spring Harb. Perspect. Med.* 3, a011718.
3. Weatherall, D.J. (1993). Thalassemia. In: Stamatoyannopoulos, G., Nienhuis, A.W., Majerus, P.W. et al. editor. *The Molecular Basis of Blood Diseases*. Philadelphia, PA: Saunders. pp. 157–206
4. Kan, Y.W. and Nathan, D.G. (1970). Mild thalassemia: the result of interactions of alpha and beta thalassemia genes. *J. Clin. Invest.* 49, 635–640.
5. Ozsoylu, S., Hiçsonmez, G., and Altay, C. (1973). Hemoglobin H-β-Thalassemia. *Acta Haemat.* 50, 184–190.
6. Loukopoulos, D., Loutradi, A., and Fessas, P. (1978). A unique thalassemia syndrome: homozygous alpha-thalassemia + homozygous beta-thalassemia. *Br. J. Haematol.* 39, 377–389.
7. Furbetta, M., Galanello, R., Ximenes, A. et al. (1979). Interaction of alpha and beta thalassaemia genes in two Sardinian families. *Br. J. Haematol.* 41, 203–210.
8. Singha, K., Tepakhan, W., Yamsri, S. et al. (2024). A large cohort of Hb H disease in northeast Thailand: a molecular revisited, diverse genetic interactions and identification of a novel mutation. *Clin. Chim. Acta* 561, 119830.

Case 39

Salt Lake and Salt Bridges

Patient Details

Age: Newborn *Sex:* M
Ethnic background: Italian

Reason for Referral

Investigation of neonatal jaundice (NNJ) and severe neonatal anaemia

History and Clinical Findings in Brief

This baby was delivered to a 29-year-old mother at 37 weeks gestation by Caesarean delivery, because of labour and previous Caesarean section. The baby had a slightly low birth weight of 2325 g. Apgar scores were 6 at 1 min and 8 at 5 min. He was the second child of a healthy unrelated couple. Maternal history included gestational diabetes treated with insulin, and lymphedema in lower limbs. During pregnancy, the mother had been on monthly benzathine penicillin G therapy, aspirin and enoxaparin. Her TORCH (Toxoplasmosis, Other infections [like syphilis], Rubella, Cytomegalovirus and Herpes Simplex Virus) serological screening was negative, and there was no evidence or history of haemolytic anaemia.

At 2 hours of life, the baby was jaundiced. There was no blood group incompatibility and the direct antiglobulin test was negative. His haematocrit was 52%. Phototherapy was started, but it was discontinued after 35 hours, because unconjugated bilirubin never rose above 205 μmol/l (12 mg/dl), although direct bilirubin (DB) had increased further; it peaked at 222 μmol/l (13 mg/dl) at 88 hours of life. There were no signs of acute bilirubin encephalopathy. Splenomegaly without hepatomegaly was detected. Intravenous immunoglobulin was administered, but there was no clinical improvement.

Laboratory Findings

At 8 hours old, the baby's haematocrit had dropped to 35% and his liver enzymes were elevated (see Table 39.1). A blood film on day of life 5 showed marked anisocytosis and poikilocytosis, some spherocytes and nucleated red cells (see Figure 39.1); by that time, the haematocrit had fallen to 32%, with marked reticulocytosis (Figure 39.2; Table 39.1), consistent with severe haemolytic anaemia. Further blood samples were drawn before a transfusion of 40 ml of packed red cells was administered. Ursodeoxycholic acid and phenobarbital were also given.

Initial Assessment

Based on the above findings, there seemed little doubt that this baby's anaemia was haemolytic. The negative direct antiglobulin test was against an autoimmune or alloimmune cause. The significant number of spherocytes

Table 39.1 Haematology and Biochemical Data

Hours of life	8	88	138
Haematocrit (%)	35	28	32
Retics ($\times 10^9$/l)	–	587	–
sTB (μmol/l)	207	402	301
DB (μmol/l)	63	222	171
AST (IU/l)	249	77	73
ALT (IU/l)	42	24	27
GGT (IU/l)[a]	119	50	52

Abbreviations: sTB, serum total bilirubin; DB, direct bilirubin; ALT, alanine aminotransferase; AST, aspartate aminotransferase; GGT, gamma glutamyl transferase.
[a] Range for age = <200 (IU/l).

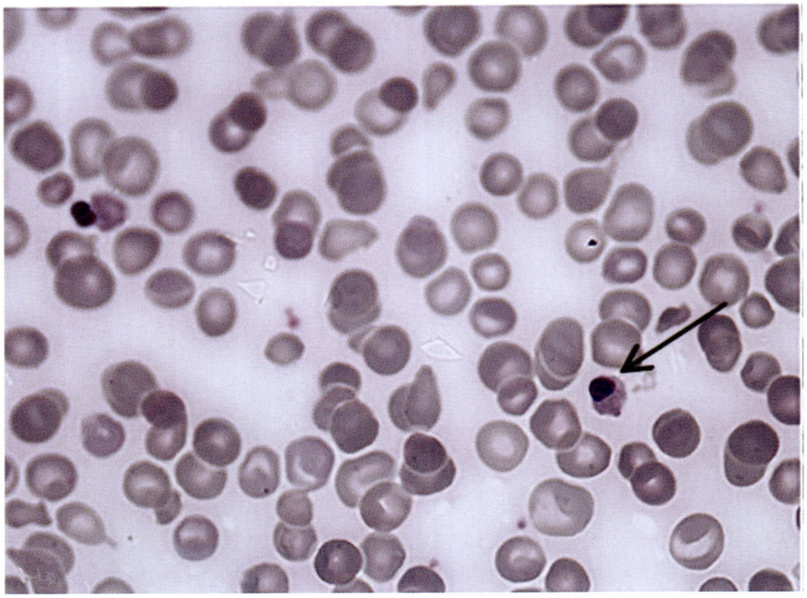

Figure 39.1 Peripheral blood film with nucleated red cell arrowed (from [5]: used with permission).

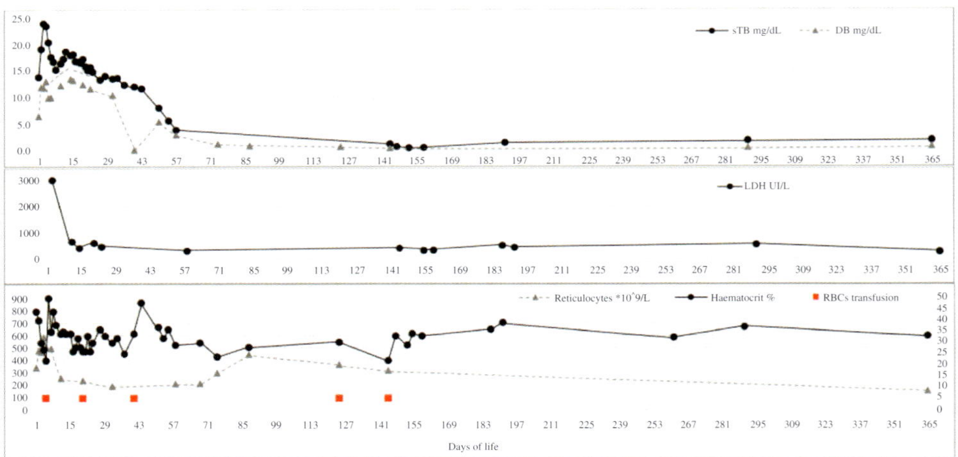

Figure 39.2 Clinical course of infant: haematological parameters (from [5]: used with permission).

on the blood film required investigation, but there was no positive family history of hereditary spherocytosis (HS). The onset of neonatal jaundice requiring phototherapy in glucose-6-phosphate dehydrogenase deficient babies is typically two days, so the clinical picture here did not fit with G6PD deficiency of a common (class B) type [1].

Further Investigations

Measurements of erythrocyte pyruvate kinase activity, α1-antitrypsin, ammonia, ceruloplasmin and thyroid hormones were normal. Screening for major metabolic diseases was negative. Molecular tests for hepatitis viruses were negative; blood cultures yielded no growth.

On abdominal ultrasound, there was no evidence of biliary atresia. Liver biopsy showed preserved architecture, cholestasis and iron-loaded hepatocytes. Portal spaces were infiltrated by lymphocytes and neutrophils; and there were foci of haematopoiesis.

The patient's red cell glucose-6-phosphate dehydrogenase (G6PD) activity was only 1.8 U/gHb. G6PD activity in his mother and grandparents (who are all from Rome) was within the normal range.

Genomic DNA was collected from peripheral blood samples of the patient, his mother and maternal grandparents and first screened for the six G6PD variants most frequent in Italy [2]. Since the patient's DNA was negative for these, bidirectional Sanger sequencing of the full G6PD gene was performed; this revealed a single base change: c.1361G>C (NM _ 0 010 42351), causing a proline for arginine amino acid replacement (p.R454P). This mutation was found in the patient's mother, who was an only child; but not in the maternal grandparents, indicating a *de novo* event.

This mutation was previously reported by Powers et al. [3] in a G6PD deficient blood sample, and it was assigned the name G6PD Salt Lake, after the area where they worked (Department of Pathology, University of Utah School of Medicine, Salt Lake City, UT). Since in their study samples were de-identified, there was no clinical information for this G6PD variant to be assigned to class A or to class B [1]. Sequencing of the *UGT1A1* gene promoter in our patient revealed homozygosity for the UGT1A1*28 (rs8175347) allele, consistent with Gilbert's syndrome. This is known to be an additional risk factor for neonatal hyperbilirubinaemia in G6PD-deficient male neonates.

Comments

There can be little doubt that the baby's anaemia, severe since hours after birth, was due to G6PD deficiency; not just because no other cause was found, but because the pattern conforms to that seen with many other class A variants; almost all present with severe NNJ [4]. In this case, the NNJ was accounted for in part by conjugated bilirubin, for which we do not have a full explanation [5].

Interestingly, two other G6PD variants affecting residue 454 were already known. G6PD Union (c.1360C>T; p.Arg- 454Cys) is a widespread polymorphic variant [6], belonging to class B (formerly class II) of the WHO classification. G6PD Andalus (c.1361G>A; p.Arg454His), instead, has been reported only in isolated instances: first, in a patient with favism in Spain [7]; later, as a class A (formerly class I) variant in Japan [8]; then, in a baby with NNJ in Malaysia [9], and in one patient in India [10]. The classification of G6PD Andalus is not clear, but it is probably in class B. The mutations involved have a dramatic impact on enzyme activity, since the residual G6PD activity in red cells is only 2.7% of normal with G6PD Union [11], and less than 1% with G6PD Andalus [6]; with G6PD Salt Lake, it was about 3% in our patient, in the face of marked reticulocytosis; and about 7% in the case of Powers et al. [3].

The finding of three different replacements of the same amino acid residue prompted comparative investigations of how they impact on enzyme structure and function (see Figure 39.3). The positively charged Arg454 residue is linked by a salt bridge to the negatively charged Asp286 [12]. The p.Arg454Pro mutation in G6PD Salt Lake would not be able to form this salt bridge, possibly thus explaining the greatly reduced activity. Arg454 is part of a cluster of polar amino acids that, in each subunit, stabilize this G6PD region through intra-molecular electrostatic interactions. Since Arg454 is the first residue in a 20 amino-acid long α-helix (residues 454–476), replacement by proline may not be excessively disruptive of the helical structure. On the other hand, since residue 454 is at 24–28 Å from both the G6P and the NADP+ binding sites, and since the intervening protein matrix consists mostly of α-helices that are rigid, and the dielectric constant of the protein core is low, loss of a positive charge at residue 454 may be perceived at both the G6P and the NADP+ sites, such that the ligands binding affinities may be altered. Based on such structural considerations, the Arg454 replacement with the non-polar residue Pro454 is expected to affect the dynamics and electrostatic interactions of the G6PD subunit in this and neighbouring regions, including the active site [5].

Follow-up

The baby required two more red cell transfusions and was discharged at the age of 8 weeks, when his haemoglobin was 9 g/dl, serum total bilirubin 65 μmol/l (3.8 mg/dl) and DB 43 μmol/l (2.5 mg/dl) (Figure 39.2). At the age of one year, the peripheral blood smear appeared normal

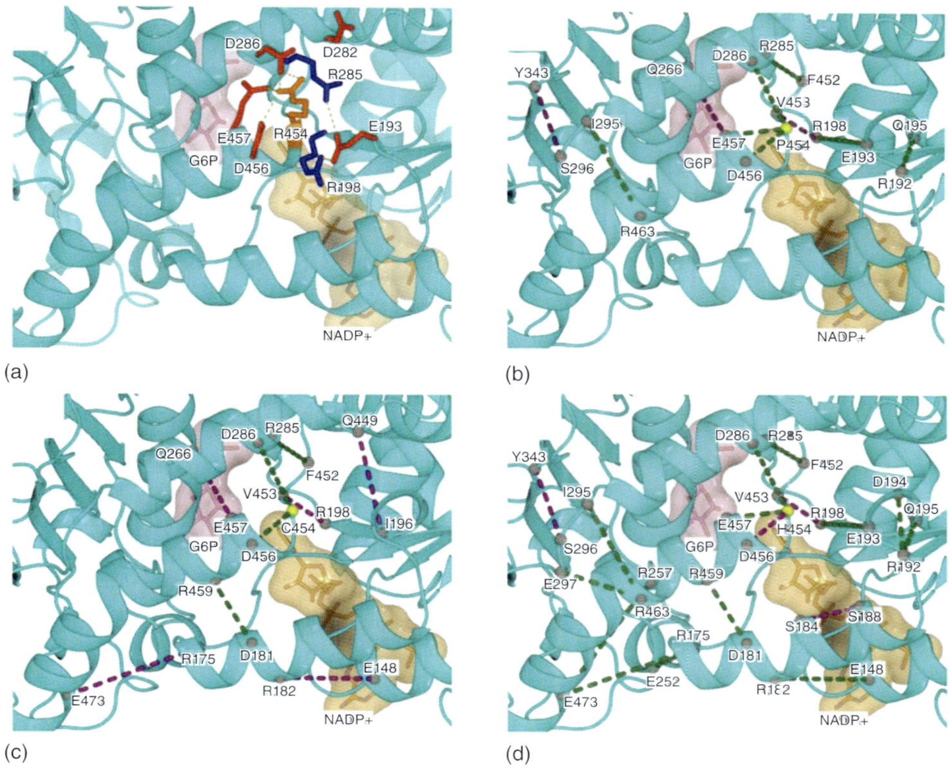

Figure 39.3 Structure of a region of the G6PD molecule surrounding amino acid 454. The image is based on cryogenic electron microscopy: individual amino acid sites are shown as small grey spheres, and residues are identified by their one-letter codes. NADP+ (light brown) and G6P (light purple) are shaped in the background. (a) Normal enzyme: arginine residue R454 (orange ball, beneath R454) is surrounded by a cluster of positively charged residues (blue sticks) and negatively charged residues (red sticks); these are highlighted because electrostatic interactions extend radially through space; dotted lines represent hydrogen bonds that provide additional local stabilization. (b) G6PD Salt Lake. (c) G6PD Union. (d) G6PD Andalus. By molecular dynamics simulations, it is seen in panels B–D that H-bond populations are different from normal, and different in each of the three variants: H-bonds that are less populated in a mutant protein compared to the wild type are shown by green-dashed lines, whereas those that are more populated compared to the wild type are shown by purple-dashed lines (from [5]: used with permission).

(Figure 39.4). The child has a persistent marked reticulocytosis and, over the first three years of life, in concomitance with urinary infections, he has experienced several further drops in haemoglobin, requiring a total of 12 red cell transfusions.

Thus, the child has a chronic non-spherocytic haemolytic disorder: confirming that we must classify G6PD Salt Lake as a class A variant.

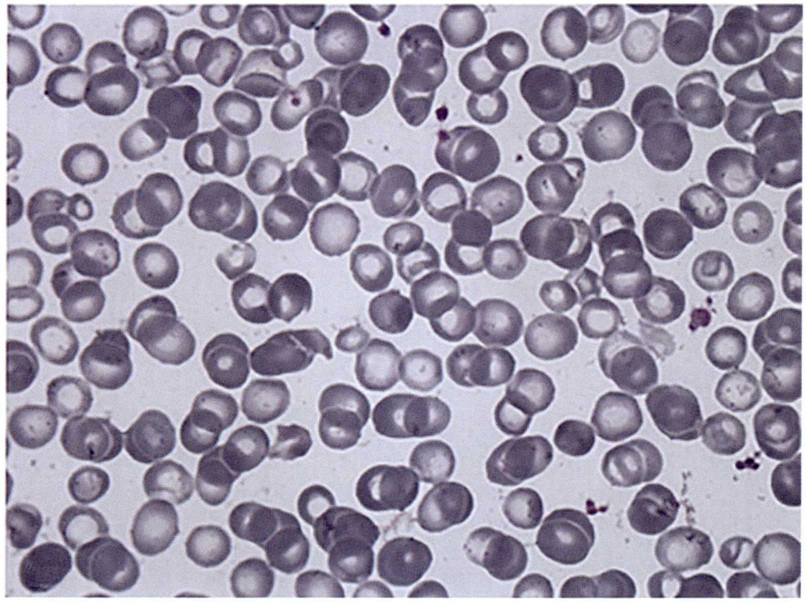

Figure 39.4 Peripheral blood film at one year of age (from [5]/John Wiley & Sons: used with permission).

The normal G6PD activity in the baby's mother is not against this classification; in fact, it is in keeping with a previous observation, namely that in heterozygotes for class A variants somatic cell selection after X chromosome inactivation favours cells having the normal G6PD allele on their active X chromosome [13].

In due course, it will be necessary to decide whether the patient may benefit from splenectomy. Or perhaps by that time G6PD gene therapy, already carried out in a mouse model [14], will be recommended for class A variants.

Conclusion

Chronic non-spherocytic haemolytic anaemia (CNSHA) due to G6PD Salt Lake.

Acknowledgements

This case has been previously published [5]. We thank particularly Angelo Minucci, Martino Bolognesi and Simonetta Costa.

References

1. Luzzatto, L., Bancone, G., Dugue, P.A. et al. (2024). New WHO classification of genetic variants causing G6PD deficiency. *Bull. World Health. Organ.* 102(8), 615–617.
2. Minucci, A., Delibato, E., Castagnola, M. et al. (2008). Identification of RFLP G6PD mutations by using microcapillary electrophoretic chips (Experion). *J. Sep. Sci.* 31(14), 2694–2700.
3. Powers, J.L., Best, D.H., and Grenache, D.G. (2018). Genotype-phenotype correlations of glucose-6-phosphate-deficient variants throughout an activity distribution. *J. Appl. Lab. Med.* 2(6), 841–850.
4. Luzzatto, L., Ally, M., and Notaro, R. (2020). Glucose-6-phosphate dehydrogenase deficiency. *Blood* 136(11), 1225–1240.
5. Costa, S., Minucci, A., Kumawat, A. et al. (2024). Pathogenic G6PD variants: different clinical pictures arise from different missense mutations in the same codon. *Br. J. Haematol.* 205(5), 1985–1994.
6. Rovira, A., Vulliamy, T.J., Pujades, A. et al. (1994). The glucose-6-phosphate dehydrogenase (G6PD) deficient variant G6PD Union (454 Arg → Cys) has a worldwide distribution possibly due to recurrent mutation. *Hum. Mol. Genet.* 3(5), 833–835.
7. Vives-Corrons, J.L., Kuhl, W., Pujades, M.A. et al. (1990). Molecular genetics of the glucose-6-phosphate dehydrogenase (G6PD) Mediterranean variant and description of a new G6PD mutant, G6PD Andalus1361A. *Am. J. Hum. Genet.* 47(3), 575–579.
8. Hirono, A., Miwa, S., Fujii, H. et al. (1994). Molecular study of eight Japanese cases of glucose-6-phosphate dehydrogenase deficiency by nonradioisotopic single-strand conformation polymorphism analysis. *Blood* 83(11), 3363–3368.
9. Ainoon, O., Yu, Y.H., Amir Muhriz, A.L. et al. (2003). Glucose-6-phosphate dehydrogenase (G6PD) variants in Malaysian Malays. *Hum. Mutat.* 21(1), 101.
10. Arunachalam, A.K., Sumithra, S., Maddali, M. et al. (2020). Molecular characterization of G6PD deficiency: report of three novel G6PD variants. *Indian J. Hematol. Blood Transfus.* 36(2), 349–355.
11. Nannelli, C., Bosman, A., Cunningham, J. et al. (2023). Genetic variants causing G6PD deficiency: clinical and biochemical data support new WHO classification. *Br. J. Haematol.* 202(5), 1024–1032.
12. Wang, X.T., Lam, V.M., and Engel, P.C. (2005). Marked decrease in specific activity contributes to disease phenotype in two human glucose 6-phosphate dehydrogenase mutants, G6PD(Union) and G6PD(Andalus). *Hum. Mutat.* 26(3), 284.
13. Filosa, S., Giacometti, N., Wangwei, C. et al. (1996). Somatic-cell selection is a major determinant of the blood-cell phenotype in heterozygotes for glucose-6-phosphate dehydrogenase mutations causing severe enzyme deficiency. *Am. J. Hum. Genet.* 59(4), 887–895.
14. Rovira, A., De Angioletti, M., Camacho-Vanegas, O. et al. (2000). Stable in vivo expression of glucose-6-phosphate dehydrogenase (G6PD) and rescue of G6PD deficiency in stem cells by gene transfer. *Blood* 96(13), 4111–4117.

Case 40
Small Red Cells with a Difference

Patient Details

Age: 55 *Sex:* M
Ethnic background: Bangladesh

Reason for Referral

Identification of abnormal haemoglobin (blood sample only).

History and Clinical Findings in Brief

There was no relevant past medical history in this patient. A blood test was prompted by an elective cataract operation.

Laboratory Findings

The patient had a normal haemoglobin but had markedly microcytic red cell indices (see Table 40.1). His reticulocyte percentage was within normal limits, but the absolute count was marginally elevated. On the blood film (see Figure 40.1), the red cells looked generally small and uniformly round

Table 40.1 Haematology Data

Hb (g/dl)	14.2
RBC ($\times 10^{12}$/l)	7.83
MCV (fl)	57.0
MCH (pg)	18.1
MCHC (g/dl)	31.8
RDW (S.D.)	40.5
Retic (%)	1.6
Retic ($\times 10^{9}$/l)	120
Hb F (%)	0.5

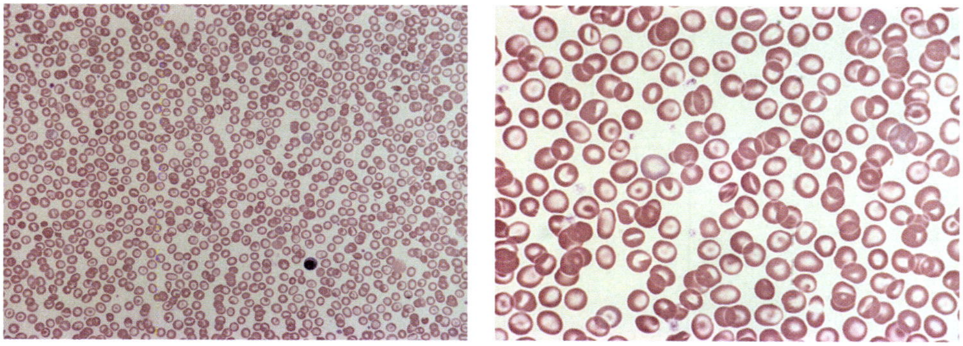

(a) (b)

Figure 40.1 Peripheral blood film: (a) medium power view; (b) high power view.

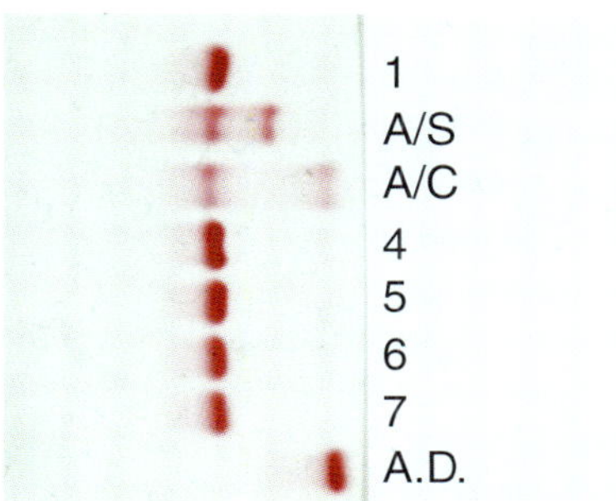

Figure 40.2 Haemoglobin electrophoresis on cellulose acetate membrane; the migration of the haemoglobin fractions is from right to left. An A/S control and A/C control are in lanes 2 and 3, respectively. The patient (A.D.) is in lane 8.

but with a high proportion of target cells. There were a few dense cells that were not quite true spherocytes, and also an occasional polychromatic cell.

Haemoglobin electrophoresis on cellulose acetate confirmed the presence of an abnormal haemoglobin (see Figure 40.2); a single band was seen in the position of Hb C and no Hb A was detected. On agar gel electrophoresis (see Figure 40.3), there was also only one band, which was in the position of Hb A: this ruled out Hb C, which by this technique is well resolved from Hb A.

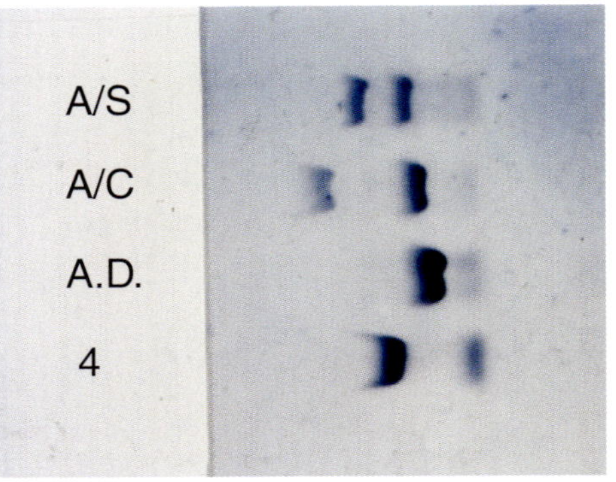

Figure 40.3 Haemoglobin electrophoresis on citrate agar gel electrophoresis. Migration of the haemoglobin fractions is from left to right. An A/S control and A/C control are in lanes 1 and 2, respectively. The patient (A.D.) is in lane 3.

Initial Assessment

The blood count data and red cell morphology suggested a thalassaemic condition. Having ruled out Hb C, and considering the ethnic origin of the patient, the most likely abnormal haemoglobin is Hb E. Therefore, the differential diagnosis was between homozygous Hb E (which is associated with microcytosis) and a heterozygote for Hb E plus β-thalassaemia; because Hb A was absent, the latter would have to be Hb E/β^0 thalassaemia. Patients with Hb E/β^0 thalassaemia almost invariably have anaemia, although this is quite variable (and it can be as severe as homozygous β-thalassaemia). A haemoglobin level of 14.2 g/dl in our patient, as well as the normal level of Hb F, were strongly in favour of homozygous Hb E [1–3].

Further Investigations

First, in view of the exceedingly low MCV and MCH, we needed to rule out superimposed iron deficiency. The ferritin level was normal (128 mg/l) and was in keeping with the normal MCHC.[1]

Because Hb A_2 cannot be resolved from Hb E, not even by HPLC, we proceeded directly to DNA analysis. A *Mnl I* digest of the PCR-amplified exon I of the β-globin gene, followed by gel electrophoresis revealed only two bands in the patient's sample; one of 198 bp and the other 80 bp. The former results from the *loss* of a restriction site, and therefore the pattern is unlike that in the normal (A/A) and heterozygous (A/E) controls, which had additional fragments of 138 bp and 60 bp. These data confirm that the patient is indeed homozygous for Hb E (see Figure 40.4).

[1] For the assessment of iron deficiency, we normally require both transferrin saturation index (TSI) and ferritin level. However, because no serum sample was available and considering that the patient had no acute disease that might have raised his ferritin we were now satisfied.

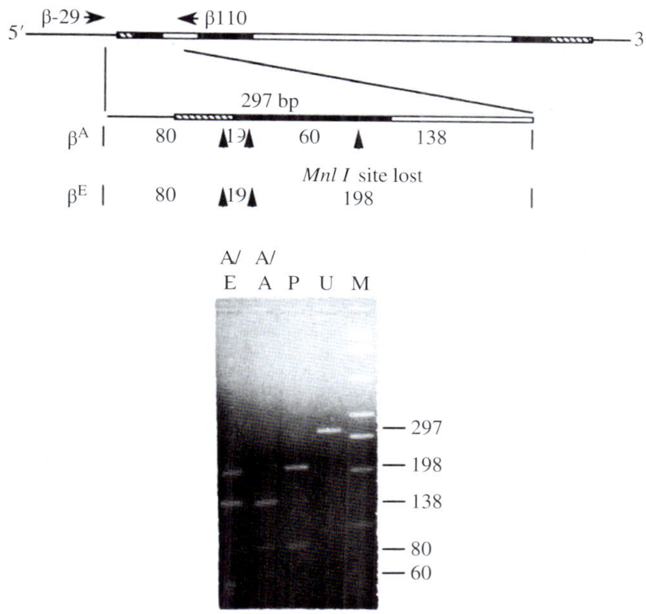

Figure 40.4 Detection of the mutation underlying Hb E by DNA analysis. A schematic representation of the β-globin gene is shown at the top; underneath, the region of the gene that was PCR-amplified by using the β(-)29 and β110 primers, with the fragment sizes (bp) expected from the normal (β^A) and from the Hb E (β^E) alleles, after digestion of the PCR product with the restriction enzyme *Mnl I*. Below, the ethidium bromide stained gel of the fragments observed with DNA from a normal control (A/A); from a heterozygote for Hb E (A/E); and from the patient (P). U: undigested fragment; M: molecular size markers.

Comments

Thus, the gentleman (who was not a patient since he was quite well) was homozygous for the haemoglobin E mutation. In this condition, like with homozygous Hb C, target cells are common; however, unlike in homozygous C, there is also a marked reduction in MCV and MCH. This can be attributed to the fact that the Hb E mutation is itself a β-thalassaemia mutation. Harvey Itano had originally formulated the "structure-rate" hypothesis, whereby he postulated that thalassaemia might arise from a qualitative change with secondary quantitative effects [4]. Subsequently, Orkin et al. [5] discovered that the base substitution at codon 26, in addition to causing a Glu→Lys amino acid replacement, also creates a new splicing site that causes abnormal mRNA processing (see Figure 40.5): hence a decrease in correctly spliced mRNA, and therefore a decrease in β^E-globin synthesis.

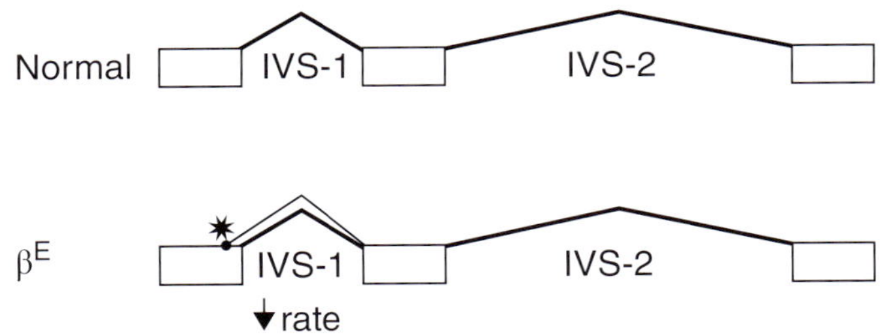

Figure 40.5 Original discovery of the β^+ thalassaemia effect of the haemoglobin E mutation. The G → A mutation (*) in codon 26, in addition to causing a Glu → Lys amino acid replacement, also creates a splice site alternative to the normal. The incorrectly spliced mRNA will have a frameshift and chain termination; the correctly spliced mRNA will make β^E globin chains, but at a reduced rate. [5]/with permission of Springer Nature.

Thus, the β^E mutation is at the same time a mild β^+ mutation [6]. Therefore, it is not surprising that a homozygote has very low MCV and MCH (lower than in most β-thal heterozygotes); indeed, the indices in our patient are very similar to those found in a homozygote for a mild β^+ mutation such as the −29 mutation in the TATA box [7] (see Case 30).

Hb E is also mildly unstable [8, 9]. This may explain why our patient did have occasional "pseudo-spherocytes" on the blood film, and a slight increase in reticulocytes. However, the haemolytic component can be fully compensated, to the extent that there is no anaemia, as in this case.

Follow-up

Once the diagnosis was fully explained to the patient, no specific follow-up seemed necessary.

Conclusion

Patient homozygous for Hb E; sometimes referred to as haemoglobin E disease.

Acknowledgements

Referred by Dr. P. Srivastava, Department of Haematology, Burton District Hospital Centre, Burton upon Trent, Staffordshire, UK.

References

1. Tatsumi, N., Tsuda, I., Funhara, Y. et al. (1992). Automatic measurement of hemoglobin F in blood obtained from patients with hemoglobin E/E and beta-thalassemia/hemoglobin-E. *Southeast Asian J. Trop. Med. Public Health*. 23(2), 91–94.
2. Imail, J.B. (1992). Thalassemia and haemoglobinopathies in Brunei Darussalam. *Med. J. Malasia*. 4, 98–102.
3. Lorey, F.W., Cunningham, G.C., Vichinsky, E. et al. (1993). Detection of E/beta-thalassemia versus homozygous EE using high-performance liquid chromatography results from newborns. *Biochem. Med. Metab. Biol*. 49, 67–73.
4. Itano, H.A. (1957). Human hemoglobins: properties and genetic control. *Adv. Protein Chem*. 12, 215–268.
5. Orkin, S.H., Kazazian, H.H., Antonarakis, S.E. et al. (1982). Abnormal RNA processing due to the exon mutation of β^E -globin gene. *Nature* 300, 768–769.
6. Luzzatto, L. (1983). Letter: thalassemia. *Nature* 301, 460.
7. Safaya, S., Rieder, R.F., Dowling, C.E. et al. (1989). Homozygous beta-thalassemia without anemia. *Blood* 73(1), 324–328.
8. Frischer, H. and Bowman, J. (1975). Haemoglobin E, an oxidatively unstable haemoglobin. *J. Lab. Clin. Med*. 85, 531–539.
9. Rees, D.C., Styles, L., Vichinsky, E.P. et al. (1998) The hemoglobin E syndromes. *Ann. N. Y. Acad. Sci*. 850, 334–343.

Case 41

Double Jeopardy When Facing Complement

Patient Details

Age: 40 *Sex:* F
Ethnic background: Italian (Sardinia)

Reason for Referral

Anaemia and thrombocytopenia.

History and Clinical Findings in Brief

This lady had presented two years previously to her local hospital with increasing thrombocytopenia (platelets 100, then 40×10^9/l), mild neutropenia and anaemia. At that time there were no signs of haemolysis, and a flow cytometry analysis did not report any glycosylphosphatidylinositol (GPI)-negative cells (PNH cells). Now she complained of increasing fatigue and occasional abdominal pain. Apart from pallor, her physical examination was essentially negative.

Laboratory Findings

The patient had a severe macrocytic anaemia with reticulocytosis (see Table 41.1); neutrophils and platelets were below the normal range. On the blood film (see Figure 41.1), there was anisocytosis and poikilocytosis with presence of macrocytes, spherocytes and hemighosts; occasional nucleated red cells were also seen. Overall, the morphology was reminiscent of oxidative damage seen in G6PD-deficient patients during a haemolytic attack (see also Case 15). Lactate dehydrogenase was elevated at about 5 × upper limit of normal, which could fit with the above. However,

Table 41.1 Laboratory Data

	Presentation	After 6 months on eculizumab	After 6 years on eculizumab	After 2 years on ravulizumab[a]
Hb (g/dl)	7.6	8.2	8.5	9.9
RBC ($\times 10^{12}$/l)	2.14	2.53	2.27	2.73
MCV (fl)	105	98	115	110
MCH (pg)	35.5	32.4	37.4	36.2
MCHC (g/dl)	33.8	33.1	32.6	32.8
RDW-CV (%)	16.8	21.2	20.0	18.4
Retic (%)	7.5	10.1	15.7	—
Retic ($\times 10^{12}$/l)	160	255	356	—
WBC ($\times 10^{9}$/l)	3.25	3.44	3.66	4.96
Neuts ($\times 10^{9}$/l)	1.64	2.0	2.39	2.73
Plt ($\times 10^{9}$/l)	85	181	199	204
Ferritin (μg/l)	84	232	1932	—
LDH (IU/l)	1517	260	295	365
Bilirubin[b] (μmol/l)	22	27	38	31
N PNH[c]	75.7	95	99.5	—
M PNH[d]	73.1	95	99.4	—
RBC PNH	19.5	37	85.7	—
PNH RBC C3+	NA	35	65.5	—

[a] 10 years from presentation.
[b] Total.
[c] PNH granulocyte population.
[d] PNH monocyte population.

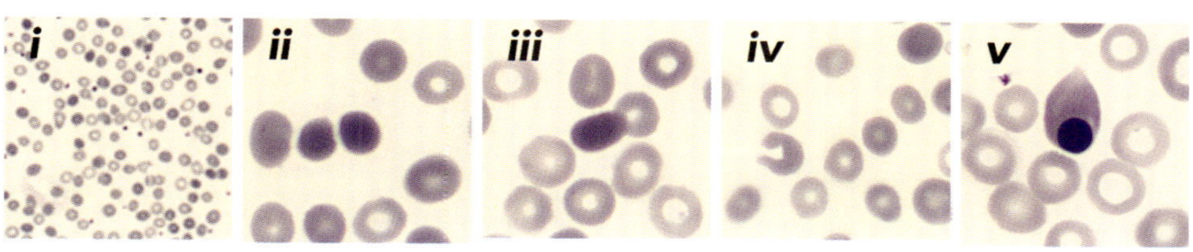

Figure 41.1 Peripheral blood film (in steady state on eculizumab). Revealing anisocytosis and conspicuous spherocytes (i), densely stained spherocytes (ii), macrocytes (iii), hemighost (iv) and a nucleated red cell (v). [1]/with permission of Elsevier.

the patient denied having eaten fava beans, and there was no other likely triggering factor for G6PD-related AHA. In view of the above, and in view of the previous pancytopenia, a flow cytometry test was repeated, and this time 59% PNH granulocytes were found.

Initial Assessment

On grounds of the above findings, clearly the patient had florid haemolytic PNH; the previous pancytopenia could be attributed to bone marrow failure, which regularly precedes and/or is associated with PNH. However, the blood film was most unusual for PNH and suggested there was something more in this patient.

Further Investigations

An assay of G6PD activity yielded a level of 5 IU/gHb (≈50% of normal), consistent with heterozygous G6PD deficiency. DNA analysis (see Figure 41.2a) confirmed that the patient was heterozygous for the G6PD Mediterranean ($G6PD^{S188F}$) mutant gene, the most common variant in Sardinia. Analysis of the *PIGA* gene (the gene that undergoes somatic mutations in PNH) revealed a deletion of nucleotide 930T in exon 4, causing a frameshift that will create a stop at codon 329, producing a truncated PIGA protein (that normally has 484 amino acids). Notably, both *G6PD* and *PIGA* are X-linked genes. Since the *PIGA* mutation must have taken place long after X chromosome inactivation, it was of interest to know which one of the two G6PD alleles was expressed in the cells belonging to the *PIGA* mutant PNH clone. Analysis of the G6PD complementary DNA (cDNA) extracted from the PNH granulocytes and monocytes exhibited only the $G6PD^{S188F}$ transcript (Figure 41.2b); in contrast, the patient's lymphocytes, most of which were non-PNH, showed expression of both the $G6PD^{S188F}$ and the normal allele (Figure 41.2b). This means that whereas the normal somatic cells of this patient had the mosaic situation typical of heterozygotes for an X-linked gene, the *PIGA* mutation must have occurred in this case, unfortunately, in a hematopoietic stem cell in which the *G6PD* normal allele was on the inactive X chromosome, whereas the $G6PD^{S188F}$ allele was on the active X chromosome. Thus, the entire PNH clone is G6PD deficient.

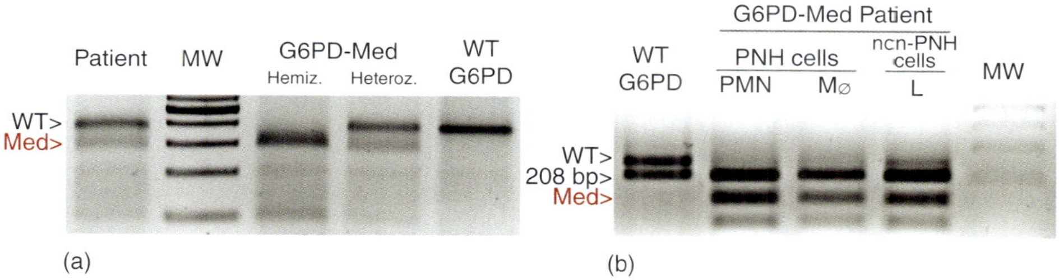

Figure 41.2 (a) Restriction analysis of genomic DNA for G6PD-Med variant (Exon 6; 563 C>T; 188Ser>Phe). After *Mbo*II digestion of an amplicon including exons 6, intron 6 and exon 7, the restriction fragments expected from wild-type (WT) G6PD (377 bp) and from mutant G6PD-Med allele (277 bp) are indicated. Controls (WT, heterozygote and hemizygote) and patient samples are shown; the patient is heterozygous for G6PD-Med. MW, molecular-weight size marker 100 bp DNA ladder; the brighter band is 500 bp. (b) Complementary DNA restriction analysis of G6PD transcripts. Granulocytes (polymorphonuclear neutrophils [PMN]) were isolated by using the double-density centrifugation method; monocytes (Mø) were obtained by using an adherence technique from peripheral blood mononuclear cells. At the time of sampling, 99% of granulocytes and 97% of monocytes were PNH. Normal (non-PNH) lymphocytes (L) were obtained after monocyte-depletion of peripheral blood mononuclear cells. G6PD complementary DNA obtained from the selected blood cell populations was amplified, and an amplicon comprising exons 4–7 was digested with *Mbo*II. The restriction fragments relevant for the identification of normal (246 bp) and mutant G6PD-Med (147 bp) transcripts are indicated (the 208 bp fragment arises from either transcript). The patient's PNH granulocytes and monocytes expressed only the G6PD-Med transcript. The patient's normal (non-PNH) lymphocytes also expressed predominantly the G6PD-Med transcript, suggesting that in this patient, X inactivation in hematopoietic cells had been highly skewed towards G6PD deficiency, regardless of PNH. MW, molecular-weight size marker 100 bp DNA ladder; the upper band is 500 bp. [1]/with permission of Elsevier.

Follow-up

Over the following six months, the PNH granulocyte population increased to 95%; at the same time neutrophil and platelet counts became normal. The patient needed red cell transfusions, and at this point treatment was started with a standard dose of the C5 inhibitor eculizumab. This anti-C5 monoclonal antibody prevents, in PNH patients, complement-mediated intravascular haemolysis and its clinical consequences. However, in almost all treated patients, a significant fraction of PNH red blood cells become coated with C3 fragments and thus opsonized, with consequent extravascular haemolysis [2]. The intensity of this process varies from patient to patient, and this may account at least in part for the fact that, whereas the normalization of LDH on eculizumab is quite uniform, with respect to raising the haemoglobin level the response is quite variable [3].

In our patient, lactate dehydrogenase levels promptly returned to normal, but reticulocytes did not (steadily above 250 × 10^9/l); and the haemoglobin level increased very little (Table 41.1).

Additional Investigations

In the latter respect, our patient was certainly a poor responder: it seemed reasonable to surmise that this might have something to do with G6PD deficiency.

To test this hypothesis, having obtained blood samples from normal and from G6PD-deficient male donors, some of the red cells were made PNH-like by blocking CD55 and CD59 with specific antibodies; the red cells were then exposed to serum with complement either active or inactivated, and reactive oxygen species (ROS) were measured (see Figure 41.3) [1].

The most important result, supported by all appropriate controls, was that with G6PD-normal red cells there was no difference in ROS levels, whether or not they were PNH-like; in contrast, with G6PD-deficient red cells, not only ROS levels were much higher than in G6PD-normal red cells, but they were further significantly elevated when the red cells were PNH-like (see Figure 41.3). This difference is of no consequence in an untreated patient, because PNH red cells will be lysed by activated complement, regardless of ROS levels (Figure 41.4a). However, when C5 is blocked

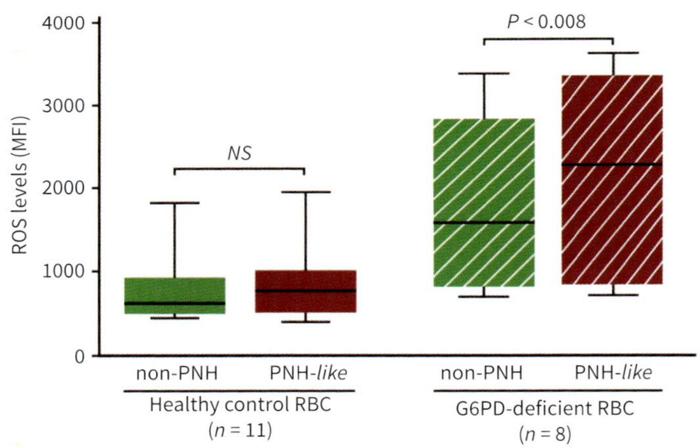

Figure 41.3 Increased ROS in G6PD-deficient red cells incubated in sera with activated complement but in the presence of eculizumab. Levels of ROS, expressed as mean fluorescence intensity (MFI), were quantitated by flow cytometry with dichlorodihydrofluorescein diacetate (400 mM) after 24 hours at 37 °C following complement activation. Statistical significance was accepted for $P \leq 0.05$. NS, not statistically significant. [1]/with permission of Elsevier.

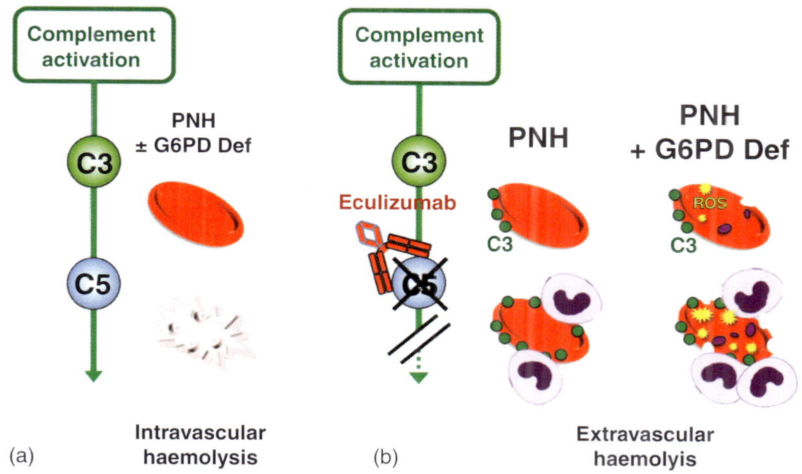

Figure 41.4 Different fate of G6PD-normal PNH red cells *versus* G6PD-deficient PNH red cells when C5 is blocked by eculizumab. (a) Complement activation results in intravascular haemolysis of PNH red cells regardless of their G6PD status. (b) Left: C5 blockade prevents intravascular haemolysis of PNH red cells, but C3 deposition results in extravascular haemolysis. Right: when PNH red cells are also G6PD-deficient, complement activation in the presence of C5 blockade causes increased production of ROS that, with C5 blocked, increases extravascular haemolysis. Adapted from [1].

by eculizumab, the high levels of ROS generated by activated complement on the surface of PNH red cells that, on account of being G6PD deficient, are defective in antioxidant defence, will cause damage and ultimately accelerate their destruction (Figure 41.4b).

Comments

The initial history of this patient illustrates well the evolution from aplastic anaemia to PNH: probably the rule rather than the exception in the natural history of PNH [4]. The gradual expansion of the PNH clone has caused increasing intravascular haemolysis, but it was associated with reversal of neutropenia and thrombocytopenia, in keeping with the notion that PNH can be "a blessing in disguise" [5].

PNH is an ultra-rare disease; on the other hand, G6PD deficiency is a relatively common X-linked genetic abnormality that in some countries may affect up to 30% of the population [6]; in Sardinia, where this patient comes from, the frequency is about 12% [7]. Therefore, the coexistence of the acquired disease with the genetic abnormality needs not to be regarded as extraordinary.

In PNH, red blood cells lyse when attacked by activated complement; in G6PD deficiency, instead, the mechanism of haemolysis is oxidative damage. It has been suggested that oxidative damage could play a role in PNH as well [8], although it is susceptibility to complement-mediated lysis that undoubtedly dominates the picture. In our patient, the red cells with the PNH abnormality are also G6PD deficient: the *in vitro* studies summarized above strongly support the hypothesis that her poor response to eculizumab results from a unique interaction, within the same red cells, between the two abnormalities. With C5 blockade, complement activation causes binding of C3 fragments to the surface of PNH red cells both *in vivo* and *in vitro*. C3 fragments on granulocytes elicit ROS formation [9]; thus, it is not unlikely that C3 fragments elicit ROS formation also on red cells [1].

Further Follow-up

Over the course of the next six years, the patient's PNH red cell population rose steadily from 20 (before eculizumab) to 86% on eculizumab; and the fraction of PNH red cells with bound C3 fragments rose to 65% (Table 41.1). After 10 years, she was switched to the C5 inhibitor ravulizumab, which has a longer half-life than eculizumab. The patient's red cells transfusion requirement remained about 10 units per year throughout.

The patient's limited response to eculizumab could not be attributed to persisting bone marrow failure, but rather to the intensity of extravascular haemolysis arising from the pathophysiological mechanism outlined above; therefore, she is a candidate for therapy with an inhibitor of the proximal complement pathway, which will prevent binding of C3 to red cells. The patient was offered pegcetacoplan [10], but she was rather awed by the prospect of subcutaneous self-administration twice a week, and she declined. The patient will be offered the oral factor D inhibitor danicopan [11], as an add-on to ravulizumab, or the oral factor B inhibitor iptacopan [12], as soon as either will become available on the Italian National Health Service.

Further Comments

For over a century, the management of PNH patients was only supportive; the introduction of eculizumab has radically improved their quality of life [13], decreased greatly the risk of thrombosis [14], and improved survival [15]. In addition, today we have the luxury of a choice of complement inhibitors [16] (with the drawback that they are all astronomically expensive). This patient's history illustrates the above, and also why in some cases proximal complement inhibition may be preferable. At the same time, we must be aware that the mode of administration has an impact and that inhibition of complement, particularly of the proximal pathway, causes a marked increase in the population of red cells that are susceptible to complement-mediated haemolysis, entailing the risk of massive "breakthrough haemolysis" [17]. Therefore, these drugs must be handled with care.

Finally, it is somewhat intriguing that half a century ago the genetic polymorphism of G6PD was key to understanding the clonal origin of PNH cells [18], and now it transpires that G6PD deficiency may influence the pathophysiology of PNH.

Conclusion

PNH and G6PD deficiency: impaired response to eculizumab.
A report on this case has been previously published [1].

Acknowledgements

Rosario Notaro and Michela Sica, Laboratory of Cancer Genetics and Gene Transfer, Core Research Laboratory–Institute for Cancer Research, Prevention and Clinical Network (ISPRO), Florence, Italy.

References

1. Sica, M., Pellecchia, A., De Angioletti, M. et al. (2020). Complement-mediated oxidative damage of red cells impairs response to eculizumab in a G6PD-deficient patient with PNH. *Blood*. 136(26), 3082–85.
2. Risitano, A.M., Notaro, R., Marando, L. et al. (2009). Complement fraction 3 binding on erythrocytes as additional mechanism of disease in paroxysmal nocturnal hemoglobinuria patients treated by eculizumab. *Blood*. 113, 4094–4100.
3. Luzzatto, L., Gianfaldoni, G., and Notaro, R. (2011). Management of paroxysmal nocturnal haemoglobinuria: a personal view. *Br. J. Haematol*. 153, 709–720.
4. Luzzatto, L. and Nakao, S. (2025). Pathogenesis of paroxysmal nocturnal hemoglobinuria. *Blood*. 145, 3077–3088.
5. Luzzatto, L., Bessler, M., and Rotoli, B. (1997). Somatic mutations in paroxysmal nocturnal hemoglobinuria: a blessing in disguise? *Cell*. 88, 1–4.
6. Nkhoma, E.T., Poole, C., Vannappagari, V. et al. (2009). The global prevalence of glucose-6-phosphate dehydrogenase deficiency: a systematic review and meta-analysis. *Blood Cells Mol. Dis*. 42, 267–278.

7. Pes, G.M., Errigo, A., Bitti, A. et al. (2018). Effect of age, period and birth-cohort on the frequency of glucose-6-phosphate dehydrogenase deficiency in Sardinian adults. *Ann. Med.* 50, 68–73.
8. Amer, J., Zelig, O., and Fibach, E. (2008). Oxidative status of red blood cells, neutrophils, and platelets in paroxysmal nocturnal hemoglobinuria. *Exp. Hematol.* 36, 369–377.
9. Hoogerwerf, M., Weening, R.S., Hack, C.E. et al. (1990). Complement fragments C3b and iC3b coupled to latex induce a respiratory burst in human neutrophils. *Mol. Immunol.* 27, 159–167.
10. Hillmen, P., Szer, J., Weitz, I. et al. (2021). Pegcetacoplan versus Eculizumab in Paroxysmal Nocturnal Hemoglobinuria. *N. Engl. J. Med.* 384, 1028–1037.
11. Lee, J.W., Griffin, M., Kim, J.S. et al. (2023). Addition of danicopan to ravulizumab or eculizumab in patients with paroxysmal nocturnal haemoglobinuria and clinically significant extravascular haemolysis (ALPHA): a double-blind, randomised, phase 3 trial. *Lancet Haematol.* 10, e955–e65.
12. Peffault de Latour, R., Roth, A., Kulasekararaj, A.G. et al. Oral iptacopan monotherapy in paroxysmal nocturnal hemoglobinuria. *N. Engl. J. Med.* 390, 994–1008.
13. Hillmen, P., Young, N.S., Schubert, J. et al. (2006). The complement inhibitor eculizumab in paroxysmal nocturnal hemoglobinuria. *New Eng. J. Med.* 355, 1233–1243.
14. Hillmen, P., Muus, P., Duhrsen, U. et al. (2007). Effect of the complement inhibitor eculizumab on thromboembolism in patients with paroxysmal nocturnal hemoglobinuria. *Blood.* 110, 4123–4128.
15. Kelly, R.J., Hill, A., Arnold, L.M. et al. (2011). Long-term treatment with eculizumab in paroxysmal nocturnal hemoglobinuria: sustained efficacy and improved survival. *Blood.* 117, 6786–6792.
16. Risitano, A.M., Peffault de Latour, R., Marano, L. et al. (2022). Discovering C3 targeting therapies for paroxysmal nocturnal hemoglobinuria: achievements and pitfalls. *Semin. Immunol.* 59, 101618.
17. Notaro, R. and Luzzatto, L. (2022). Breakthrough hemolysis in PNH with proximal or terminal complement inhibition. *N. Engl. J. Med.* 387, 160–166.
18. Oni, S.B., Osunkoya, B.O., and Luzzatto, L. (1970). Paroxysmal nocturnal hemoglobinuria: evidence for monoclonal origin of abnormal red cells. *Blood.* 36, 145–152.

Case 42

Camden Town: Not Just the Market

Patient Details

Age: 32 *Sex:* F
Ethnic background: Cameroon

Reason for Referral

Anaemia and query abnormal haemoglobin (blood sample only).

History and Clinical Findings in Brief

The patient had a long history of menorrhagia for which she had been investigated at her local hospital. Examination had revealed uterine fibroids.

Laboratory Findings

The patient had a moderate microcytic hypochromic anaemia (see Table 42.1). The red cell indices MCV, MCH and MCHC were all very low. On the blood film (see Figure 42.1), there was a moderate degree of anisocytosis, with hypochromic microcytes, as well as cells with normal haemoglobinization, giving an overall dimorphic appearance. Large target cells and polychromatic cells seemed to stand out. There were a few poikilocytes, including some elliptocytes.

Table 42.1 Haematology Data

	Initial	Follow-up[a]
Hb (g/dl)	10.0	14.0
RBC ($\times 10^{12}$/l)	7.04	4.71
MCV (fl)	57.1	85.1
MCH (pg)	14.2	29.7
MCHC (g/dl)	24.9	34.9
RDW (S.D.)	41.8	—
Retic (%)	1.2	—
Retic ($\times 10^9$/l)	87	—
Hb A_2 (%)	2.3	—
Hb F (%)	0.6	—

[a] Supplied by the referring hospital.

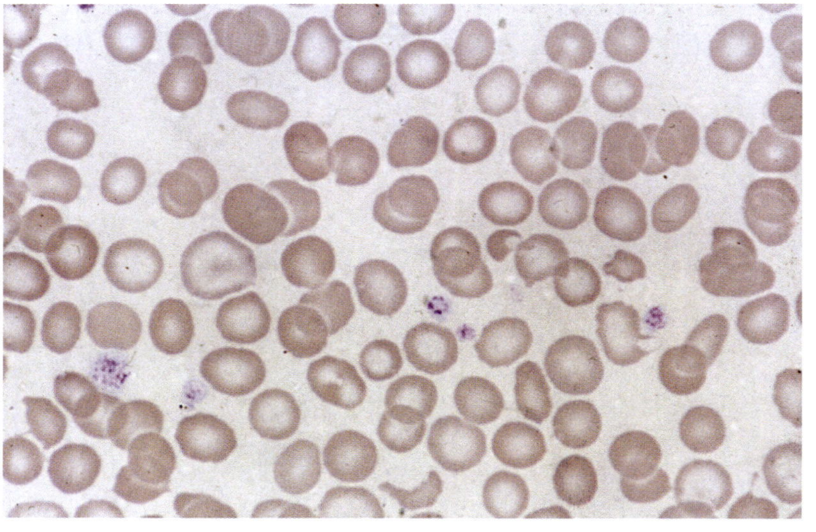

Figure 42.1 Peripheral blood film; high power view.

Haemoglobin electrophoresis (see Figure 42.2) revealed two abnormal bands: one just ahead of the position of Hb A (but slower than Hb J); the other was in the position of Hb S; no Hb A was seen. A solubility test confirmed the presence of sickle haemoglobin. The MCH (<27) triggered our computer to calculate discriminant function (DF) values[1] for

[1] DF values are derived from mathematical formulae applied to the blood count data to help differentiate the two very common causes of low red cell indices, namely iron deficiency anaemia {IDA} and β-thalassaemia trait. Two formulae we routinely use are based on the England-Fraser [1] algorithm (MCV – RBC – (5 × Hb) – 8.4) and the Shine and Lal [2] algorithm ([MCV × MCV × MCH] ÷ 100).

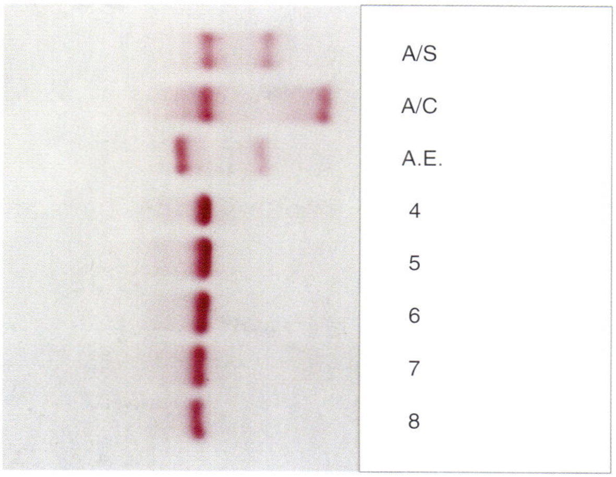

Figure 42.2 Haemoglobin electrophoresis on cellulose acetate membrane; the migration of the haemoglobin fractions is from right to left. An A/S control and an A/C control are in lanes 1 and 2, respectively. The patient (A.E.) is in lane 3.

this patient. According to the computer, the results were in keeping with β-thalassaemia trait.

Initial Assessment

The red cell morphology and the extremely low MCHC were strongly indicative of iron deficiency (not surprisingly in view of her clinical history, and we had to disagree with the computer here): the dimorphic appearance suggested that perhaps the patient had already started taking iron. At the same time, there was clearly a genetic haemoglobin abnormality, on which we assumed the iron deficiency was simply superimposed. The abnormality seemed to be complex. Since one band must be Hb S (based on the solubility test) and since there was no Hb A, we inferred that the other band was another β-chain variant.

Further Investigations

The ferritin level was 8 μg/l, confirming iron deficiency. Quantitation of the haemoglobins gave a level of 2.3% for the Hb A_2 (therefore not in keeping with β-thalassaemia trait); a level of 28% for the Hb S; a level of 69% for the other variant haemoglobin. On citrate agar gel electrophoresis (see Figure 42.3), the variant haemoglobin still had a fast mobility, ahead of the position of Hb A. Conversely, on globin chain (alkaline) electrophoresis (see Figure 42.4), a band was detected with a very slow mobility (the globin barely moved away from the point of application), in addition to bands in the β^S and α^A position. This was in keeping with the variant haemoglobin being a β-chain variant.

Next, we proceeded to DNA analysis Upon sequencing her β-globin gene, we found that the patient was heterozygous for the β-S mutation at codon 6. In addition, at codon β131, we found a band in both the C and the G tracks, showing that the patient was heterozygous for a C→G replacement (see Figure 42.5). This predicts the substitution in that position of Gln by Glu, which has been previously reported in an abnormal haemoglobin called Hb Camden [3]. Because of the uneven proportions of the two haemoglobins, we tested for an alpha thalassaemia; restriction enzyme analysis did not reveal any evidence of alpha thalassaemia due to an α-globin gene deletion.

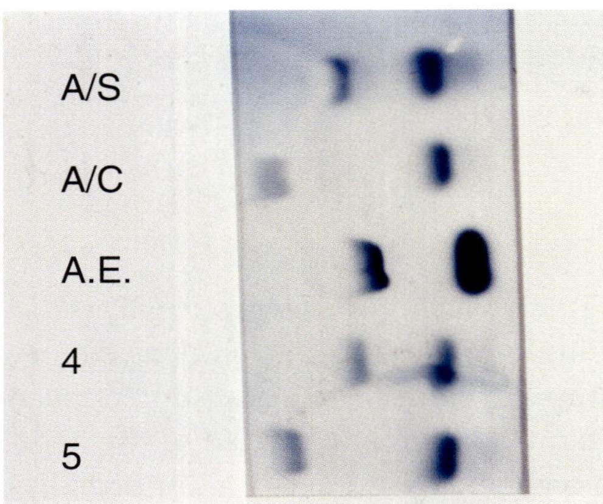

Figure 42.3 Citrate agar gel; the migration of the haemoglobin fractions is from left to right. An A/S and A/C control are in lanes 1 and 2, respectively. The patient (A.E.) is in lane 3.

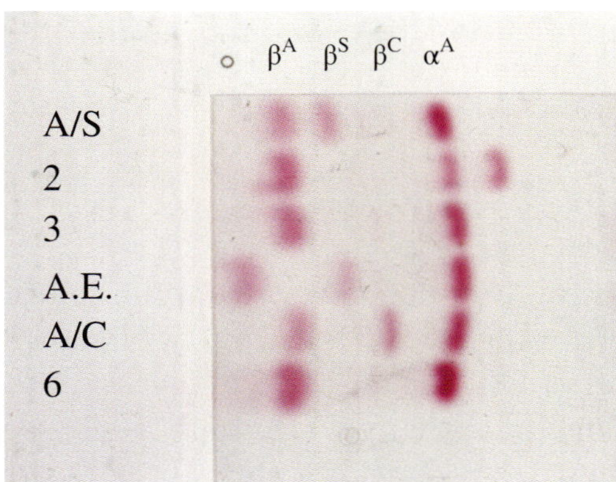

Figure 42.4 Globin chain (alkaline) electrophoresis on cellulose acetate membrane; the migration of the globin chains is from left to right. An A/S and A/C control are in lanes 1 and 5 respectively. The patient (A.E.) is in lane 4.

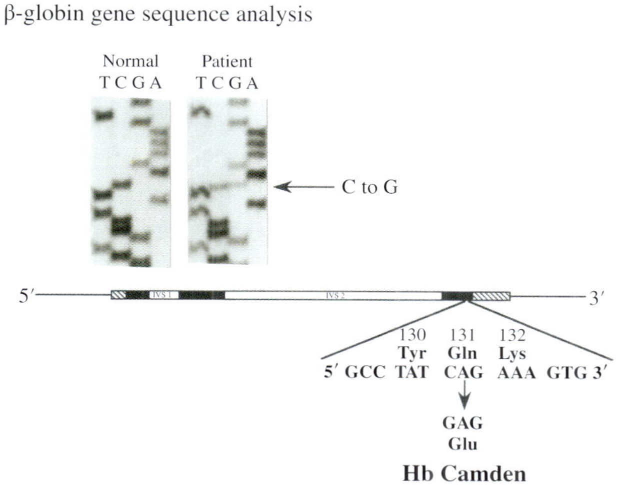

Figure 42.5 At the bottom is a schematic representation of the β-globin gene: exons and introns are indicated by black and white boxes, respectively; the shaded areas represent the 5′ and 3′ untranslated regions. Above the diagram, the results of direct sequence analysis of PCR products are shown. Within codon β131, a band in both C and G tracks is seen in the patient's DNA (highlighted by the arrow on the right), showing the patient to be heterozygous for a mutation in codon β131.

Comments

Hb Camden is a rare β-chain variant, on which we were able to find only nine *clinical* references in the literature. Interestingly, although the first description was of a patient of African ancestry living in Camden [3], other examples have been discovered in African American persons [4–7], Japan [8–10] and Russia [11].

The simple heterozygous state for Hb Camden is asymptomatic. A patient who had Hb Camden in combination with Hb Hope had chronic haemolytic anaemia, not surprisingly, since Hb Hope is itself unstable.

We found in the literature two precedents for the biallelic combination of Hb Camden with Hb S. The first report described a healthy three-year-old African–American girl from Washington, D.C., who had 66% Hb Camden and 34% Hb S [4]. Honig et al., [7] reported a patient who also had α-thal trait; his S level was 19.5%, and he was clinically asymptomatic. In our patient, the Hb S level was 28%, and she too had no manifestations reminiscent of sickle cell disease.

The most common combination of two abnormal haemoglobins is, of course, in Hb S/C disease, where, characteristically, Hb S and Hb C are usually very close to 50:50. By comparison, S/D and S/O are relatively rare, and in most of these, the ratio is still even. In the case of the S/Camden combination, the ratio is instead markedly in favour of haemoglobin Camden, and even in an A/Camden heterozygote, haemoglobin Camden was in excess of haemoglobin A [9]. These data suggest that β-Camden globin chains compete more effectively with β-S or even β-A globin chains for available α-chains. Interestingly, a correlation has been observed between the electrostatic charge of a β-chain and its percentage in heterozygotes [12], and β-Camden globin has an extra negative charge; in addition, the β-131 residue is part of the α1β1 interface [13].[2]

Follow-up

The patient has two sisters who also have this Hb S/Hb Camden combination, and they were clinically and haematologically normal. As for our patient, with iron therapy her blood count became completely normal, including normal red cell indices (see Table 42.1). Iron repletion did not affect the Hb S level.

Conclusion

Iron deficiency anaemia due to blood loss in a patient who is a genetic compound for Hb S and Hb Camden.

Acknowledgements

Martin Jarvis, Haematology Department, North Middlesex Hospital, London, UK.
Dr. Yardumian, Haematology Department, North Middlesex Hospital, London, UK.

References

1. England, J.M. and Fraser, P.M. (1973). Differentiation of iron deficiency from thalassaemia trait by routine blood-count. *Lancet* 1, 449–452.
2. Shine, I. and Lal, S. (1977). A strategy to detect beta-thalassaemia minor. *Lancet* 1, 692–694.

[2] Today a *Haemoglobinopathies NGS Panel* would promptly return for this patient the two mutations *HBBE6V* and *HBBQ131E*. However, it would not tell us whether they are in *cis* or in *trans:* i.e., it would not provide the important genetic information as to whether there is one doubly mutant gene or two allelic singly mutant genes: to find out would require e.g. nanopore sequencing with appropriate primers as an additional test.

3. Wade Cohen, P.T., Yates, A., Bellingham, A.J. et al. (1973). Letter: amino-acid substitution in the alpha 1 beta 1 intersubunit contact of haemoglobin-Camden beta 131 (h9) g1n → g1u. *Nature* 243, 467–468.
4. Blackwell, R.Q., McCurdy, P.R., Liu, C.S. et al. (1975). Double heterozygosity for hemoglobin Camden (beta 131 Gln yields Glu) and hemoglobin S in an American negro. *Vox Sang.* 28(1), 50–56.
5. Hubbard, M., Wilson, J.B., Wrightstone, R.N. et al. (1975). Hb Camden and Hb Hope found during routine testing. *Acta Haematol.* 54, 53–58.
6. Natta, C., Cassey, R., and Lehman, H. (1978). Double heterozygosity for hemoglobin Camden (beta131 Gln replaced by Glu) and alpha thalassemia. *Hemoglobin* 2(5), 463–468.
7. Honig, G.R., Mason, R.G., Shamsuddin, M. et al. (1980). Two new sickle cell syndromes: Hb S, Hb Camden, and alpha thalassaemia; and Hb S in combination with Hb Tacoma. *Blood* 55, 655–660. PMID: 7357091.
8. Ohba, Y., Miyaji, T., Matsuoka, M. et al. (1975). Hemoglobin Toluchi: beta 131 glutamine leads to glutamic acid, an example of Hb Camden in Japan. *Nihon Ketsueki Gakkai Zasshi.* 38(1), 1–7. PMID: 1173714.
9. Harano, T., Harano, K., Shibata, S. et al. (1982). Hemoglobin Camden (beta 131 (H9) Gly→Glu): the second instance in Japan. *Haemoglobin* 6, 427–432.
10. Shiwa, M., Fukuda, K., Kawata, Y. et al. (1988). Abnormal hemoglobin (Hb Camden) detected by interference in the determination of glycosylated hemoglobin with high performance liquid chromatography. *J. Clin. Pathol.* 36, 866–870. PMID: 3236471.
11. Aseeva, E.A., Lutsenko, I.N., Fivnik, A.V. et al. (1993). The first case of Hb Camden carriage in Russia. *Ter. Arkh.* 65, 49–51.
12. Thom, C.S., Dickson, C.F., Olson, J.S. et al. (2015). Normal and abnormal hemoglobins. In: Orkin, S.H., Fischer, D.E., Ginsburg, D. et al. editor. *Nathan and Osli's Hematology and Oncology of Infancy and Childhood*. 1 ed. Philadelphia: Elsevier Saunders. pp. 630–672.
13. Chang, C.K., Simplaceanu, V., and Ho, C. (2002). Effects of amino acid substitutions at beta 131 on the structure and properties of hemoglobin: evidence for communication between alpha 1 beta 1- and alpha 1 beta 2-subunit interfaces. *Biochemistry* 41(17), 5644–5655.

See also related Case 24.

Case 43

Mutating Again Gives You a High on Oxygen

Patient Details

Age: 31 *Sex:* F
Ethnic background: Nigeria

Reason for Referral

Identification of abnormal haemoglobin (blood sample only).

History and Clinical Findings in Brief

The patient gave no past history of anaemia or jaundice and had no relevant family history. She had been pregnant on four previous occasions in her hometown in Lagos, Nigeria, before her arrival in England in 1987. She was referred to the Haematology department at the North Middlesex Hospital because during her fifth pregnancy, on a routine antenatal investigation, she was found to have an abnormal band on electrophoresis. It was reported that on examination, the patient was well, with no jaundice or splenomegaly.

Laboratory Findings

The blood count was normal apart from a borderline low MCV, contrasting with an MCHC at the upper limit of normal (see Table 43.1). On the blood film (see Figure 43.1), most of the cells looked normal and very well haemoglobinized, but there was slight anisocytosis. Occasional cells appeared quite dense but still retained a small area of central pallor. A few target cells could be seen in which the central area was not round and isolated but like a bar across the diameter of the cell (not unlike a "no-entry" road sign).

Haemoglobin electrophoresis (see Figure 43.2) revealed, in addition to the normal haemoglobin components (Hb A and Hb A_2), a very slow-moving component migrating *behind* the haemoglobin C control, i.e. between the origin and the major band of carbonic anhydrase. On citrate agar gel electrophoresis (see Figure 43.3), the normal band of Hb A was present, plus a band situated at the point of application, i.e. it did not migrate; this was unlike the Hb C control that was cathodic to the origin. Interestingly, on a commercially available citrate/maleate agar gel, both the variant Hb and C control show a different mobility (see Figure 43.3b), still different from each other.

Table 43.1 Haematology Data

Hb (g/dl)	12.4
RBC ($\times 10^{12}$/l)	4.58
MCV (fl)	79.0
MCH (pg)	27.1
MCHC (g/dl)	34.3
RDW (S.D.)	38.9
Retic (%)	1.0
Retic ($\times 10^{9}$/l)	46
Hb A_2 (%)	2.8
Hb F (%)	1.1

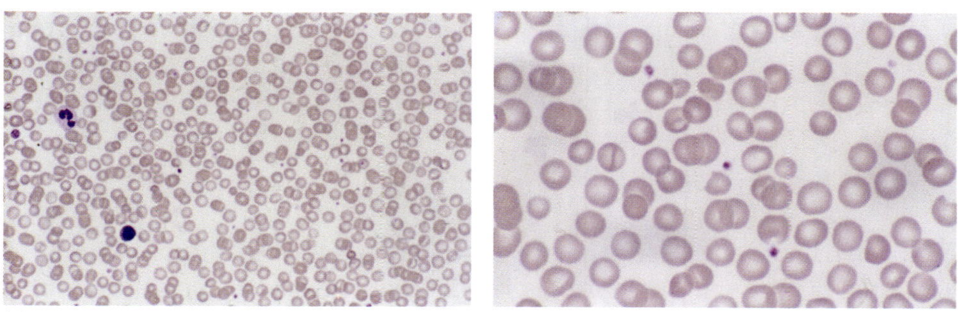

(a) (b)

Figure 43.1 Peripheral blood film: (a) medium power view; (b) high power view.

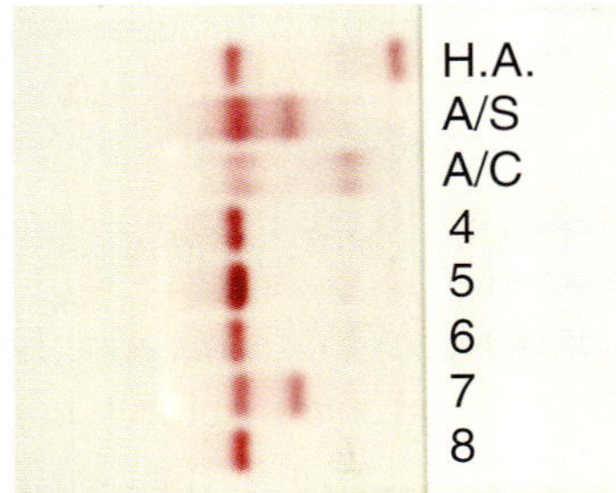

Figure 43.2 Haemoglobin electrophoresis on cellulose acetate membrane; the migration of the haemoglobin fractions is from right to left. An A/S control and an A/C control are in lanes 2 and 3, respectively. The patient (H.A.) is in lane 1.

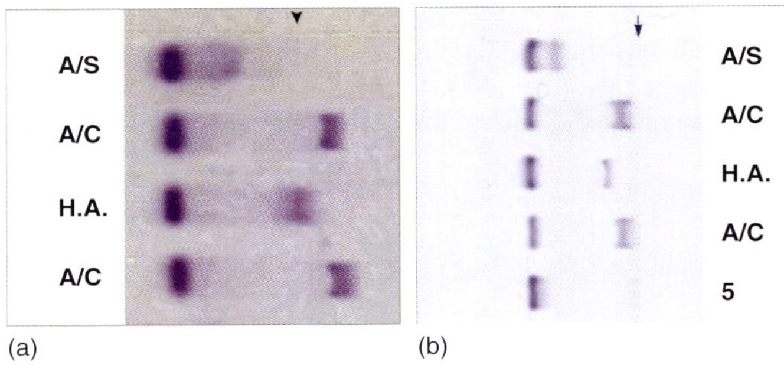

Figure 43.3 Haemoglobin electrophoresis: (a) on citrate agar gel; (b) on citrate/maleate agar gel. Migration of the haemoglobin fractions is from right to left: The point of application is marked. An A/S control is in lane 1 and A/C controls are in lanes 2 and 4. The patient (H.A.) is in lane 3.

Initial Assessment

The data were suggestive of a heterozygous state for a haemoglobin variant with an amino acid substitution that produces a molecule containing one additional negative charge in comparison with Hb C, something which we had never seen before. In fact, no single amino acid replacement can give a net change in charge greater than 2, which is the case with Hb C. Therefore, we had to postulate that either an unknown amino acid replacement produced an anomalous electrophoretic behaviour or there must be two amino acid replacements in the same molecule.

Further Investigations

First of all, in order to verify that we were dealing with a genetic abnormality, we tested the patient's daughter, and we obtained exactly the same results. Next, globin chain electrophoresis revealed bands in the normal positions of α^A and β^A only (see Figure 43.4). At first sight, this was very surprising. However, we noticed that compared to the band in the β^A position, the band in the α^A position was of much greater intensity; therefore, it was tempting to imagine that the abnormal globin was a β variant co-migrating with α^A.

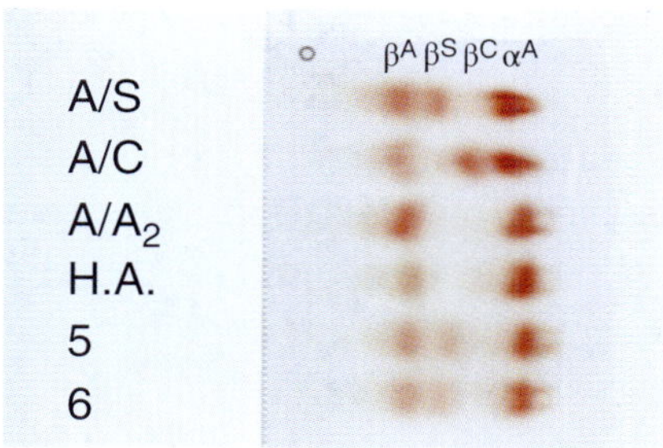

Figure 43.4 Globin chain (alkaline) electrophoresis on cellulose acetate membrane; the migration of the globin chains is from left to right; "o" indicates the application point. A/S, A/C and A/A_2 controls are in lanes 1, 2 and 3, respectively. The patient (H.A.) is in lane 4.

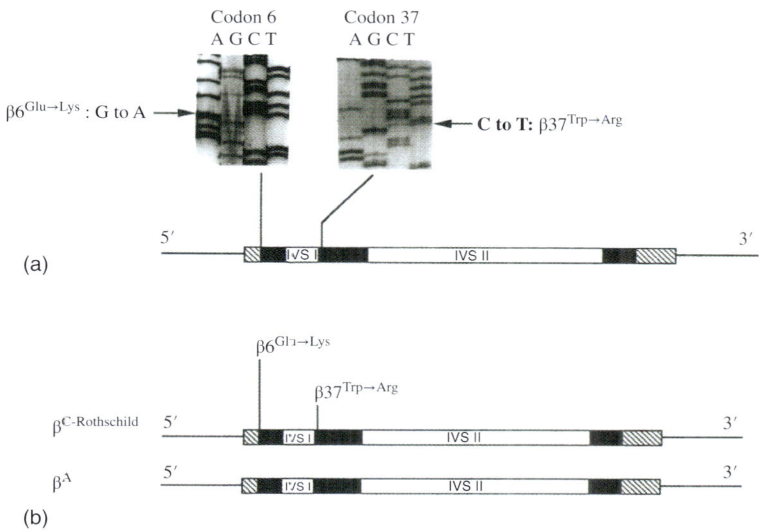

Figure 43.5 (a) A schematic representation of the β-globin gene is shown: exons and introns are indicated by black and white boxes, respectively. The shaded areas represent the 5′ and 3′ untranslated regions. Above the diagram, the results of direct sequence analysis of PCR products are shown, and the position of the mutation within the β-globin gene. Within codon β6, a band in both G and A tracks is seen in the patient's DNA (highlighted by the arrow on the left), showing the patient to be heterozygous for the Hb C mutation in codon β6. In addition, the sequence analysis revealed the patient to be heterozygous for another mutation in codon β37, whereby C is replaced by T (as indicated by the arrow on the right). (b) The β-globin genotype of the patient is illustrated diagrammatically, showing both the β^A and $\beta^{C\text{-Rothschild}}$ alleles. The $\beta^{C\text{-Rothschild}}$ allele has two mutations in *cis*.

The patient's haemoglobin level was on the lower side of the reference range. In view of this and of the borderline decreased MCV, we obtained a ferritin level, which was normal. We inferred that the slight microcytosis was probably due to her abnormal haemoglobin. An oxygen dissociation curve was normal (not shown).

Next, we proceeded to sequencing the patient's β-globin gene (see Figure 43.5). The patient was heterozygous for the (C→G) mutation of Hb C. In addition, we found another nucleotide change (C→T) in codon β37, predicting the replacement of Trp by Arg. This substitution has previously been reported, on its own [1], in Hb Rothschild.

Comments

If the two mutations in codons β6 and β37 had been in *trans*, i.e. one on each of the β-globin alleles, we would have seen on electrophoresis two bands (Hb C and Hb Rothschild) in addition to that of normal Hb A. Since on electrophoresis there was instead only a single variant haemoglobin, the two mutations must have been in *cis*, i.e. on the same allele. At first sight it may appear surprising that another mutation has occurred on a β^C globin gene; however, in southwestern Nigeria (from where this person came) the frequency of A/C heterozygotes is as high as 6%; interestingly, it is instead only 0.4% in southeastern Nigeria [2], as though the Niger river has been a major obstacle to the spread of this gene.

Hb Rothschild was named after the hospital in Paris where the first case was discovered. The amino acid substitution occurs within the $\alpha_1\beta_2$ contact area (see Figure 43.6), and it is involved in the structural transition that occurs on oxygenation: in fact, Hb Rothschild has a reduced oxygen affinity. In our case, the oxygen dissociation curve was reported by the clinical lab as normal; however, it was carried out on the total haemoglobin, of which we estimate only 30% was the abnormal component; therefore, we must interpret this result with caution.

While there are numerous examples of double mutants in the β-globin gene where a second mutation coexists with β-S, there seems to be only one previous example of a double mutant including the Hb C mutation, namely Hb Arlington-Park [3] (β6 {A3} Glu→Lys {Hb C} and β 95 {FG2} Lys→Glu {N-Baltimore}). In this variant, the charge change produced by the two amino acid replacements compensate each other,

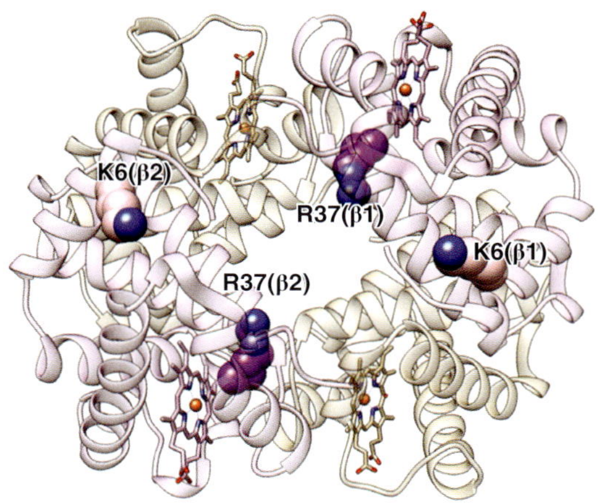

Figure 43.6 Image of Hb North Middlesex. α-chains in grey; β-chains in light violet. The amino acid replacements of Hb C are highlighted in pink; the amino acid replacements of Hb Rothschild are highlighted in purple. Courtesy of Francesco Angelucci.

and therefore the electrophoretic mobility is normal (indeed, this unique haemoglobin was discovered accidentally when the patient's sample was used as a control in a fingerprint analysis!). In our patient, instead, both amino acid replacements displace migration in the same direction, thus explaining the extraordinarily slow electrophoretic mobility. From the hospital that referred this patient, the appropriate name for this new haemoglobin is Hb North Middlesex.

Follow-up

Over the next seven years, the patient and her daughter have both remained well.

By this time, first-line haemoglobinopathy screening was being performed by HPLC. Not surprisingly, the patient's chromatogram revealed a late-eluting fraction within the designated Hb C "window" (see Figure 43.7).

TECH ID# 1
VIAL# 26
SAMPLE ID# 00000000000000000026

ANALYTE ID	%	TIME	AREA
F	2.8	1.06	67131
P2	3.0	1.26	75464
P3	4.9	1.62	122818
Unknown 1	0.7	1.93	17854
Ao	46.0	2.38	1162512
A2	2.9	3.56	69690
Unknown 2	2.3	4.82	58365
Unknown 3	3.6	5.02	90111
C-WINDOW	33.9	5.24	857128
	TOTAL AREA		2521073

F 2.8% A2 2.9%

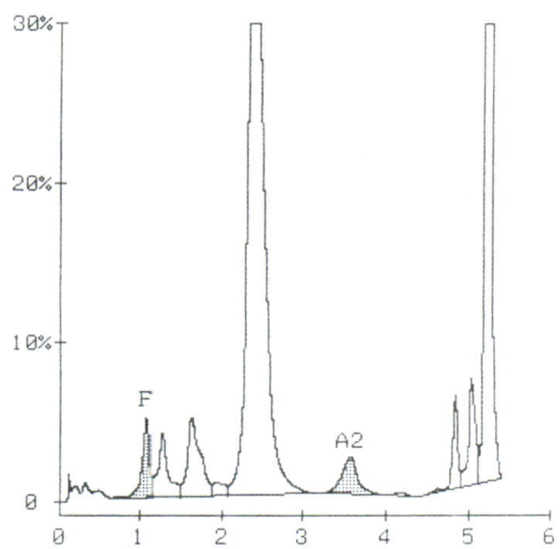

Figure 43.7 HPLC chromatogram of patient. The horizontal axis shows the retention (elution) time, and the vertical axis is the area (expressed as a percentage) for each haemoglobin. Haemoglobin A (A_0) is eluting at 2.38 minutes and the variant within the C-window.

However, this technique would not have revealed on its own that there was in this patient a new haemoglobin, with different physiologically relevant properties. With respect to contemporary methodologies, we also note that NGS would have detected both mutations, but not whether they were in the same allele; this would be revealed instead by nanopore sequencing.

Conclusion

Heterozygous for haemoglobin North Middlesex$^{(\beta 6\ \mathrm{Glu \rightarrow Lys:}\ \beta 37\ \mathrm{Try \rightarrow Arg})}$, a new haemoglobin arising from two β-globin mutations in *cis*.

Acknowledgements

Dr. I. Dokal, Haematology Department, Hammersmith Hospital, London, UK.
Martin Jarvis, Haematology Department, North Middlesex Hospital, London, UK.
Dr. J. Reeve, Haematology Department, North Middlesex Hospital, London, UK.
Francesco Angelucci (for Figure 43.6).

References

1. Gacon, G., Belkhodja, O., Wajcman, H. et al. (1977). Structural and functional studies of Hb Rothschild β37 (C3) Trp→Arg: a new variant of the α1 β2 contact. *FEBS lett*. 82(2), 243–246.
2. Usanga, E.A., Andy, J.J., Ekanem, A.D. et al. (1996). Haemoglobin C gene in south eastern Nigeria. *East Afr. Med. J.* 73(9), 566–567.
3. Adams, J.G. and Heller, P. (1977). Hemoglobin Arlington Park. A new hemoglobin variant with two amino acid substitutions in the beta chain. *Hemoglobin* 1(5), 419–426.

Case 44

Epigenetic Upheaval Can Make You Alpha-broke

Patient Details

Age: 57 *Sex:* M
Ethnic background: Sierra Leone

Reason for Referral

Investigation of anaemia.

History and Clinical Findings in Brief

The patient presented to another hospital because of a feeling of "fullness in his stomach." Recently, he also felt short of breath, and he experienced gradual loss of appetite; over the last three months he had been losing weight. There was no other significant medical history. There was no personal or family history of anaemia. The patient has four children who are all well. On examination, the patient appeared very pale; he had signs of superficial thrombophlebitis in his left leg and mild heart failure. His spleen was just palpable.

Laboratory Findings

The patient had a moderate to severe microcytic, hypochromic anaemia (see Table 44.1). The red cell morphology (see Figure 44.1) showed a very considerable variation in cell size and in haemoglobinization (anisocytosis and anisochromasia). There was a dimorphic appearance to the film, although (rather unusually) many of the hypochromic cells were larger than their fully haemoglobinized counterparts: some of the cells appeared hyperchromic, but they did not look spherocytic. Numerous target cells could be seen. There was also marked polychromasia, and some of the presumably young red cells were prominent, as though a deep blue shade was lurking under the pink. Other cells contained either a single Howell–Jolly body or multiple small inclusions (Pappenheimer bodies). While performing a white cell differential, we counted 136 nucleated red cells per 100 white cells. The platelets were increased in number and a proportion of them, in size also; some were extremely large and had a foamy structure: these were probably megakaryocyte fragments.

Table 44.1 Haematology Data

Hb (g/dl)	7.5
RBC ($\times 10^{12}$/l)	4.69
MCV (fl)	75.1
MCH (pg)	16.0
MCHC (g/dl)	21.3
RDW (S.D.)	+++
Retic (%)	21.0
Retic ($\times 10^{9}$/l)	984
WBC ($\times 10^{9}$/l)	27.2
PLT ($\times 10^{9}$/l)	1048

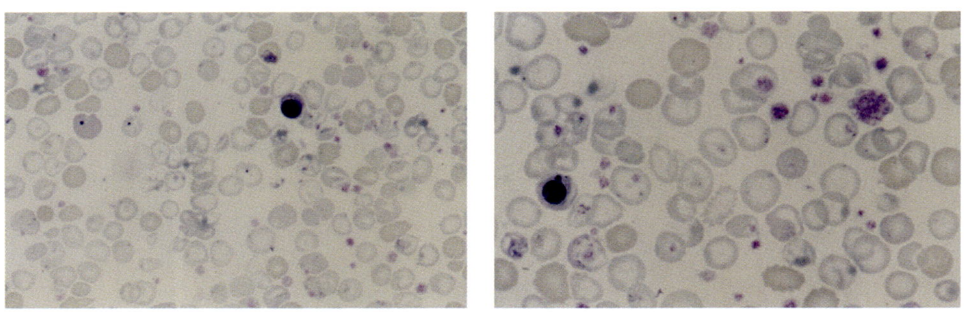

(a) (b)

Figure 44.1 Peripheral blood film: (a) medium power view; (b) high power view.

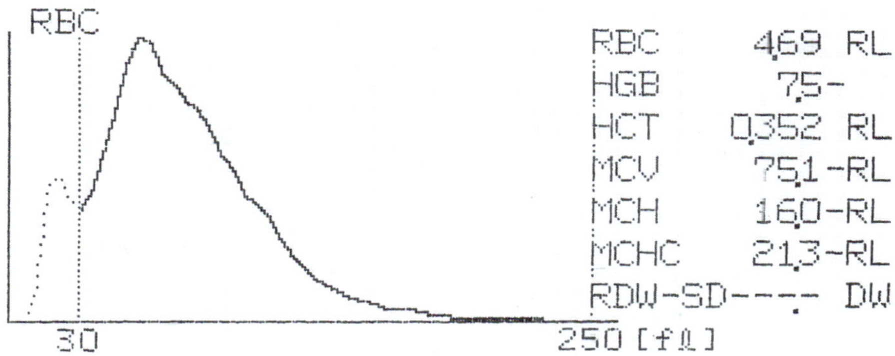

Figure 44.2 Red cell profile.

There was an overlap in size between the platelets and the microcytic red cells (see Figure 44.2), and as a result, the analyzer failed to give an RDW value, which otherwise would have been hugely increased.

A bone marrow aspirate was hypercellular. There was erythroid hyperplasia and hypogranular myeloid cells; megakaryocytes were markedly increased in number and had abnormal morphology, with numerous micro-megakaryocytes. There was abundant iron in the marrow fragments but no ring sideroblasts.

Unfortunately, the slides are no longer available, but the picture was similar to that in Figure 44.3.

Initial Assessment

There is severe microcytic hypochromic anaemia with marked reticulocytosis and thrombocytosis. The bone marrow appearance shows three-lineage dysplasia, consistent with a myelodysplastic syndrome (MDS); thrombocytosis is uncommon in MDS, but it can occur.

Further Investigations

Haemoglobin electrophoresis (see Figure 44.4) revealed normal components in the positions of Hb A and Hb A_2. In addition, we saw a minor band with a very fast mobility (had we left the electrophoresis running for just a little longer, this abnormal band would have migrated off the end of the cellulose membrane, and therefore it would have been missed). When

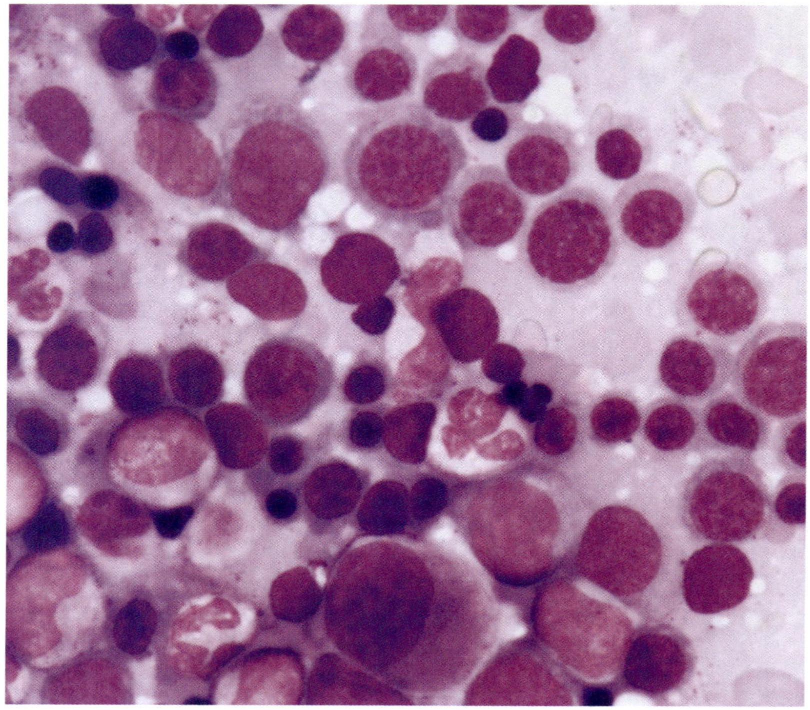

Figure 44.3 Bone marrow aspirate. One sees erythroid hyperplasia and hypogranular myeloid cells. Megakaryocytes were increased in number, most of them were micro-megakaryocytes or otherwise dysplastic, as the one in this photo. Courtesy of Dr. Prashant Sharma [1].

Figure 44.4 Haemoglobin electrophoresis on cellulose acetate membrane; the migration of the haemoglobin fractions is from right to left. An A/S control and A/C control are in lanes 1 and 2, respectively. The patient (L.G.) is in lane 5; his Hb H fraction is indicated by the arrow.

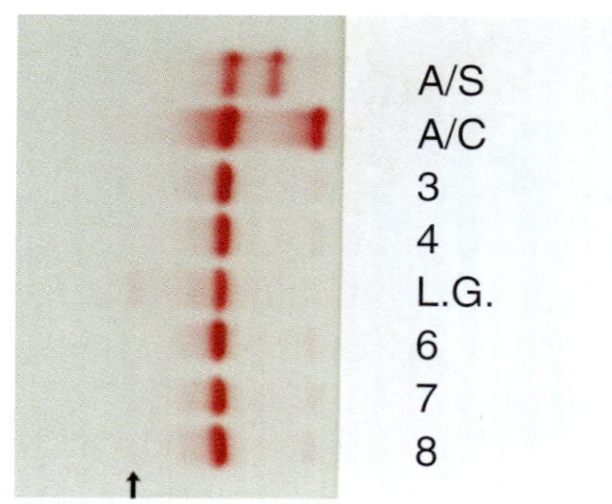

azure-B was used to supravitally stain the red cells (see Figure 44.5), this highlighted, of course, the high reticulocytosis and also revealed a large number of the "golf-ball" cells, typically seen with Hb H.

In view of the very low MCH and MCHC in the face of apparently normal iron stores, a ferrokinetic study was also performed (see Table 44.2).

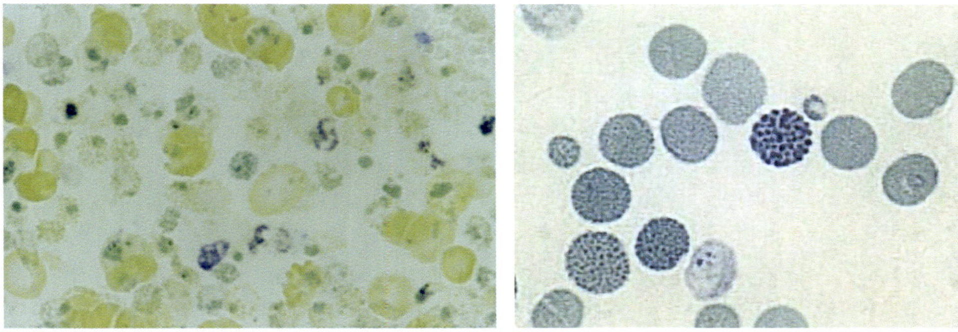

(a) (b)

Figure 44.5 Hb H prep: (a) Hb H inclusions generated after supravital staining in azure-B solution for 2 hours at 37 °C in the patient; (b) Hb H inclusions in a patient with Hb H disease (α–/—).

Table 44.2 Radioisotope Studies

Plasma iron[a] (μmol/l)	31.5	(N 11–30)
Transferrin (g/l)	2.49	(N 1.5–3.0)
Plasma Fe clearance (min)	32	(N 60–140)
Plasma Fe turnover (μmol/l/day)	659	(N 100–150)

[a] Patient had been started on iron in the preceding week.

The very rapid plasma clearance (approximately three times normal) and markedly increased plasma iron turnover (approximately five times normal) were consistent with erythroid hyperplasia. These findings, together with the high plasma iron concentration, are implying ineffective erythropoiesis.

Comments

Haemoglobin H (β_4 tetramer) is formed whenever there is a significant deficit of α-chain synthesis compared to β-chain synthesis; when the α/β imbalance is mild, little Hb H is formed, and it can be only visualized by supravital staining (Hb H inclusion bodies in "golf-ball" cells). If the imbalance is more severe, Hb H can accumulate sufficiently to show up as a discrete band on electrophoresis. This happens typically when three out of four α-genes are either deleted or non-functional, causing moderate to severe anaemia, as in classic Hb H disease.

Our patient had no anaemia when he was a young man, but now, in his late 50s, he has severe anaemia, thrombocytosis and an abnormal bone marrow: he clearly fits the picture originally described as acquired Hb H disease [2], which has since become known as the alpha thalassaemia myelodysplasia syndrome (ATMDS) [3]. This syndrome is due to somatic mutations of the *ATRX* gene [4] (mapping to Xp13.3), germ-line mutations of which were already known to underlie α-thalassaemia with mental retardation [5]: we did not test for *ATRX* mutations when our patient was seen; in the similar case (whose bone marrow is shown in Figure 44.3), a missense mutation was found in exon 31, causing a lysine to threonine replacement (p.K2883T), regarded as potentially pathogenic. The ATRX protein is a chromatin remodelling gene that contains an ATPase-helicase domain and has several important epigenetic functions [6]: among these, to provide a configuration of the α-globin genes conducive to their expression (see Figure 44.6). Thus, loss of function (LOF) mutations of *ATRX* will

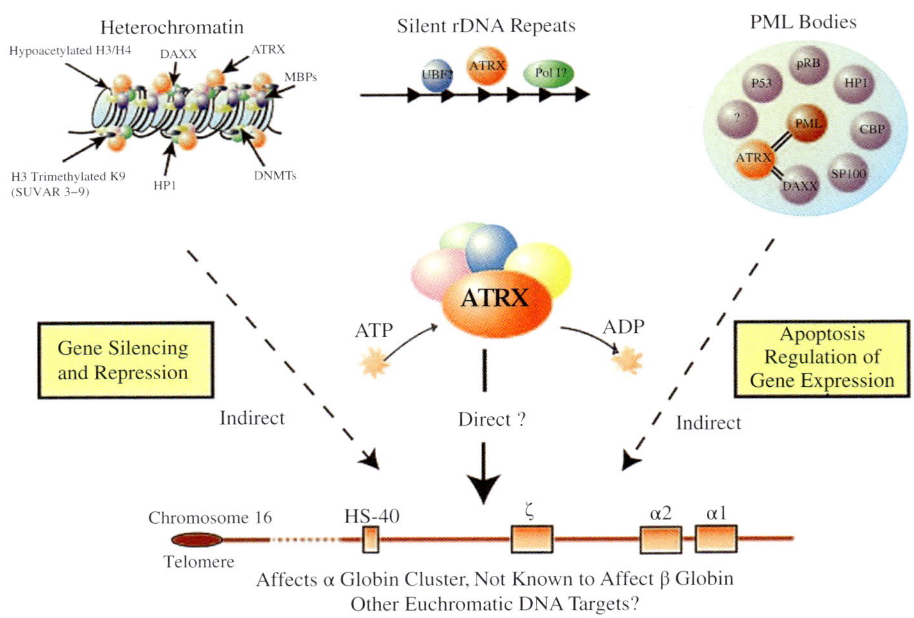

Figure 44.6 Model for how ATRX might influence gene expression. ATRX is part of a multiprotein complex that uses the energy of ATP to remodel chromatin or its associated DNA in a way that affects transcriptional activity at euchromatic loci, including the α-globin gene cluster. ATRX function may be associated with its presence at one of its target nuclear locations (e.g. heterochromatin, ribosomal DNA repeats, PML bodies) in addition to euchromatic sites. The multiprotein complex, of which ATRX is a part, causes epigenetic modifications of histone-associated DNA, leading to alterations in local chromatin conformation, required for α-globin gene expression. [8]/with permission of Elsevier.

cause a severe decrease in output of all four α-globin genes [7], causing a much more severe α/β chain imbalance than in most cases of conventional α-thalassaemia (in ATMDS the α/β biosynthetic ratio is often about 0.2 [8]). Our patient had in fact also an α-globin gene deletion (genotype α −/αα), but this must have been greatly overshadowed by the effect of the *ATRX* mutation. Some case reports have associated acquired Hb H with various forms of myeloproliferative disorders [9, 10].

In our patient, MCV was low; MCH and MCHC were very low: this is interesting, since more often in MDS there is instead macrocytosis. Indeed, hypochromic, microcytic red blood cells and striking anisopoikilocytosis were a feature of the original characterization of ATMDS [3]; and in a subsequent study the frequency of *ATRX* mutations was less than 1% in unselected MDS cases, but 43% in those who were microcytic [11]. Since before they had MDS, these patients had presumably normal red cells, we infer that haemoglobin synthesis itself is a strong determinant of MCV. It seems as though the size of the red cell is not predetermined, and then filled with haemoglobin; rather, the red cell is shaped to some extent by the amount of haemoglobin that has been produced. As is often the case, pathology informs us about physiology.

The large majority of ATMDS patients have been male, as in our case, although a few authentic cases have also occurred in women [12]. In considering possible reasons for this strong gender bias, an obvious departure point is that *ATRX* is on the X chromosome: therefore, in a male cell, a LOF somatic mutation will inactivate the only *ATRX* allele, and the result will be an acquired α-thalassaemia phenotype. In females, since *ATRX* is not one of the genes that normally escape X inactivation (not even in elderly women [12]), if a mutation occurs on the *ATRX* allele on the inactive X-chromosome, it will have no phenotypic consequence; if the mutation occurs on the *ATRX* allele on the active X-chromosome, the phenotype will be α-thalassaemia, like in a male (except it may be milder because in fewer cells). The situation would be different if *ATRX* escaped X inactivation[1]: in this case the un-mutated allele on the other X chromosome would greatly mitigate the effect of a LOF mutation. There is evidence, albeit thus far indirect, that in neoplastic cells *ATRX* may escape inactivation [15].

It is not yet clear whether in MDS and related disorders *ATRX* mutations are passengers or drivers. The former view seems to be favoured in the literature; however, this would imply that in ATMDS there are regularly

[1] In the multisystem inflammatory disease known as VEXAS [13], there is also marked male gender bias. VEXAS is caused by LOF somatic mutations in the X-linked *UBA1* gene, which regularly escapes X inactivation: the presence, in female cells, of a normal *UBA1* allele on the other X chromosome directly explains, in this case, the gender bias [14].

other mutations, and there are no systematic data in this respect. We must also consider that the ATRX protein is involved in genome maintenance and in alternative telomere maintenance and that *ATRX* mutations have been found in a variety of tumours, for instance gliomas [16]. Therefore, the matter of driver *versus* passenger mutations is still open [6].

Follow-up

Just as further investigations were planned, we were saddened to learn about the patient's sudden death, attributed to a pulmonary embolism.

Conclusion

Alpha thalassaemia-myelodysplastic syndrome (ATMDS) with acquired haemoglobin H.

Acknowledgements

Referred by Dr. U. Hegde, Haematology Department, Ealing Hospital, London, UK.
Dr. S.M. Lewis, Haematology Department, Hammersmith Hospital, London, UK.
Dr. H. McMichael, Consultant Physician, Ealing Hospital, London, UK.
Dr. Prashant Sharma, Haematology Department, Postgraduate Institute of Medical Education and Research (PGIMER), Chandigarh, India.

References

1. Mallik, N., Singh, N., Jamwal, M. et al. (2022). A novel ATRX splice variant causing acquired HbH disease in myelodysplastic syndrome with excess blasts-1. *Cancer Genet.* 260–261, 53–56.
2. Higgs, D.R., Wood, W.G., Barton, C. et al. (1983). Clinical features and molecular analysis of acquired hemoglobin H disease. *Am. J. Med.* 75, 181–191.
3. Steensma, D.P., Higgs, D.R., Fisher, C.A. et al. (2004). Acquired somatic ATRX mutations in myelodysplastic syndrome associated with alpha thalassemia (ATMDS) convey a more severe hematologic phenotype than germline ATRX mutations. *Blood* 103, 2019–2026.
4. Gibbons, R.J., Pellagatti, A., Garrick, D. et al. (2003). Identification of acquired somatic mutations in the gene encoding chromatin-remodeling factor ATRX in the alpha-thalassemia myelodysplasia syndrome (ATMDS). *Nat. Genet.* 34, 446–449.
5. Gibbons, R.J., Picketts, D.J., Villard, L. et al. (1995). Mutations in a putative global transcriptional regulator cause X-linked mental retardation with alpha-thalassemia (ATR-X syndrome). *Cell* 80(6), 837–845.

6. Clynes, D., Higgs, D.R., and Gibbons, R.J. (2013). The chromatin remodeller ATRX: a repeat offender in human disease. *Trends Biochem. Sci.* 38, 461–466.
7. Anagnou, N.P., Ley, T.J., Chesbro, B. et al. (1983). Acquired alpha-thalassaemia in preleukaemia is due to decreased expression of all four alpha-globin genes. *Proc. Natl. Acad. Sci. USA*. 80, 6051–6055.
8. Steensma, D.P., Gibbons, R.J., and Higgs, D.R. (2005). Acquired alpha-thalassemia in association with myelodysplastic syndrome and other hematologic malignancies. *Blood* 105, 443–452.
9. Yoo, D., Schechter, G.P., Amigable, A.N. et al. (1980). Myeloproliferative syndrome with sideroblastic anemia and acquired hemoglobin H disease. *Cancer* 45, 78–83.
10. Abbondanzo, S.L., Anagnou, N.P., and Sacher, R.A. (1988). Myelodysplastic syndrome with acquired hemoglobin H disease. Evolution through megakaryoblastic transformation into myelofibrosis. *Am. J. Clin. Pathol.* 89, 401–406.
11. Herbaux, C., Duployez, N., Badens, C. et al. (2015). Incidence of ATRX mutations in myelodysplastic syndromes, the value of microcytosis. *Am. J. Hematol.* 90, 737–738
12. Haas, P.S., Roy, N.B., Gibbons, R.J. et al. (2009). The role of X-inactivation in the gender bias of patients with acquired alpha-thalassemia and myelodysplastic syndrome (ATMDS). *Br. J. Haematol.* 144, 538–545.
13. Beck, D.B., Ferrada, M.A., Sikora, K.A. et al. (2020). Somatic mutations in UBA1 and severe adult-onset autoinflammatory disease. *N. Engl. J. Med.* 383, 2628–2638.
14. Luzzatto, L., Risitano, A.M., and Notaro, R. (2021). Mutant UBA1 and severe adult-onset autoinflammatory disease. *N. Engl. J. Med.* 384, 2164.
15. Dunford, A., Weinstock, D.M., Savova, V. et al. (2017). Tumor-suppressor genes that escape from X-inactivation contribute to cancer sex bias. *Nat. Genet.* 49, 10–16.
16. Yuan, K., Tang, Y., Ding, Z. et al. (2024). Mutant ATRX: pathogenesis of ATRX syndrome and cancer. *Front. Mol. Biosci.* 11, 1434398.

List of Diagnoses